HUMAN MUSCLE POWER

Edited by
Norman L. Jones, MD, Neil McCartney, PhD,
and Alan J. McComas, MB

McMaster University
Hamilton, Ontario

Human Kinetics Publishers, Inc.
Champaign, Illinois

Library of Congress Cataloging-in-Publication Data

These proceedings are from the McMaster International Symposium on Human Muscle Power, held July 15-17, 1984 at McMaster University, Hamilton, Ontario, Canada.

Human muscle power.

Includes bibliographies.
1. Muscle strength--Congresses.   2. Muscle contraction--Congresses.   3. Muscle contraction--Regulation--Congresses.   4. Muscle tone--Congresses.
I. Jones, Norman L.   II. McCartney, Neil, 1952-
III. McComas, Alan J.   IV. Symposium on Human Muscle Power (1984: McMaster University) [DNLM: 1. Exertion--congresses.   2. Muscles--physiology--congresses.
3. Physical Fitness--Congresses.   WE 103 H9183]
QP321.H86   1986   612'.74   85-30240

ISBN 0-87322-004-8

Developmental Editor: Sue Wilmoth, PhD
Production Director: Ernest Noa
Copy Editor: Steve Davenport
Typesetter: Theresa Bear
Text Design: Julie Szamocki
Text Layout: Denise Mueller
Cover Design: Jack Davis
Printed By: Braun-Brumfield, Inc.

ISBN 0-87322-004-8

Printed in the United States of America

10 9 8 7 6 5 4 3 2 1

Human Kinetics Publishers, Inc.
Box 5076, Champaign, IL 61820

Dedicated to the memory of

Lars Hermansen, PhD
(1933-1984)

Director of the Institute of Muscle Physiology
Oslo, Norway.

Scientist, Teacher, Friend and Colleague.

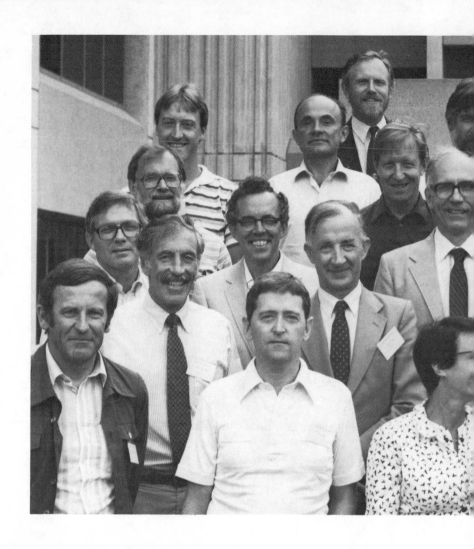

Group Photograph Legend of Contributors

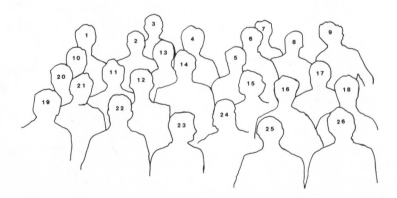

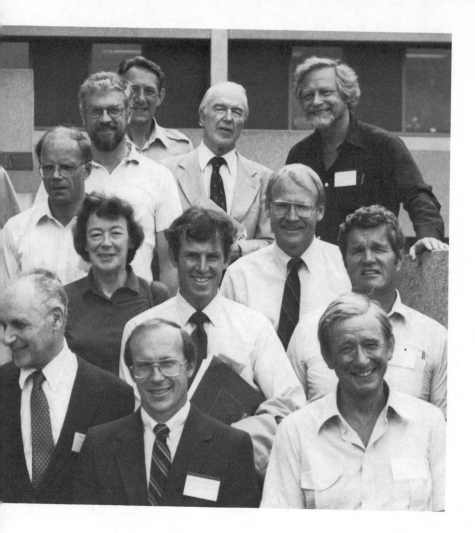

McMaster International Symposium on Human Muscle Power
July 15-17, 1984

Primary Authors

Dr. Michael Bárány
The University of Illinois
College of Medicine at Chicago
Department of Biological
  Chemistry
1853 West Polk Street,
  A-312 CMW
Box 6998
Chicago, Illinois 60680

Dr. Robert E. Burke
National Institutes of Health
Public Health Service
Laboratory of Neural Control
Bethesda, Maryland 20205

Dr. B. Chance
University of Pennsylvania
Department of Biochemistry and
  Physiology
Philadelphia, Pennsylvania 19104

Professor V. Reggie Edgerton, Ph.D.
University of California
Department of Kinesiology
2864 Slichter Hall
Los Angeles, California 90024

Dr. John A. Faulkner
University of Michigan Medical
  School
Department of Physiology
Ann Arbor, Michigan 48109

Dr. Philip D. Gollnick
Washington State University
Department of Physical Education
  for Men
Pullman, Washington 99164

Dr. William J. Gonyea
The University of Texas Health
  Sciences Centre
5323 Harry Hines Blvd.
Dallas, Texas 75235

Dr. Howie Green
Faculty of Human Kinetics and
  Leisure Studies
Department of Kinesiology
University of Waterloo
Waterloo, Ontario
Canada, N2L 3G1

Dr. Lennart Grimby
Department of Neurology
Karolinska Hospital
S-104 01 Stockholm, Sweden

Dr. H. Howald
Head of Institute
Research Institute of the SSPES
Magglingen 2532
Switzerland

Dr. Eric Hultman
Department of Clinical Chemistry
11
Huddinge University Hospital
S-141 86 Huddinge, Sweden

Dr. C.D. Ianuzzo
Department of Physical Education
& Biology
4700 Keele Street
Downsview, Ontario
Canada M3J 1P3

Dr. N.L. Jones
Director
Cardiorespiratory Unit-3U1
McMaster University Health
Sciences Centre
1200 Main Street West
Hamilton, Ontario
Canada L8N 3Z5

Dr. Paavo V. Komi
University of Jyvaskyla
Department of Biology of Physical
Activity
Seminaarinkatu 15
SF-40100 Jyvaskyla 10, Finland

Dr. J.D. MacDougall
School of Physical Education &
Athletics
PEC-AB 117
McMaster University
Hamilton, Ontario
Canada L8S 4K1

Dr. Neil McCartney
Cardiorespiratory Unit-3U
McMaster University Health
Sciences Centre
1200 Main Street West
Hamilton, Ontario
Canada L8N 3Z5

Dr. A.J. McComas
Department of Medicine-4U7
McMaster University Health
Sciences Centre
1200 Main Street West
Hamilton, Ontario
Canada L8N 3Z5

Dr. Eric A. Newsholme
Merton College
Oxford, England
OX1 4JD

Mr. Jim Perrine
98 Buckskin Road
Canoga Park, California 91307

Dr. Brenda Bigland-Ritchie
John B. Pierce Foundation
Laboratory
290 Congress Avenue
New Haven, Connecticut 06519

Dr. D.G. Sale
School of Physical Education &
Athletics
PEC-AB 123
McMaster University
Hamilton, Ontario
Canada L8S 4K1

Dr. B. Saltin
Laboratory for the Theory of
Gymnastics
August Krogh Institute

University of Copenhagen, 13
Universitetsparken
2100 Copenhagen, Denmark

Dr. Richard B. Stein
Professor, Department of
Physiology
The University of Alberta
Edmonton, Alberta
Canada T6G 2H7

Dr. D.A. Winter
Faculty of Human Kinetics and
Leisure Studies
Department of Kinesiology
University of Waterloo
Waterloo, Ontario
Canada N2L 3G1

Dr. D.R. Wilkie
Department of Physiology
University College London
Gower Street
London, England
WC1E 6BT

Contents

Acknowledgments

We received generous grants from the Ontario Department of Recreation and Tourism (Minister—The Honourable Reuben Baetz) and the National Science and Engineering Research Council. The conference could not have been held, and this book would not have been written, without this support.

The conference was organized with great efficiency and enthusiasm by Ms. Liz McCormick and Mrs. Ruth McHugh of the Department of Continuing Education at McMaster. Drs. Duncan MacDougall and Digby Sale served on the Organizing Committee and many other colleagues provided help at the meeting, and also helped in recording the discussion periods—John and Nancy Kowalchuk, Lawrence Spriet, Graham Jones, Mike Lindinger, Anthony Vandervoort. Audrey Hitchcock, Dorothy Agnew, and Marjorie Young were instrumental in the preparation of the manuscript. Thanks also go to Dr. Rainer Martens and his staff at Human Kinetics Publishers for their expertise in publishing the book.

Preface

A number of ideas provided the stimulus for us to organize a symposium on human muscle power at McMaster University in 1984. Meeting in Hamilton, Ontario, close to the Olympic Games, was partly for practical reasons so that as many international exercise scientists as possible could more easily attend. The nearby Olympic Games also inspired the symposium's theme, focusing on the mechanisms that allow humans to achieve very high power outputs in dynamic exercise. This focus was in part a reaction to recent symposia on muscle fatigue. Our goal, however, was to examine the factors that allow high levels of power to be generated and maintained.

Physiologist Sir Joseph Barcroft had once said, "Every adaptation is an integration." In drawing the analogy to a great steam locomotive, composed of many complex parts, each of which are needed to function well for the entire system to generate maximum power, Barcroft (1933) stated, "The condition of exercise is not a mere variant of the condition of rest, it is the essence of the machine." Our attempt, therefore, was not only to review the mechanisms individually, but to also obtain a sense of the integration among all of them. This integration may perhaps allow us to explain the feats of Olympians in relationship to all the complex parts of the human locomotive.

In organizing the symposium we were fortunate to obtain a stellar group of speakers, imaginative financial support, and an excellent organization group. Very few of our invited speakers were unable to attend. Tragically, Dr. Lars Hermansen died shortly before the conference. As a modern physiologist, Dr. Hermansen exemplified the classical integrative approach in his work. Dr. Hermansen's achievements were reviewed in a lecture by Dr. Bengt Saltin, his long time colleague and friend. In addition, this volume is dedicated in his memory. Dr. Martin Kushmerick, Harvard University, and Professor Richard Edwards, University College, London, could not attend. To all our contributors—speakers, chairmen, and discussants—we extend our grateful thanks. We hope this book not only serves as a report of the proceedings of our symposium, but also provides a summary of the most current information and research in human muscle power.

Section **1**

Mechanics

1

Muscle Function: A Historical View

D.R. Wilkie
University College, London

W e are far more likely to arrive at our destination if we know what it is. For those of us who are interested in how muscles work, the destination is the progressive unification of our knowledge of the physics, chemistry, and structure—at all levels—of muscular systems. The same integration is needed to understand other organs, but in my opinion the field of muscle research has progressed further than the others. Optimists that we are, our goal seems almost within our grasp. Perhaps it is just at the rainbow's end.

The Early Years

The need to relate muscular structure to its mechanical function has been apparent for centuries. Certainly it was clear to Galileo and Borelli, both of whom understood dimensional analysis, and to Leonardo da Vinci, who understood most things. To my mind, William Harvey is preeminent in this regard because he added the stern discipline of *experimentation*—with all its cussedness—to control the somewhat easier task of speculation.

By the late 18th century, the relation between living function and the then new subject of chemistry was emerging from the work of geniuses like Priestley and especially Lavoisier. As early as 1807 the great Berzelius "convinced himself that the amount of free lactic acid in a muscle is proportional to the extent to which it has been previously exercised" (Lehmann, 1851). With a few refinements, this conclusion remains valid today.

The great achievements of the 19th century seem to be, though not in order of importance, as follows:

1. The perfection of our knowledge of gross anatomy.
2. A great increase in our knowledge of chemistry and physics. This leads to the dismissal of "vital forces" (i.e., the notion that living processes were in some essential way different from nonliving ones). Leibig and Pasteur were among the giants who debated this issue.
3. The demonstration of the continuity of life (i.e., the absence of "spontaneous generation"). In this Pasteur also played a key part.
4. Methods of light microscopy were brought almost to their modern state of perfection. However, the amazing things Leeuwenhoek saw 200 years before, using a simple lens and a sharp mind, should never be forgotten. The observations made on living muscle during the 19th century were in fact more accurate than the ones that dominated the scene in my youth. This salutary warning story is brilliantly told in the 1957 review by Andrew Huxley.

The Twentieth Century

Every so often the synthesis between the chemistry and physics of muscle has seemed to be within our grasp. For example, during the "lactic acid era," roughly 1920 to 1930, it was believed by many that the formation of lactic acid was the primary event that powered muscular contraction. This view disintegrated from the blow struck by Lundsgaard in 1931 (i.e., muscle contraction can take place in the absence of lactic acid formation). At a dinner to celebrate his retirement in about 1969, Lundsgaard talked wryly to me about the great difficulties he had after his initial success in Copenhagen in reproducing his experiments in Meyerhof's laboratory.

My own interest in muscle began abruptly on the Friday afternoon of August 22, 1941, during a practical class in a converted barn. (University College had been severely damaged in the bombing of October 1940.) I became fascinated by a routine class experiment on free and afterloaded muscle twitches. I spent such time as a medical student's life would permit in doing more experiments and reading what I could find about muscle. An ironical consequence was that I did badly at the problem set in my practical examination, which was on muscle. I could not understand then, any more than I can now, how the work output in an isometric muscle twitch could be force × length ÷ 6.

Unknown to me, the stage was already set for the new revolution in which we live. The electron microscope was already waiting in the wings, and, during the next two decades, our knowledge of the structure, chemistry, and mechanics of muscle would be brought together in the sliding-filament theory of contraction. At the same time crossbridges between actin and myosin, powered by the free-energy change for ATP hydrolysis, were shown to be the most probable site of force generation. These theories seem to be surviving well, though one should never be overconfident about this strange machine that, unlike those made by man, transforms chemical energy into mechanical energy at constant temperature. Muscle biology may still have a few tricks up its sleeve.

The elements that contribute to our current theories of muscle contraction come from diverse sources. A.V. Hill's classic paper (1938) had shown a seemingly clear and certainly intriguing relation between the force-velocity curve and the heat production of muscle. Some years before, he and his co-workers had established many of the ideas still current in exercise physiology, such as that of "oxygen debt." I've always wondered whether Hill's interest in muscle and exercise physiology arose from his own fine athletic abilities.

I first met A.V. Hill in 1945, bringing the results of my research done as a student. Hill gave these not a glance, which was discouraging, but proposed that I get to work on the force-velocity curve of human muscle, which I duly did with results (Wilkie, 1950b) that may be familiar to some of you. Calculations of the way in which velocity rose with time that are shown in my 1950b paper took more than two weeks of solid hand-cranking on a Brunsvega calculator. I thought that there must be a better way and devised the analog circuit shown in Figure 1 (Wilkie, 1950a). The editors of the *Journal of Physiology* excluded it from my manuscript on the ground that it was "too technical," so I take the excuse to publish it here. I think that it was the first computer simulation of muscular contraction.

On the biochemical front, Lippman, Lohmann, Lundsgaard, and many others had established by 1940 in "test tube" studies that ATP is indeed the prime fuel for muscular contraction. The first step towards closing the gap between the chemical and the physical had been made in 1939 by V.A. Engelhardt and his wife, M.N. Lyubimova, in Moscow when they showed that muscle protein had ATP-ase activity. According to Dorothy Needham (1971), "the idea of the enzymic activity of the muscle machinery itself was an entirely new one, and the Russian workers fully realized its implications." They went on to examine the effect of ATP on muscle-protein threads. Perversely, the threads relaxed.

Quite soon the next great step was made by Albert Szent-Gyorgyi. In what seems to have been a flash of inspired imagination, Szent-Gyorgyi had devised the glycerinated rabbit psoas preparation that has been a steady and sturdy contributor to muscle research ever since. Under the action of ATP, these fibres contract as strongly and as fast as living muscle does.

In retrospect it seems strange that it took so long for the biophysical and the biochemical approaches to link up. Partly it was a matter of mutual ignorance, but there was also an element of aversion: Some of the key (and correct) biochemical experiments seemed very messy to the precise-minded biophysicists. The real coming-together of biophysics and biochemistry occurred in a

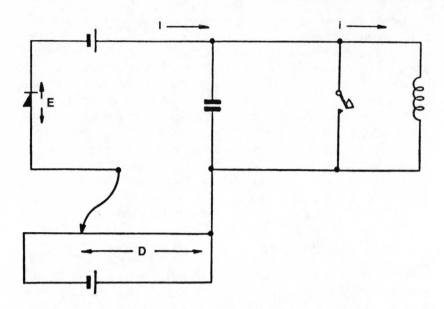

Figure 1. An analogue circuit having voltage-current characteristics that mimic the force-velocity curve of muscle. This was used to calculate how the velocity rises as a function of time during a single contraction of a muscle pulling against a force, an inertia and a compliance, in series. A single solution of the nonlinear differential equation concerned previously took several days using numerical methods and a hand-cranked calculator. The current i through the inductance on the right is proportional to the velocity of the load. For details see Wilkie (1950a, 1950b).

new field, that of ultrastructure, when Hugh Huxley and Jean Hanson (1954) showed how the long-demonstrated biochemical processes actually operate at ultramicroscopic level. Initially, Hugh Huxley obtained the first low-angle, X-ray diffraction studies of muscle. Then through a mastery of the electron microscope in the days when it was extremely difficult to use, he progressed to his latest studies of time-resolved changes in X-ray diffraction as observed using the powerful X-ray beams derived from a synchrotron.

An almost unknown and, for me, very sad story concerns the way in which Annemarie Weber and I could in principle have discovered in 1951 that muscle shortening results from sliding movement of actin relative to myosin filaments. At least we had assembled in my laboratory all the essential apparatus: polarizing microscope, glycerinated rabbit psoas, ATP and Mg solutions. It never occurred to either of us, however, to look critically at contraction down the microscope: We measured the force-velocity curve instead, and because of our blinkers a golden opportunity was lost.

In those days we were obliged to make much of our own apparatus, often out of government surplus bits and pieces. This was highly educational and at least spared us the present harassment over grant applications. Nevertheless, I cannot help regretting the time spent in trying to build stable DC amplifiers (especially in the Plymouth laboratory, where *everything* conducted electricity) and in making calculations. In some ways I do think the old days were more suited to accurate experimentation. Wallace Fenn once observed to me that in his youth there were few laboratory assistants and every scientist performed all aspects of experiments, including all the critical washing of glassware. On the other hand, at that time one could hire servants to look after the house. Today we have technicians in the laboratory and at home we must do our own washing up.

By 1960 even I was forced to realize the importance of biochemistry as a result of thinking and writing about thermodynamics (Wilkie, 1960b). This showed among other things that the measurements of heat and work that we had made up until then could not be interpreted without parallel chemical measurements. You will be spared details of the next 15 years' work, the chief conclusion of which (Gilbert, Kretzschmar, & Wilkie, 1972; Curtin, Gilbert, Kretzschmar, & Wilkie, 1974) was that although all the *work* could be accounted for by measured chemical changes, a large early element of the *heat production* was unaccounted for. That remains the situation today.

In the meantime I had developed a parallel interest in man-powered flight. This arose from an approach by some members of the Royal Aeronautical Society in 1958: They were forming a committee to promote the subject and wanted physiological advice. My first approach was by dimensional analysis (see Figure 2), which indicated that man-powered flight was just marginally possible, so I gladly agreed to provide the specification of "Man as an Aeroengine." I thought mistakenly that this would merely involve spending a couple of afternoons in the library. How mistaken! It must be a familiar experience that one often takes ages to assemble the information required and seldom finds exactly what one wants (Wilkie, 1960a).

Physiologists had provided numberless measurements of oxygen consumption, but the most complete measurements of mechanical power production were the work of a German engineer, Otto Ursinus (1936), who had made them in connection with an earlier burst of interest in man-powered flying machines. The human engine has the characteristics shown in Figure 3. These results, obtained by direct measurement on a single subject, confirm the conclusions of the earlier literature survey. The mechanical power that can be produced varies, at first very steeply, with the duration for which it must be maintained. The physiological reason for this is that a fixed amount of *work* can be obtained from anaerobic sources (hydrolysis of phosphocreatine, formation of lactic acid) over a variable period of time. This is added to the steady *power* production from oxidative metabolism, which can be maintained for long periods of time. Not surprisingly, we have found that sprinting athletes show a very high ability to produce anaerobic work, while endurance athletes are able to maintain a high steady aerobic power output.

Clearly the region of interest in designing man-powered aircraft is from about 3 min onwards, where the very shallow negative slope means that a

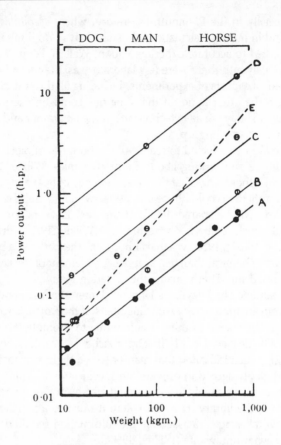

Figure 2. The way in which the power output of an animal varies with its body weight. The experimental points are for dogs, men, and horses. Line A (black spots) represents the basal metabolic rate in the resting animal, line B effort of the kind that can be kept up all day, line C the effort when the animal is really working hard, and line D the maximum output that can be maintained for a few seconds only. The dashed line E represents the power needed to fly. These data suggest that dogs and men are physically capable of flying—though it would be really hard work—but horses are not. See Wilkie (1959).

large increase of duration will be obtained from a small decrease in power requirement. On the basis of quite inadequate information, we had to draw up regulations for the first Kremer competition to make the task difficult but not impossible. I think that our figure-of-eight course must have been about right because the prize was not won for 20 years.

The first straight flights took place in England in 1961 and were repeated and extended over a period of years, mostly in England and Japan. However, the prize was not actually won until 1977 when a brilliant team from California, led by Dr. Paul McCready, adopted a totally novel approach to the problem,

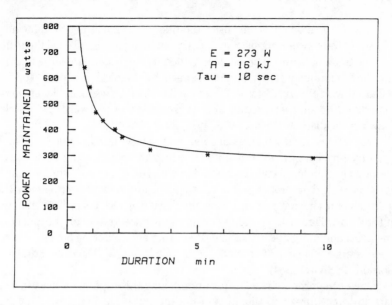

Figure 3.   A special bicycle ergometer was designed and constructed at the request of the Royal Aeronautical Society. Both force and speed could be freely adjusted to suit the task and the performer. Our subject was asked to maintain a given constant power output for as long as he was able. Circles are experimental points. The line is the theoretical curve plotted on the basis of a constant anaerobic *work* (A) that can be produced for a variable period of time, together with an aerobic *power* production (E) that rises exponentially ($T_{1/2}$ = 0.1 min) to a maximum value (Wilkie, 1980; Wilkie, 1981).

ending up with a machine (the Gossamer Condor) that resembled in many ways the original design of the Wright brothers (Grosser, 1981). Among many brilliant ideas was the one to fly at the very slow speed of 9 mph, about half that of the other contestants. Because air resistance increases as the square of the speed, the earlier aircraft had not been able to use the extensive system of bracing wires that made such an important contribution to the success of the California aircraft.

A successor to the original aircraft, the Gossamer Albatross, flew the English Channel. The team wore T-shirts with the message "If it hasn't broken, it's too heavy." Somehow for me this sums up the charm of the very many outstanding engineers and others with whom I was associated for more than 20 years. As Grosser (1981, p. viii) writes, "Anyone who has lost faith in the kindness and altruism of humanity should try building a human-powered airplane." For the latest news about this activity, read the article by Drela and Langford (1985).

My most recent interest concerns the application of nuclear magnetic resonance spectroscopy to intact tissues, which became possible in the early 1970s. I was fascinated by this technique. Radio had been one of my hobbies as a schoolboy, and now I could use radio-frequency signals to determine non-invasively the concentrations of metabolites in living muscle. To tell the truth, I was getting a bit weary after more than a decade of quick-freezing frog muscles and then laboriously analyzing their extracts by chemical methods. Working at Oxford with our collaborator, David Gadian, Joan Dawson and I were fairly soon able to obtain useful results from oxygenated and anaerobic frog muscles (Dawson, Gadian, & Wilkie, 1976, 1977, 1978, 1980).

By 1980 technical advances allowed us to study human muscle as well. The first physiological experiments on a human subject using NMR spectroscopy were undertaken in collaboration with colleagues at Oxford Research Systems using their prototype Topical Magnetic Resonance Spectrometer. The spectrum of resting forearm muscle obtained that day, October 8, 1980, is shown in Figure 4A; Figure 4B shows the changes in concentration of phosphocreatine (PCr) and inorganic phosphate (Pi) during and following 58 min of complete arterial occlusion (Cresshull, et al., 1981; Wilkie, Dawson, Edwards, Gordon, & Shaw, 1984).

One of the primary reasons for undertaking this experiment was to validate our procedures for calibration of the spectral peaks in terms of metabolite concentrations. Notice that while PCr and Pi changed markedly during

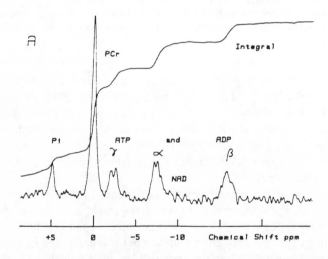

Figure 4A. ³¹P nuclear magnetic resonance spectrum obtained from approximately 20 cm³ of human forearm muscle using a surface coil in the 20 cm TMR 32 spectrometer at Oxford Research Systems on October 8, 1980. The spectrum was accumulated in 26 min (800 pulses at 2 s intervals) and enhanced by convolution differencing. The spectrum itself shows peaks arising from the mobile phosphorus-containing metabolites. The "staircase" curve is the integral of the spectrum. The heights of the steps are proportional to the concentrations of the metabolites.

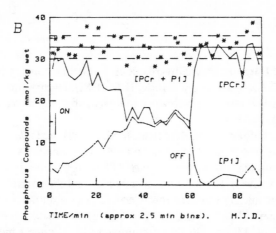

Figure 4B. The changes in concentration of phosphocreatine and inorganic phosphate during and following 58 min of complete arterial occlusion. Stars indicate the sum of [PCr] + [Pi] with solid and dashed lines representing mean ± S.D. See Wilkie (1983); and Wilkie, Dawson, Edwards, Gordon and Shaw (1984).

the course of the experiment, the sum PCr + Pi remained unchanged, as we know it must. An important physiological result concerning the mechanism of activation of glycolysis emerged from this experiment as well. It has been widely believed that glycolysis is regulated by concentrations of phosphorous metabolites or by calculated quantities dependent upon them, such as "phosphate potential" or "adenylate charge." These theories are presented as facts in well-known textbooks (Lehninger, 1975; Stryer, 1981). The results obtained in living muscle are inconsistent with these theories. In spite of the large changes in phosphorous metabolites that accompany ischaemia in the resting muscle, the intracellular pH (indicated by the position of Pi on the X-axis) goes slightly *alkaline*. Similar changes in phosphorous metabolites as a result of contraction rather than ischaemia are accompanied by a large *acid* shift in pH, indicating lactic acid formation through the glycolytic pathway. We concluded that whatever switches glycolysis on is closely associated with contraction and does not directly involve changes in phosphorous metabolite levels (Dawson, 1983; Wilkie, 1983).

I suppose that I should end by peeping into the future, but almost everyone is (fortunately perhaps) so bad at this endeavor that I shall not even attempt it. I hope that the future will *not* contain too much wasteful discovery of facts that were actually perfectly plain many years ago. Our predecessors were not fools, and we should take our satisfaction from adding a brick or two to an existing edifice, not in imagining that we built the whole thing ourselves.

References

Cresshull, I., Dawson, M.J., Edwards, R.H.T., Gadian, D.G., Gordon, R.E., Radda, G.K., Shaw, D., & Wilkie, D.R. (1981). Human muscle analysed by ^{31}P nuclear magnetic resonance in intact subjects. *Journal of Physiology* (London), 317-318.

Curtin, N.A., Gilbert, C., Kretzschmar, K.M., & Wilkie, D.R. (1974). The effect of the performance of work on total energy output and metabolism during muscular contraction. *Journal of Physiology* (London), **238**, 455-472.

Dawson, M.J. (1983). Phosphorous metabolites and the control of glycolysis studied by nuclear magnetic resonance. In H.G. Knuttgen, J.A. Vogel, & J. Poortmans (Eds.), *Biochemistry of Exercise: International series of sports sciences* (Vol. 13, pp. 116-125). Champaign, IL: Human Kinetics.

Dawson, M.J., Gadian, D.G., & Wilkie, D.R. (1976). Living muscle studied by ^{31}P nuclear magnetic resonance. *Journal of Physiology* (London), **258**, 82-83.

Dawson, M.J., Gadian, D.G., & Wilkie, D.R. (1977). Contraction and recovery of living muscle studied by ^{31}P nuclear magnetic resonance. *Journal of Physiology* (London), **267**, 730-735.

Dawson, M.J., Gadian, D.G., & Wilkie, D.R. (1978). Muscular fatigue investigated by phosphorous nuclear magnetic resonance. *Nature,* **274**, 861-866.

Dawson, M.J., Gadian, D.G., & Wilkie, D.R. (1980). Mechanical relaxation rate and metabolism studied in fatiguing muscle by phosphorous nuclear magnetic resonance. *Journal of Physiology* (London), **299**, 465-484.

Dawson, M.J., & Wilkie, D.R. (1977, March). Theoretical and practical considerations in harnessing man power. *Royal Aeronautical Society Symposium on Man-Powered Flight.*

Drela, M., & Langford, J.S. (1985, November). Human-powered flight. *Scientific American,* pp. 122-129.

Gilbert, C., Kretzschmar, K.M., & Wilkie, D.R. (1972). Heat, work, and phosphocreatine splitting during muscular contraction. *Cold Spring Harbor Symposium on Quantitative Biology,* **37**, 613-618.

Grosser, M. (1981). *Gossamer odyssey: The triumph of human-powered flight.* London: Michael Joseph.

Hill, A.V. (1938). The heat of shortening and the dynamic constants of muscle. *Proceedings of the Royal Society of London: Series B,* **126**, 136-195.

Huxley, A.F. (1957). Muscle structure and theories of contraction. *Progress in Biophysics and Biophysical Chemistry,* **7**, 255-318.

Huxley, A.F., & Hanson, J. (1954). Changes in the cross-striations of muscle during contraction and stretch and their structural interpretation. *Nature,* **173**, 973-976.

Lehmann, C.G. (1851). *Physiological Chemistry* (G.E. Day, Trans.). London, Harrison & Son.

Lehninger, A.L. (1975). *Biochemistry* (2nd ed.). New York: Worth Publishers.

Needham, D.M. (1971). *Machina Carnis* [The biochemistry of muscular contraction in its historical development]. Cambridge University Press.

Stryer, L. (1981). *Biochemistry* (2nd ed.). San Francisco: W.H. Freeman.

Ursinus, O. (1936). Grundung des Muskelflug. Instituts Frankfurt a.M., etc., Flugsport, 1-28.

Ursinus, O. (1937). Versuche mit Energie-speichern, etc., Flugsport, pp. 33-40.

Wilkie, D.R. (1950a, October). The circuit analogue of muscle. *Electronic Engineering,* pp. 435-438.

Wilkie, D.R. (1950b). The relation between force and velocity in human muscle. *Journal of Physiology* (London), 110, 249-280.

Wilkie, D.R. (1959). The work output of animals: Flight by birds and by manpower. *Nature,* 183, 1515-1516.

Wilkie, D.R. (1960a). Man as a source of mechanical power. *Ergonomics,* 3, 1-8.

Wilkie, D.R. (1960b). Thermodynamics and the interpretation of biological heat measurements. *Progress in Biophysics,* 10, 259-298.

Wilkie, D.R. (1980). Equations describing power input by humans as a function of duration of exercise. *Elsevier/North Holland Biochemical Press, Exercise bioenergetics and gas exchange,* 25-34.

Wilkie, D.R. (1981). Shortage of chemical fuel as a cause of fatigue: Studies by nuclear magnetic resonance and bicycle egometry. In R. Porter & J. Whelan (Eds.), *Human muscle fatigue: Physiological mechanisms* (Ciba Foundation Symposium 82, pp. 102-119). London: Pitman Medical.

Wilkie, D.R. (1983). The control of glycolysis in living muscle studied by nuclear magnetic resonance and other techniques. *Biochemical Society Transactions,* II, 244-246.

Wilkie, D.R., Dawson, M.J., Edwards, R.H.T., Gordon, R.E., & Shaw, D. (1984). ^{31}P NMR studies of resting muscle in normal human subjects. In G.H. Pollack & H. Sugi (Eds.), *Contractile mechanisms in muscle* (pp. 333-347). New York: Plenum.

2

The Biophysics of Maximal Muscle Power Outputs: Methods and Problems of Measurement

James J. Perrine
University of California, Los Angeles

My interest in the amazing dynamic force-developing capabilities of muscle tissue became serious in 1962 when I became curious about the possible functional advantages of exercising muscles at maximum power output, rather than simply at maximum force capacity. Also, it seemed clear that there was a need for an improved method to measure a muscle's dynamic force potentials that could be applied in research and training. That was the start of 10 years of work on the isokinetic loading power dynamometer. I will review some of the theoretical and practical considerations related to its design and use in the measurement of maximal power output by human muscles in vivo.

Until recently much of the interest and attention in muscle testing and training has been on the absolute maximum force or strength potential of muscles. The functional relevance of the maximum rate that a muscle can generate and transfer mechanical energy has not been generally appreciated. Furthermore, many have assumed that strong muscles are also capable of achieving high instantaneous power factors. However, this is not always the case for a number of reasons, some of which I will refer to later.

Another basic functional property of muscle—that of endurance—is tied directly to the muscle power factor, in that the amount of time a muscle is capable of performing a given task depends on the rate of energy expenditure, in relation to the amount of energy available and the rate at which it is replaced. However, many methods that measure local muscle endurance control neither the power factor nor the contraction/rest interval "duty cycle."

If muscles behave similarly to other mechanical energy generation systems having a low volume, intermediate energy storage medium, the maximal rate that a muscle can generate and transfer mechanical energy (first) to its integral elastic component (i.e., develop a primary, internal power factor) will determine how well the muscle is able to handle two basic types of functional demand. First is the demand associated with a rapidly developing muscle contraction, in which the requirement is to build up an effective force quickly. In this situation, a high internal energy generation rate/power factor is required even when there is little or no external shortening, and thus little or no external energy/power output. An example occurs when stabilizing muscles must contract quickly to prevent undesirable movement. The second demand is the maintenance of dynamic force, when a muscle needs to rapidly replace mechanical energy in its elastic component and maintain force against a moving load. This is the case in activities such as jumping, when it is important to continue to apply accelerative force as vertical velocity increases before leaving the ground. Note that for both of these dynamic demands, a muscle's (immediate) internal power capacity is a limiting factor to the relative amount of external force it can apply.

If muscles behaved in vivo according to Hill's (1938) classical in vitro relationship, one could assess muscle power potentials by simply measuring the maximal static or isometric force capacity and use the characteristic equation to derive the force potentials for various velocities, including the velocity associated with the maximal instantaneous power output. However, it appears that the in vivo force-velocity relationship varies considerably from individual to individual in the lower velocity region, thus requiring more complex methods to measure the maximum power output capabilities of muscle in vivo.

Measurement of Muscle Versus Machine Power

Mechanical engineers use both preloading and afterloading methods to measure the power output of motors and engines. The advantage of simpler loading mechanisms associated with preloading methods is offset by the complexity of instrumentation required to measure acceleration, inertial forces, and position. Afterloading methods are more flexible in their usage and application as long as their operating speed range is adequate. The measurement of power outputs generated by continuous operation motors and engines is a relatively simple task for mechanical engineers. But physiologists attempting to measure the power factors achieved in individual muscle contractions are at a disadvantage because muscles have only a small range of shortening and combine mechanical energy generation and storage. It is impossible to measure the rates at which muscles produce and transfer mechanical energy internally. Only the external manifestations of the energy are capable of measurement. Knowledge of the specific amount of mechanical energy that is absorbed and dissipated internally would be required to even calculate the internal power factor developed transiently during explosive isometric contractions. This amount is unknown, so we wait until a muscle's elastic component is saturated with mechanical energy and is transferring the energy externally at a steady state.

Because the shortening range of muscles is finite, high velocity contractions are often brief in relation to the characteristics of mechanical force measuring instruments. A further restriction on muscle testing time comes from the necessity, in dynamic in vivo testing, of beginning both the muscle contraction and the movement from a static start. This requires a measurement time delay while the muscle builds up energy and force in its elastic component. The "contract and release" method used with isolated muscles is not practical in vivo: The unavoidable fall in force following the release and the later redevelopment of the force consume too much time during dynamic contractions.

It appears that most subjects also have difficulty reproducing true maximal position-specific forces at very low velocities, efforts in which maximal contractions are maintained longer than about 500 ms. In our studies the maximal force generation capacities at the lower velocities were found by instructing subjects to delay the onset of full maximal effort until near the joint angle of interest. It is possible that some of the maximal in vivo force-velocity data obtained in earlier studies may be inaccurate if the testing method did not allow for this phenomenon.

The choice of the measurement position is important in obtaining a series of position-specific forces at various velocities. The position has to be sufficiently distal in the range of movement to enable the muscle to attain its full force capability. Otherwise, time may also become a limiting factor to the muscle's force development capability if the limb passes the chosen position before full force potential has been developed at high velocities.

In obtaining valid measurements of power potential, both tester and subject should understand the difference between maximum strength efforts and maximum power efforts. High power output efforts typically involve high movement velocities that are coupled with brief contraction times. In rapid movements lasting only half a second or less, there is little kinesthetic feedback regarding the amount of force generated, and the majority of subjects grossly underestimate the actual force produced. Many athletes who have trained with weights become conditioned to make their best efforts when they can sense the force that they are developing. In the laboratory these individuals commonly misunderstand the type of effort required for maximum power generation compared to static or low velocity maximum strength efforts. Successful athletes in power-dependent activities may be those who have learned to use upper motor centers for performing maximum power contractions without relying on any kinesthetic feedback; such athletes make good subjects for the study of muscle power potentials. Notwithstanding the aforementioned difficulties, comprehensive dynamic in vivo force data may be obtained with isokinetic loading methods.

The Cybex Isokinetic Dynamometer

The Cybex dynamometer, a velocity-specific isokinetic afterloading instrument, overcomes many of the problems inherent in muscle power testing. A basic mechanical feature is a rotary torque input that simplifies the task of isolating muscle groups according to their joint functions. Extraneous muscle contributions to the effort may be prevented by supplemental stabilization means, and by avoiding unfavorable measurement positions. For example, if the knee extensors are tested at a position earlier than about 60° before full extension, then at or near zero speed some subjects may use their trunk muscles to lever their pelvis and thigh slightly forward, producing a spuriously high knee extensor torque value in that position. This tendency invariably disappears at higher test velocities because time is restricted.

The main feature of isokinetic testing is the controlled constant velocity loading, which simplifies position, time, and velocity determinations by establishing a linear relationship between time and position. Of course, if the velocity of a limb is held constant, the shortening velocity of the muscles may still vary because of leverage effects. But when the measurement position is fixed, the muscle is frozen in time at various instantaneous relative shortening velocities. By comparison, when the measurement position is allowed to change in simple peak force-velocity measurements, both the muscle's actual shortening position and its relative velocity may be expected to change also.

Another feature of the apparatus is the virtual absence of resistance below the test velocity, which allows muscles to contract at their optimal power development velocities for a maximum possible time. This may lead to a momentary velocity control lag due to mechanical and system compliance, manifested as a brief initial overspeed and subsequent torque overshoot caused by rapid deceleration of the limb and lever arm mass back down to the control speed. However, this inertial force does not interfere with maximal power testing because it occurs only at the start of a muscle's initial force development period. The apparatus has a maximal loading velocity of 300°/s, which is well under the maximal unloaded velocities of some joints. However, this is not a practical limitation because even the most powerful muscles can barely complete force development before reaching the limit of the range of movement.

Isokinetic dynamometers provide immediate readout of the applied position and velocity-specific forces, allowing the tester to see whether or not the subject's effort has been optimal, and thereby providing an opportunity to encourage the subject to try harder if the preceding value appears to be too low. In determining a full force-velocity profile, an upward progression of test velocity is preferable, with one return to the previous lower velocity for verification of its validity. It is also preferable to control the time interval between successive efforts to about 10 to 15 s.

A number of observations made during the last 20 years may be helpful to others in choosing the design of maximum power testing or training methods. When subjects perform multirepetition contractions at low speed over an extended duration, there is a characteristic sequence of events: an initial brief period of progressive torque improvement, followed by a period of sustained peak output, a progressive decline in torque, and finally a drop off to almost zero, or a leveling off at an apparently self-determined work rate that can be continued indefinitely. Also through the work bout, a cyclical pattern may be seen in the peak force values. However, when conducting multirepetition tests at or near maximum power output velocities, most subjects take three contractions to reach their peak, but this peak cannot be reproduced for more than a single contraction before a progressive decline occurs. Clearly, the energy requirements associated with generating maximum power exceed energy supply and prevent the reproduction of maximum power without a recovery interval of at least several seconds.

It is also clear that muscles do not seem to follow, at least at low velocities, the force-velocity relationship established for isolated muscles. In 1968 I alluded to this possibility, but it was not until 10 years later that I collected data from a diverse subject population in collaboration with V.R. Edgerton. In 1978 we reported that when the maximal in vivo force potential of the knee extensors is measured at a 30° angle of knee flexion, the in vitro relationship is apparently followed from limb velocities of 288° down to about 192°/s, but at this point there is an abrupt change in the curve (see Figure 2). This finding, corroborated in three other studies (Gregor, Edgerton, Perrine, Campion, & DeBus, 1979; Caiozzo, Perrine, & Edgerton, 1981; Wickiewicz, Roy, Powell, Perrine, & Edgerton, 1984) suggests that the force at zero velocity may be less than 50% of that expected if the muscles were stimulated maximally in vitro. This theory is based on the close fit obtained between the curves in our studies spanning the three highest test velocities and those of Hill (1970) between the relative in vitro velocities of 0.37 and 0.56. Also, if our velocity values are extended up the curve for isolated muscle, a mean maximal unloaded velocity capability of 832°/s is projected; this value agrees with the maximal "unloaded" knee extensor velocity of a number of investigators.

The maximal instantaneous power in our study exhibited a peak at 240°/s. This corresponds to a relative velocity of 0.46 on the isolated muscle scale, and is close to the 0.52 relative velocity for peak power by those maximally stimulated muscles. Furthermore, it is possible that the mean in vivo force value recorded at 288°/s was slightly low because some nonathletic subjects found

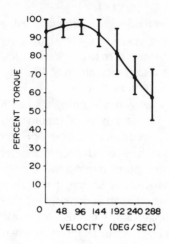

Figure 1. Force-velocity performances of 15 subjects normalized with respect to maximum torque attained by each subject. Dots represent means and vertical bars the range of values for all subjects.

it difficult to make consistent high quality efforts at this velocity. The discrepancy between the force values obtained in vivo and those of isolated muscle at low velocities may be due to the action of a tension-limiting neural regulatory mechanism.

Our work has shown that there is generally little deviation from the isolated muscle curve at high test velocities, but that large individual differences may exist in the lower velocity portion of the curve. From this it may seem necessary to conduct a force velocity test over the whole range of velocities in order to determine a given muscle's power output capacity. However, it seems likely that velocity-specific force measurements made anywhere above the apparent inhibitory zone—more than 200°/s for knee extensors—will closely follow the characteristic equation for force velocity relationships, and thus provide a reasonably good index of power potential when studying a population.

A relative index of maximum power may also be determined from the relative peak force attained in a single, high speed, velocity-specific test as long as the starting point for the movement is controlled for all the subjects to be compared. We used this method in 1976 (unpublished observations) to study the total leg extensor power capabilities of several groups of athletes, and demonstrated good correlations to leg performance measures obtained during natural activities. A correlation coefficient of 0.87 was found between the peak total leg power per unit body weight and the vertical jump heights of a collegiate volleyball team. A similar correlation was obtained between the peak total leg power per unit body weight and the 100-yd dash times of a

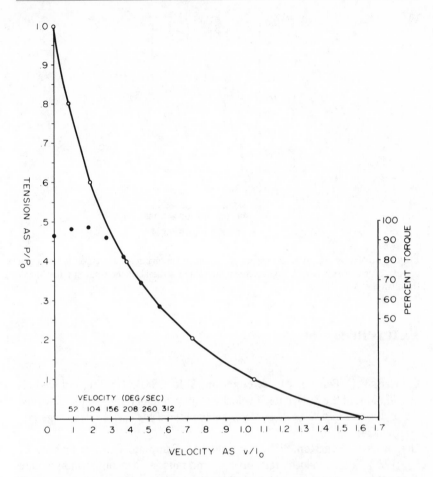

Figure 2. Force-velocity relationships of isolated animal and in-vivo human muscles as determined in two separate experiments under similar loading conditions. Curve drawn through open circles from V = .42 (P^o – P)/P + .26, as determined for isolated muscles in 1968 by Hill. Curve drawn through dots from human in-vivo muscle data of Perrine and Edgerton (1978) scaled to yield best fit with isolated muscle curve.

women's track team. As the maximal velocity and instantaneous power output of athlete's muscles are likely to be higher than those of the general population, natural measures of maximal power may become more popular in the assessment of athletic performance. From a practical standpoint, a natural vertical jump test provides a good index of current leg power, and may also be used on a regular basis to improve the skill factor in jumping, along with the leg muscle power capacity. Such a method was used by the 1984 USA Men's Olympic Volleyball team with good results.

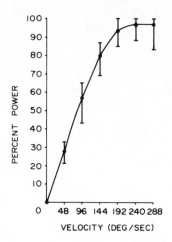

Figure 3.   Power-velocity performances of 15 subjects, normalized with respect to maximum power attained by each subject. Dots represent means and vertical bars the range of values for all subjects.

References

Caiozzo, V.J., Perrine, J.J., & Edgerton, V.R. (1981). Training induced alterations of the in-vivo force-velocity relationship of human muscle. *Journal of Applied Physiology: Respiratory, Environmental and Exercise Physiology, 51,* 750-754.

Gregor, R.J., Edgerton, V.R., Perrine, J.J., Campion, D.S., & DeBus, C. (1979). Torque-velocity relationships and muscle fiber composition in elite female athletes. *Journal of Applied Physiology: Respiratory, Environmental and Exercise Physiology, 47,* 388-392.

Hill, A.V. (1938). The heat of shortening and the dynamic constants of muscle. *Proceedings of Royal Society of London,* B, **126,** 136-195.

Hill, A.V. (1970). *First and last experiments in muscle mechanics.* London: Cambridge University Press.

Perrine, J.J. (1968). Isokinetic exercise and the mechanical energy potentials of muscle. *Journal of Health, Physical Education, Recreation, 39,* 40-44.

Perrine, J.J., & Edgerton, V.R. (1978). Muscle force-velocity and power-velocity relationships under isokinetic loading. *Medicine and Science in Sports,* **10,** 159-166.

Wickiewicz, T.L., Roy, R.R., Powell, P.L., Perrine, J.J., & Edgerton, V.R. (1984). Muscle architecture and force-velocity relationships in humans. *Journal of Applied Physiology: Respiratory, Environmental and Exercise Physiology,* **57,** 435-443.

Discussion

Mr. Perrine was asked whether there was any advantage in exercising at a constant velocity. In slow jogging and running there is a marked power reversal in both the knee and ankle that is almost entirely due to velocity changes, with angular velocity constantly changing in a positive and negative direction. He replied that there are increases in power that can be transferred to specific skills. For example, volleyball players have increased their vertical jump height by training with a constant velocity leg press exercise. By increasing maximal power at a constant velocity, power is also increased in an accelerating movement. There was no evidence to show that training under accelerating conditions is any better.

Dr. Stauber described studies carried out using a method in which force was measured at the point of application rather than through a lever system. In much slower velocities of 5°/s, the forces began to drop to levels below the isometric values. He wondered whether there was a force:time integral that, once exceeded, was associated with central nervous inhibition. Mr. Perrine agreed that this phenomenon could be demonstrated easily, and he suspected that the effect could be overcome somewhat in well-trained and motivated individuals. In his studies of athletes such as weight lifters, who are used to low velocity activity, many did better at lower velocities; however, he had not been able to come close to the classical Hill curve that characterizes isolated muscle. Attempts to obtain a reproducible EMG index to assess this phenomenon have proved difficult, and the available data did not allow one to even speculate.

Dr. Faulkner pointed out that in comparing data to the classical in vitro muscle force velocity curve the findings did not agree with the studies of forearm flexors done many years ago by Dr. Wilkie, who did obtain the classical relationships. Mr. Perrine replied that Dr. Wilkie did not directly measure force output but calculated it using equations in which inertial corrections had to be applied. Many of the movements involved accelerative forces and thus cannot be compared directly to studies in which constant loads are applied. Dr. Wilkie pointed out that he had measured the horizontal component of velocity as in the work of Braune and Fischer (Wilkie, 1950). This is much easier to interpret in terms of functioning muscle; instead of measuring torque or angular velocities, he reported the horizontally resolved component in his paper. This could be the explanation for the difference between the results.

Dr. Stein wondered whether the difference between Mr. Perrine's results and Dr. Wilkie's might be due to the muscle groups employed; he asked whether other muscle groups had been studied and whether the same results were obtained. Mr. Perrine replied that many different muscle groups had been studied, and they all seemed to demonstrate the same general behavior.

Dr. Winter enquired whether the force velocity curve was studied at similar lengths of muscle for all velocities; he wondered whether a length-tension effect was occurring, with the force falling dramatically as a result of changes in length. Mr. Perrine replied that length tension effects were negated in examining the force-velocity curve. Although the torque output at a joint does not reflect what is going on in the linear axis of the muscle in terms of tension, there is a certain geometry of a joint system that is not altered with changes in velocity. Thus, if a muscle can do better or worse at different velocities, it will show that relationship at various specific positions. By measuring at an angle of 30° from full extension, the muscle has a chance to reach sufficient velocity to generate its full force potential.

Dr. Bigland-Ritchie wondered if it was only at very low velocities, and not during isometric contractions, that a large inhibition of force was produced, and if there was any fall in the force during isometric contractions without shortening. Mr. Perrine replied that no difference between zero velocity and low velocities was found in the way that his experiments were carried out. Dr. Bigland-Ritchie mentioned that a maximal voluntary contraction of the quadriceps may be matched by supramaximal stimulation of the femoral nerve. In this type of study a very good relationship was found to indicate that the rate of metabolic heat production between a maximal voluntary contraction and supramaximal stimulation is identical, which was extremely persuasive evidence that all the muscle fibers in a well-practiced subject are activated by a voluntary contraction. These findings are thus incompatible with an inhibitory process. Mr. Perrine said he was unable to see how these findings would confirm that the muscles had been maximally activated because losses may occur in the external excitation, just as internal attenuations may be due to the body's own inhibitory process. He did not know whether Dr. Bigland-Ritchie's results proved that if one were to take the muscle out of the body, it could not produce more force.

Dr. Heigenhauser pointed out that in using a Cybex apparatus the rotatory component of force development in the leg is being mainly measured; the other component of force is in the same direction as the leg and results in a compressive force at the joint. He wondered what happened to the compression component of force at different velocities as this might significantly influence the interpretation of the results. Mr. Perrine conceded this possibility but felt that losses of this type were small; also because all his results had been obtained at a position of 30° from horizontal, the knee extensor's compression force should have been relatively low.

There was further discussion regarding the validity of studying force velocity characteristics with the Cybex apparatus applied to the knee joint. Because the torque measured depends in part on the position of the knee, and anterior and posterior displacement of the tibia may occur, knee joint kinematics are very sensitive to loads applied to the tibia, which might be altered by the relative points of contact between the femur and the tibia. This effectively, if only slightly, changes the length of the lever arm; in a position in which there is anterior displacement of the tibia, the anterior cruciate ligaments will be loaded and the tibia pulled forward in the isometric condition through stretching of the cruciates. However, in a high speed contraction the force on the ligaments is much less. These relative positional changes will be influenced by the resistive load that is applied to the tibia.

Mr. Perrine was also asked whether the increases in torque observed with multiple repetitive contractions were due to increases in activation and whether this phenomenon was observed at all testing speeds, to which he replied that the maximal voluntary power output of a muscle occurs quite consistently after two or three contractions. Apart from its consistency he was not sure what the behavior represented, although it has interesting implications for human performance, such as in a maximal high jump.

Dr. Wilkie felt that the emphasis of studies on the knee was misplaced, and more valid information may be obtained by studies of the upper arm in which the effect of changes in muscle length is more easily studied. It depends on whether one is trying to examine a muscle in situ or during athletic events; both are important but they are different. It was shown by Braune and Fischer in about 1895 that if the muscles of the upper arm are examined and the measurements of force made in terms of the components parallel with the upper arm, then it is possible to measure the properties of the muscles themselves (Wilkie, 1950). The knee joint is much more complicated due to the patella tendon rotating around a cone. This was the reason that he had used the upper arm and examined the horizontal component of the force rather than torque. However, nowadays with the use of on-line computers, forces and torques may be expressed in either way relatively simply. Mr. Perrine replied that he was aware of the value of looking at the actual tension along the linear axis of the muscle. No one purported that the torque moment measured on the Cybex apparatus is the tension along the axis of the muscle, but that it was a useful index of the linear tension. He wondered whether one can ever measure the tension in a muscle in situ. Even if a strain gauge is placed on the Achilles tendon, the actual placement of the instrument would perhaps ruin the evaluation. In terms of human muscle power he did not feel that it made any difference whether one measures torque moments or the tension in the muscle along the linear axis.

Reference

Wilkie, D.R. (1950). The relation between force and velocity in human muscle. *Journal of Physiology (London)*, **110**, 240-280.

3

The Stretch-Shortening Cycle and Human Power Output

Paavo V. Komi
University of Jyväskylä

Research strategies to explore the phenomenon and mechanisms of normal human movement must include two important elements. One requirement is that the exercise conditions cover a considerable portion of the physiological range. The other is that the exercise should be as natural as possible with regard to muscle function. This paper is concerned primarily with the natural type of muscular contraction—stretch-shortening cycle—and attempts to describe how mechanical parameters of muscle and also efficiency may differ from the results demonstrated in isolated muscle contraction. The power output of the human skeletal muscle will be included in this discussion.

Types of Muscle Contraction

The term contraction may be thought of as the state of muscle when tension is generated across a number of actin and myosin filaments. Depending on the external load, the direction of action, and the magnitude (see Table 1), contraction may be concentric, in which the muscle shortens (i.e., the net muscle moment is in the same direction as the change in joint angle, and mechanical work is positive); eccentric, in which the muscle is lengthened (i.e., net muscle moment is in the opposite direction to the change in joint angle, and mechanical work is negative); and isometric, in which neither muscle length nor joint angle changes and mechanical work is zero.

Table 1. Classification of Contraction and Exercise Types

Type of Contraction	Function	External Mechanical Work
Concentric	Acceleration	Positive (W = F [+D])
Isometric	Fixation	Zero (no change in length)
Eccentric	Deceleration	Negative (W = F [−D])

It is in the eccentric mode that the force and power capacities of the skeletal muscle are greatest. According to the force-velocity curve, the maximum force decreases (concentric contraction) or increases (eccentric contraction) as a function of the shortening or stretching velocities, respectively. The increase in force output in eccentric contraction is primarily of chemomechanical origin. This was demonstrated by Edman, Elzinga, and Noble (1978), who showed that the force of an isolated sarcomere increases beyond Po when the fibril is being stretched after the isometric maximum is reached with a constant tetanic stimulation. This "mechanical" origin of the high force in eccentric contraction was also emphasized in studies with human forearm flexors (Komi, 1973) when the maximum integrated EMG (IEMG) was similar in both eccentric and concentric contractions at relatively slow velocities. On the other hand, it has been suggested that when human skeletal muscle is stretched after the maximum isometric force has been reached, EMG activity is also increased, perhaps through increased activation of Ia afferents (Bührle, Schmidtbleicher, & Ressel, 1983). Although the contribution of this additional motor unit activation to the eccentric force is probably a small part of the entire force enhancement, it emphasizes the important role of the nervous system in influencing the force and stiffness characteristics of the contracting muscle. As will become evident, this role is also important in the stretch-shortening cycle.

Two additional differences between eccentric and concentric contractions need to be mentioned. First, it is well documented that the slopes representing IEMG and force relationships are different in these two types of contraction (Bigland & Lippold, 1954; Komi, 1973; see Figure 1A). To attain a certain force level requires much less motor unit activation in eccentric than concentric contraction. Secondly, oxygen consumption is much lower during eccentric exercise than in comparable concentric exercise (Asmussen, 1952; see Figure 1B). These findings indicate quite clearly that input/output relationships of the two exercise types are very different and that the mechanical efficiency of eccentric exercise may be several times higher than that of pure concentric exercise. This can also be seen for Figure 1C, which shows Margaria's (1938) findings that in higher stretch-velocity conditions the mechanical efficiency of eccentric exercise (negative work) may reach a constant value of −1.2 (120%).

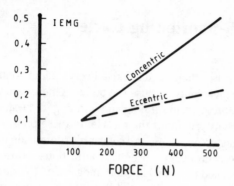

Figure 1A. Relationship between integrated electromyographic (IEMG) activity of the bicep brachii muscle and the elbow flexor force under concentric and eccentric contraction performed with comparable velocities of shortening and stretching, respectively (Komi, 1973).

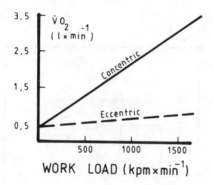

Figure 1B. Relationship between oxygen uptake ($\dot{V}O_2$) and work rate during positive (concentric) and negative (eccentric) work (Asmussen, 1952).

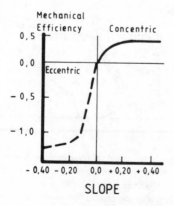

Figure 1C. Mechanical efficiency of negative (eccentric) and positive (concentric) work during treadmill walking at different downhill and uphill inclinations, respectively (Margaria, 1938).

The Stretch-Shortening Cycle

The types of contraction listed in Table 1 very seldom occur alone in normal human muscle movements because the body segments are periodically subjected to impact forces, as in running and jumping, or because some external force such as gravity lengthens the muscle. In these phases the muscles are usually contracting eccentrically, and concentric contraction follows. Thus, the combination of eccentric and concentric contractions forms a natural type of muscle function called the "stretch-shortening cycle" (Norman & Komi, 1979; Komi, 1984). This behavior allows the final action (concentric contraction) to take place with greater force or power output than a movement initiated by concentric contraction alone. Figure 2 characterizes the nature of the stretch-shortening cycle in relation to the impact loads associated with walking or running.

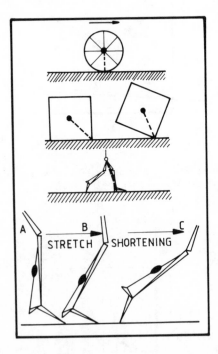

Figure 2. Human walking and running do not resemble the movement of a rotating wheel, where the center of gravity is always directly above the point of contact and perpendicular to the line of progression. Instead they resemble the action of a "rolling" cubic box and have considerable impact loads when contact takes place with the ground. Before contact the muscles are preactivated (A) and ready to resist the impact, during which they are stretched (B). The stretch phase is followed by a shortening (concentric) contraction. The lower part of the figure demonstrates the stretch-shortening cycle, the natural form of muscle function (Komi, 1984).

The modifications in mechanical and metabolic performance associated with a preceding high efficiency eccentric contraction have been studied in experiments performed with isolated fibrils, isolated muscles, and intact human muscles. Edman et al. (1978) demonstrated that especially at greater lengths the sarcomere force-velocity curve is shifted to the right when shortening follows an active stretch. Also, Cavagna, Saibene, and Margaria (1965) demonstrated in isolated frog sartorius muscle that the performance of muscle in concentric contraction was potentiated when preceded by an active stretch. Similar phenomena have been demonstrated in human leg extensor muscles (Komi, 1983; see Figure 3). Of importance in this potentiation is close coupling between stretch and shortening phases.

Enhancement of performance through prestretching can be seen both in the force-length and force- (or work-) velocity curves (Cavagna, Dusman, & Margaria, 1968). When the force-velocity (F-V) curve is measured during a complex movement involving several joints, as in vertical jumping, preparatory countermovement shifts the F-V curve to the right, thus causing the leg ex-

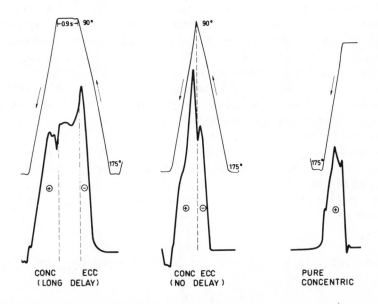

Figure 3. The coupling time between the eccentric and concentric phases of the stretch-shortening cycle influences the potentiation of the force in the concentric phase. (Middle) Concentric contraction is preceded by eccentric (−) contraction and no delay is allowed when contraction is changed. The eccentric phase begins somewhere in the middle of the quadriceps muscle lengthening from the 175° (knee extended) position to the 90° position. Note the clear force potentiation in the concentric (+) phase as compared to the condition on the right. (Right) Pure concentric contraction of the knee extensors is from approximately 100° to 175°. (Left) A longer delay (0.9 s) was allowed between the eccentric and concentric phases, and the potentiation effect on the concentric phases was reduced (Komi, 1983).

tensor muscles to exert much higher forces at any angular velocity of the knee in the concentric phase (Bosco & Komi, 1979). Similarly, the power-angular velocity curve is also displaced so that a greater power output is recorded at any angular velocity in countermovement jumps than in squatting jumps. As the original study of Cavagna et al. (1965) was in isolated frog sartorius muscle, the performance potentiation of the stretch-shortening cycle may have been due solely to the effects of elastic potentiation. Later, Cavagna et al. (1968) were able to obtain similar results with intact human elbow flexor muscles. The experiments of Edman, Elzinga, and Noble (1982) with isolated fibrils also argue in favor of pure elastic (chemomechanical) potentiation. However, because the stretching of muscles in the eccentric phase must activate muscle spindles, some potentiation via reflex loops may also occur. Myoelectrical activity of the leg extensor muscles may be potentiated during the contact phase of the running cycle (Dietz, Schmidtbleicher, & Noth, 1979). Thus, it is likely that when the nervous connections are intact, the enhancement of performance in the stretch-shortening cycle can be attributed to the combined effects of restitution of elastic energy and stretch reflex potentiation of muscle.

Estimation of the relative contributions of the two mechanisms has also been made in jumps performed with plantar flexion when the knee and hip joints were fixed (Bosco, Tarkka, & Komi, 1982). The calculations suggested that the elasticity accounts for slightly more than 2/3 of the total potentiation. It must be emphasized, however, that while these calculations are only estimates, the *elastic* and *myoelectrical* components should not be separated because any increase in myoelectrical potentiation results in elastic potentiation. Also, when active muscle is under stretch, the activity from both the muscle spindles and the Golgi tendon organs will increase. The magnitude of the stretch load will then determine which of these reflexes—facilitatory or inhibitory—will dominate, and thus the magnitude of the potentiation. Reflex potentiation has been demonstrated by Schmidtbleicher (personal communication) in well-trained athletes; preactivation before contact on the ground occurs very late but rapidly and is followed by a pronounced increase of EMG activity via a stretch reflex.

Mechanical Efficiency of Stretch-Shortening Cycle Exercise

If the potentiation of performance in the concentric phase after prestretching can be attributed mainly to mechanical factors, then the mechanical efficiency of positive work may be increased as well. In order to answer this question, it is important to determine the efficiency of the eccentric exercise. When satisfactory answers to this question have been obtained, it is easier to examine the problem in a combined eccentric-concentric contraction.

Based primarily on studies by Margaria (1938) and Davies and Barnes (1972), negative work (eccentric exercise) has been accorded a standard efficiency value of −1.2 or −120% (see Figure 1C). However, although the isolated eccentric exercise has very high efficiency, it is very seldom constant and exhibits both interindividual and intraindividual differences that depend primarily on the stretch velocity of the eccentric contraction.

To study concentric or eccentric exercise a special "sledge" apparatus (see Figure 4) was constructed. The apparatus consists of (a) a sledge (m = 33 kg) to which the subject is fixed in a sitting position; (b) a slide of slow friction aluminum tracks on which the sledge runs; and (c) a force-plate perpendicular to the sliding surface. To investigate the mechanical efficiencies of isolated concentric or eccentric exercises, several submaximal exercises are selected. In concentric exercise the subject extends his or her legs so that the sledge slides uphill to a certain distance corresponding to the specified energy level. When the sledge starts its movement downwards, two assistants retard its motion to the starting position (e.g., 90° knee angle) to avoid resistive muscular movement when foot contact with the force-plate is resumed. No countermovement is allowed at the initiation of each contraction. A sufficient number of concentric contractions (e.g., 80 times) can be performed with a constant intercontraction interval. Isolated eccentric contractions may be performed with the sledge being released from a distance corresponding to the required energy level, and the subject resists the downward movement. A rope is attached to the end of the sledge and fixed so that the movement of the sledge stops when the knee angle of 90° is reached. The assistants then pull the sledge back to the release distance for the next contraction. The force-plate reaction forces are used to calculate the mechanical work, and expired air collected during

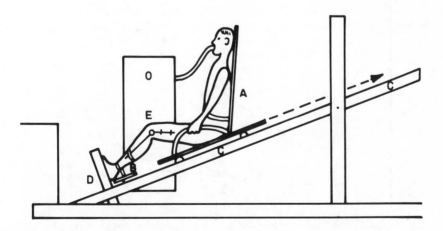

Figure 4.   The special "sledge" ergometer for eccentric and concentric exercises (Kaneko et al., 1984; Komi et al., 1985).

exercise is used to obtain energy expenditure (Kaneko, Komi, & Aura, 1984; Aura & Komi, in press).

This procedure has shown the relationship between energy expenditure and mechanical work to be linear in concentric exercise, but in eccentric exercise the energy expenditure remained relatively low with increasing mechanical work (Kaneko et al., 1984; see Figure 5). The same study also demonstrated that mechanical efficiency of eccentric exercise increased with increasing mechanical work approaching, in some individuals, values of over −1.5 (150%) (see Figure 6). In a similar study, Komi, Kaneko, and Aura (in press) also performed EMG analysis and determined that, despite increasing mechanical work, the integrated EMG (IEMG) of the leg extensor muscles was relatively constant. In concentric exercise, on the other hand, IEMG increased linearly with increasing mechanical work.

The following conclusions may be drawn from the mechanical efficiency studies of isolated eccentric and concentric exercises:

1. Mechanical efficiency of eccentric exercise is very high but not constant.
2. This high efficiency may be increased by increasing stretch velocity.
3. Efficiencies above 100% may be obtained with low motor unit activation in eccentric exercise.

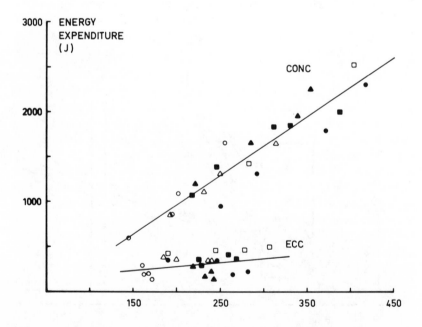

Figure 5. Relationship between net energy expenditure (J/contraction) and mechanical work in concentric (Conc) and eccentric (Ecc) exercises (Kaneko et al., 1984).

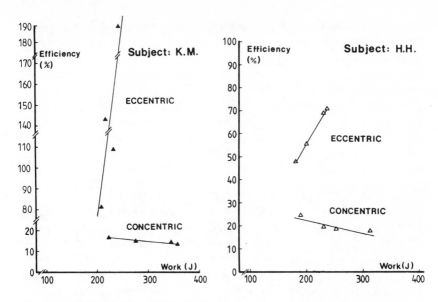

Figure 6. Mechanical efficiency of isolated concentric and eccentric exercises in two male subjects (Kaneko et al., 1984).

4. In concentric exercise the change in EMG, energy expenditure, and mechanical work is parallel.

In normal locomotion where the stretch-shortening cycle is the fundamental form of muscle action, the positive work efficiency has been calculated from the Margaria "constant" of -1.2 for negative work efficiency. From the observations above, it is clear that the efficiency of the prestretch (negative) work phase has both intra- and interindividual differences. Thus, efficiency values presented in our recent reports (Komi, Ito, Sjödin, Wallenstein, & Karlsson, 1981; Bosco et al., 1982b; Ito, Komi, Sjödin, Bosco, & Karlsson, 1983) of positive work should be considered approximations only.

It is also possible with the sledge apparatus described earlier to measure quite accurately the efficiency of the positive work phase in stretch-shortening cycle conditions. The assumption must be made, however, that when eccentric contractions are performed separately, without allowance for any positive work phase, the efficiency of that exercise is the same as in the eccentric phase of the stretch-shortening exercise where the impact conditions are comparable (i.e., with the subject being dropped against the force-plate from the same height). In the study by Aura and Komi (in press), the experimental conditions were arranged so that the concentric work level was always kept constant at 60% of the maximum concentric effort. The preceding eccentric load differed in the various test situations, with minimum time being allowed between eccentric and concentric phases, and the hopping frequency in each series was constant at 0.33 Hz. The efficiency of the positive work for the various stretch-shortening cycle exercises was calculated according to the following formula:

$$\eta^+ = \frac{W_{pos}}{\dfrac{\Delta E_n - W_{neq}}{\eta^-}} \times 100$$

Where η^- denotes the efficiency of the comparable negative work obtained in a separate eccentric exercise situation for each subject. As in the previous studies the individual values for negative work efficiency varied considerably between 72% and 209%. The efficiency value for the 60% positive work was 22.4%. This value was increased considerably when positive work was preceded by negative work. The potentiation effect was greater, the greater the dropping height (i.e., the level of the negative work). The result was similar when the negative work phase was expressed as the mean flexion velocity of the knee joint.

EMG activities from the knee extensor muscles were also integrated separately for negative and positive work phases in each exercise condition. The integrated EMG value for the constant 60% concentric work decreased significantly when the preceding eccentric work level was changed from 20% to 80% maximum. Assuming that the amount of the recorded EMG activity reflects the expenditure of metabolic energy, one can understand the increase in the mechanical efficiency of positive work with higher preceding stretches or mechanical energy levels.

Conclusions

The results presented in this paper should not be taken to indicate that our understanding of the stretch-shortening cycle is clear and that the mechanism for potentiation has been explained. Future research should examine more closely the role of the nervous system in potentiation of performance in this natural form of muscle function. For example, there is a need for better understanding of the stretch reflex activity during the stretch-shortening cycle. Facilitatory and inhibitory reflexes with increasing stretch-loads should be identified. One of the challenging tasks facing researchers is the identification of the sites in the muscle-tendon complex where storage of elastic energy takes place.

References

Asmussen, E. (1952). Positive and negative muscular work. *Acta Physiologica Scandinavica*, **28**, 364-382.

Aura, O., & Komi, P.V. (in press). The mechanical efficiency and EMG activity in stretch-shortening cycle exercises. *Acta Physiologica Scandinavica*.

Bigland, B., & Lippold, O.C.J. (1954). The relation between force, velocity and integrated electrical activity in human muscles. *Journal of Physiology* (London), **123**, 214-224.

Bosco, C., Ito, A., Komi, P.V., Luhtanen, P., Rahkila, P., Rusko, H., & Viitasalo, J.T. (1982b). Neuromuscular function and mechanical efficiency of human leg extensor muscles during jumping exercises. *Acta Physiologica Scandinavica*, **114**, 543-550.

Bosco, C., & Komi, P.V. (1979). Potentiation of the mechanical behavior of the human skeletal muscle through prestretching. *Acta Physiologica Scandinavica*, **106**, 467-472.

Bosco, C., Tarkka, I., & Komi, P.V. (1982). Effect of elastic energy and myoelectrical potentiation on triceps surae during stretch-shortening exercise. *International Journal of Sports Medicine*, **3**, 137-140.

Bührle, M., Schmidtbleicher, D., & Ressel, H. (1983). Die spezielle Diagnose der einzelnen Kraftkomponenten im Hochleistungssport. *Leistungssport* 3/83, 11-16.

Cavagna, G.A., Dusman, B., & Margaria, R. (1968). Positive work done by the previously stretched muscle. *Journal of Applied Physiology*, **24**, 31-32.

Cavagna, G.A., Saibene, P.F., & Margaria, R. (1965). Effect of negative work on the amount of positive work performed by an isolated muscle. *Journal of Applied Physiology*, **20**, 157-158.

Davies, C.T.M., & Barnes, C. (1972). Negative (eccentric) work: Physiological responses to walking uphill and downhill on a motor driven treadmill. *Ergonomics*, **15**, 121-131.

Dietz, V., Schmidtbleicher, D.S., & Noth, J. (1979). Neuronal mechanisms of human locomotion. *Journal of Neurophysiology*, **42**, 1212-1222.

Edman, K.A.P., Elzinga, G., & Noble, M.I.M. (1978). Enhancement of mechanical performance by stretch during tetanic contractions of vertebrate skeletal muscle fibres. *Journal of Physiology* (London), **281**, 139-155.

Edman, K.A.P., Elzinga, G., & Noble, M.I.M. (1982). Residual force enhancement after stretch of contracting frog single muscle fibers. *Journal of General Physiology*, **80**, 769-784.

Ito, A., Komi, P.V., Sjödin, B., Bosco, C., & Karlsson, J. (1983). Mechanical efficiency of positive work in running at different speeds. *Medicine and Science in Sports and Exercise*, **15**, 299-308.

Kaneko, M., Komi, P.V., & Aura, O. (1984). Mechanical efficiency of concentric and eccentric exercises performed with medium to fast contraction rates. *Scandinavian Journal of Sports Sciences, 6*, 15-20.

Komi, P.V. (1973). Relationship between muscle tension, EMG and velocity of contraction under concentric and eccentric work. In J. Desmedt (Ed.), *New Developments in Electromyography and Clinical Neurophysiology* (Vol. 1, pp. 596-606). Basel: Karger.

Komi, P.V. (1983). Elastic potentiation of muscle and its influence on sport performance. In W. Baumann (Ed.), *Biomechanics and Performance in Sport* (pp. 59-70). Schorndorf: Verlag Karl Hoffman.

Komi, P.V. (1984). Physiological and biomechanical correlates of muscle function: Effects of muscle structure and stretch-shortening cycle on force and speed. In R.L. Terjung (Ed.), *Exercise and Sport Sciences Reviews* (Vol. 12, pp. 81-121). Lexington, MA: The Collamore Press.

Komi, P.V., Ito, A., Sjödin, B., Wallenstein, R., & Karlsson, J. (1981). Muscle metabolism, lactate breaking point, and biomechanical features of endurance running. *International Journal of Sports Medicine, 3*, 148-153.

Komi, P.V., Kaneko, M., & Aura, O. (in press). EMG activity of the leg extensor muscles with special reference to mechanical efficiency in concentric and eccentric work. *Scandinavian Journal of Sport Sciences.*

Margaria, R., (1938). Sulla fisiologia e specialmente sul consumo energetico della marcia e della corsa a varia velocia ed inclinazione del terreno. *Atti Reale Acc. Naz. Lincei, 7*, 299-368.

Norman, R.W., & Komi, P.V. (1979). Electromechanical delay in skeletal muscle under normal movement conditions. *Acta Physiologica Scandinavica, 106*, 241-248.

Discussion

Dr. Winter welcomed a discussion on the negative work and negative power aspects of human movement. That they had received relatively little emphasis in the literature is surprising when one considers that over the course of a day roughly equal amounts of power are expended in negative work as in positive work. The major work done in walking and jogging is during plantar flexor push off; negative power is absorbed by the plantar flexors as the leg rotates over the foot, and as the plantar flexors are stretched, more power is generated during the positive work phase. He wondered whether it was possible to quantify the energy absorbed during the negative work phase in the series elastic component, the viscous component (as heat), and in metabolic events in the contractile elements. Dr. Komi was unable to answer in specific terms; he emphasized, however, that one should be cautious when dividing negative work into its various components without considering the contribution of reflexes and also of mechanical potentiation in the entire stretch-shortening cycle. At the present time the calculations can be applied only to studies in isolated muscle rather than in limb movement.

Mr. Perrine wondered whether the assumption of higher EMG activity indicating higher energy output should be questioned. Was it possible that motor and sensory electrical signals were being detected? If higher force was being applied to muscle, one would expect a higher sensory EMG signal. Dr. Komi thought that the finding of increases in EMG activity during a muscle stretch following an isometric contraction supported the possibility of reflex potentiation. As this potentiation can come only from reflex sources, mechanical factors and EMG potentiation from muscle spindle activity probably both contribute. In addition to reflex activity increasing with increasing stretching loads, inhibitory influences also increase, and at some point these two factors may become equal. This may occur in an impact loading situation in which the load or the velocity is large enough to produce a decrease in performance. During a slow stretch-shortening cycle, the potentiation of EMG activity could be "tied" to the concentric phase. In running, the stretch-shortening cycle is short and impact loads high. More EMG activity has been recorded in the eccentric phase (Komi, 1983). The concentric phase can therefore take place in a recoil manner with lowered EMG activity. There is more EMG activity in the eccentric phase, and the same EMG activity will be associated with higher forces in the eccentric phase than in the concentric phase (see Figure 1).

Reference

Komi, P.V. (1983). Elastic potentiation of muscle and its influence on sport performance. In W. Baumann (Ed.), *Biomechanics and Performance in Sport* (pp. 59-70).

Section **2**

Morphology

4

Morphological Basis of Skeletal Muscle Power Output

V.R. Edgerton, R.R. Roy, R.J. Gregor, and S. Rugg
University of California, Los Angeles

The power produced by a skeletal muscle is the product of the force it generates and the velocity at which it shortens. In turn, the force and velocity potential of a muscle is a function of the biochemical properties of its sarcomeres (Barany, 1967) and how these sarcomeres are arranged with respect to one another (Gans & Bock, 1965; Partridge & Benton, 1981; Spector, Gardiner, Zernicke, Roy, & Edgerton, 1980; Bodine et al., 1982). Because a muscle's force potential is proportional to the number of active sarcomeres *in parallel* and its velocity potential is proportional to the number of active sarcomeres *in series*, this sarcomere arrangement must influence the power potential of different muscles and muscle groups at varying velocities of shortening.

Muscle Architecture and Contractile Properties

The two theoretical muscle designs shown in Figure 1 will be used to illustrate the significance of the sarcomere arrangement. Muscle A has two sarcomeres *in series*; muscle B has two sarcomeres *in parallel*. Assuming that these two muscles have identical masses and the same biochemical features that dictate the force and velocity characteristics of a sarcomere, the differences in their contractile responses can be attributed to the sarcomere arrangement. Isometric twitch contraction and relaxation times will be similar in muscles A and B because the time of onset and termination of activation, and thus a peak twitch tension, will be reached at the same time. But muscle A will have developed

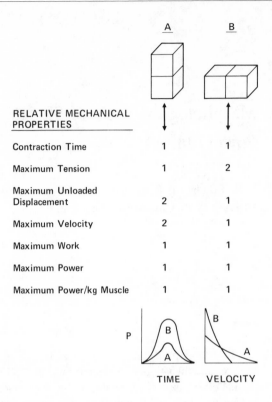

<table>
<tr><td></td><td>A</td><td>B</td></tr>
</table>

RELATIVE MECHANICAL PROPERTIES		
Contraction Time	1	1
Maximum Tension	1	2
Maximum Unloaded Displacement	2	1
Maximum Velocity	2	1
Maximum Work	1	1
Maximum Power	1	1
Maximum Power/kg Muscle	1	1

Figure 1.   Two theoretical ways of arranging two sarcomeres, *in series* and *in parallel*, are shown. The relative effects of these arrangements on the mechanical properties are listed. In addition, the relative isometric and isotonic properties are graphically illustrated at the bottom of the figure for condition A and condition B.

only half the tension in the same period of time as B. On the other hand, when maximally stimulated and unloaded, muscle A will shorten twice as much as B in the same period of time; therefore, the maximal velocity of shortening (V_{max}) of A will be two times higher than B's.

If each muscle is loaded to the same percentage of its respective maximum tetanic tension potential, then both will yield similar amounts of work in the same period of time. Therefore, maximal power and power potential per unit of muscle mass will be the same in both muscles. However, the velocity at which peak power can be produced will differ significantly between muscles A and B (see Figure 2). The peak power of A will occur at twice the velocity as the peak power of B. Further, the range in velocities through which muscle A can produce power will be twice that of B. This power-velocity difference will be significant when two muscles have a common insertion, but one has longer fibers than the other.

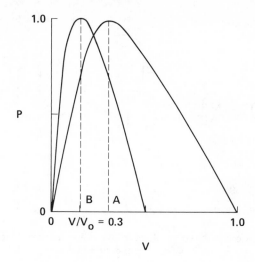

Figure 2. The theoretical power potentials of conditions A and B from Figure 1 are shown. The dashed lines identify the velocity at which peak power was assumed to have occurred relative to the maximum velocity of shortening.

Muscle Architecture, Contractile Properties, and Energy Cost

Differences in energy cost of contraction also are expected of muscles A and B (see Figure 3). For example, when the muscles are fully activated, the same amount of ATP will be utilized, but B will produce twice as much force; therefore, the ATP cost per unit of force will be twice as high in A as in B. The opposite will be true of the energy cost of displacement; that is, half as much shortening will occur in B as in A, although both will have consumed the same amount of ATP when activated similarly. Theoretically, the unit of energy cost per unit of work and power will be similar in muscles A and B. The advantage that muscle A has for displacement (and thus, velocity) will be countered by a similar advantage in muscle B for force production (see Figure 3).

Another way to assess the physiological significance of the two muscle models in Figures 1 and 3 is to estimate the energy cost when both muscles produce the same absolute tensions (see Figure 4). When only half of B and all of A are activated, for example, both muscles will yield identical tensions. In this situation (see Figure 4), twice as much energy will be used in A as in B to produce the same force. The net effect mimics the situation in the previous figure. In contrast, the energy cost of displacement illustrated in Figure 4 is

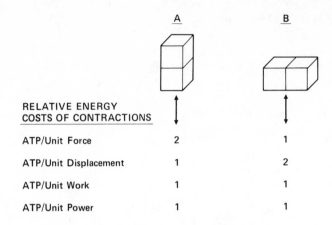

Figure 3. Relative energy costs of muscle models A and B as described in Figure 1 are shown. It is assumed that the two muscle models are maximally activated.

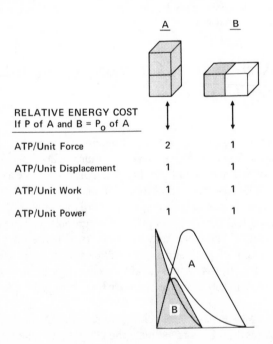

Figure 4. The comparisons made between muscle models A and B are the same as in Figure 3 except that both are "recruited" to produce the same absolute force. Therefore, only one sarcomere is activated (shaded) in B, though both are activated in A.

similar in A and B, as is the cost of power. In this case, A utilizes twice as much ATP as B does, but produces twice as much displacement and power. Perhaps one of the most significant effects of the different muscle designs of A and B is A's higher power over a greater range in velocities (see Figure 2).

Muscle Architecture and Physiological Measurements of Force

The comparisons made in Figures 1-4 represent the theoretical relative effects of the arrangement of sarcomeres *in series* and *in parallel*. Does experimental evidence corroborate these predictions? Powell, Roy, Kanim, Bello, and Edgerton (1984) have shown a remarkably similar maximum tension per physiological cross-sectional area for guinea pig muscles that vary widely in mass and design (see Figure 5). The only muscle that did not produce approximate-

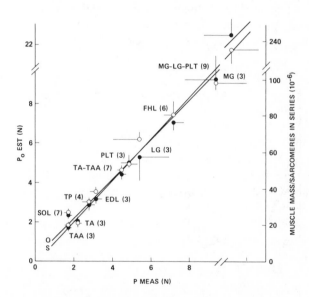

Figure 5. A plot demonstrating the relationship between (1) the measured maximum tetanic tension (Po MEAS) and the estimated Po (Po EST) of selected muscles and muscle groups in the guinea pig hindlimb (o), and (2) the Po MEAS and a ratio of muscle mass to the number of sarcomeres *in series* (•). Linear regressions are plotted for each comparison. The number of muscles tested is in parentheses. The bars represent standard errors.

ly 22.5 N.cm⁻² when maximally stimulated was the homogeneously slow soleus, which produced about 15.7 N.cm². It is likely that this lower specific tension in the muscle is due to differences in the intrinsic biochemical characteristics of the sarcomeres.

Muscle Architecture and Physiological Properties of the Cat Semitendinosus

There also are experimental data that support the contention that a muscle's displacement and V_{max} is proportional to muscle fiber length or number of sarcomeres *in series*. This relationship was illustrated quite clearly by Bodine et al. (1982) when one or both ends of the cat semitendinosus, a muscle that has two anatomically distinct compartments arranged *in series*, were stimulated. Each compartment has fibers that extend the length of the compartment, and the fiber type population is similar in both ends. The distal end has fibers that are twice as long as those in the proximal end, and its V_{max} is twice as fast (see Figure 6). Also, when both ends are stimulated simultaneously, the whole muscle's V_{max} approximates the sum of their respective velocities. This experi-

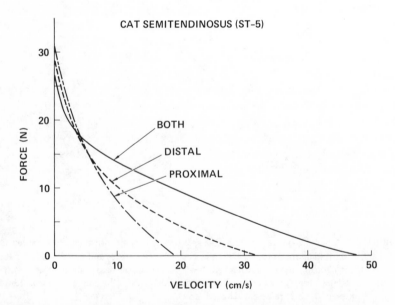

Figure 6. Force-velocity relationships are plotted for the three stimulation conditions in the cat semitendinosus (i.e., when the distal and proximal ends are stimulated independently or together). Maximum forces are similar while maximum velocities of shortening are proportional to functional fiber lengths. The lines are based on data points obtained from one adult cat.

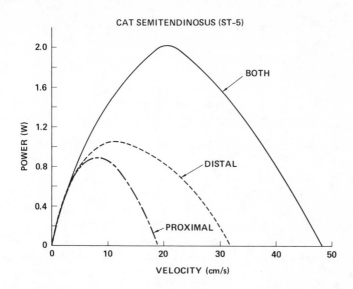

Figure 7. Power curves for the cat semitendinosus under the same three stimulation conditions and for the same muscle shown in Figure 6. Absolute peak power (W) occurs at a shortening velocity relative to functional fiber length.

ment also provides further evidence that fiber length has little effect on maximum tetanic tension because similar tensions are produced when either end is stimulated individually and when both ends are stimulated simultaneously.

The power outputs of the semitendinosus under each of the three stimulating conditions are shown in Figure 7. These experimental conditions are comparable to the theoretical paradigms shown in Figure 4. That is, the active physiological cross-sectional areas are similar under each circumstance, but the effective lengths of the fibers differ. As one would predict, based on the previously discussed concepts, the power potential is proportional to the length of muscle fibers activated (see Figure 7). Similarly, the more sarcomeres *in series* that are activated, the greater is the range in velocities over which the muscle is capable of producing power.

Muscle Architecture and Physiological Properties of the Cat Soleus and Medial Gastrocnemius

A combination of architectural and biochemical characteristics of the cat soleus and medial gastrocnemius muscles account for their large differences in force, V_{max}, and power (see Figure 8). When V_{max} is normalized to an equivalent number of sarcomeres *in series*, a 2.5-fold velocity difference remains

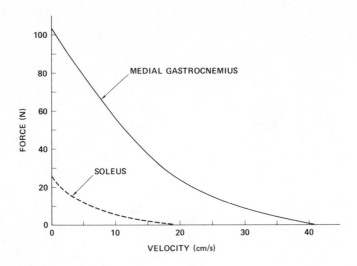

Figure 8. Absolute force-velocity relationships of an adult cat soleus and medial gastrocnemius muscle are shown.

(Spector et al., 1980). This difference corresponds to the 2-3 fold higher potential of fast to slow muscle for hydrolysis of ATP (Buller, Mommaerts, & Seraydarian, 1969). In addition, the functional cross-sectional area and maximum tetanic tension of the medial gastrocnemius is about five times larger than that of the soleus (Sacks & Roy, 1982). Consequently, the large differences in peak power potential between the soleus and medial gastrocnemius muscles are due to a combination of architectural and intrinsic biochemical properties. Perhaps as important as peak power with respect to *in vivo* function of these synergists is the fact that the shortening velocity at which the soleus can produce significant power is restricted to very low rates of ankle plantarflexion. Theoretically, when the medial gastrocnemius functions at peak power, the soleus can produce only a small percentage of its peak power (see Figure 9).

Muscle Architecture and Physiological Properties of Human Muscle Groups

It is possible to make reasonable estimates of physiological properties of human muscles similar to those previously discussed for other mammalian muscles. By combining a series of muscle architectural measurements on human cadavers (Wickiewicz, Roy, Powell, & Edgerton, 1983) and *in vivo* physiological mea-

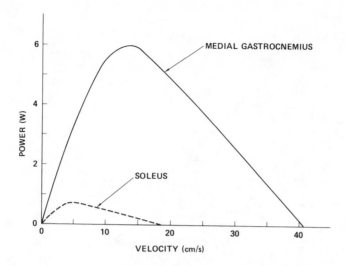

Figure 9. The relationship between power and velocity for cat soleus and medial gastrocnemius muscles is shown. The lines represent data points from the same muscles for which force and velocity are plotted in Figure 8.

surements on normal subjects (Wickiewicz, Roy, Powell, Perrine, & Edgerton, 1984), estimates of maximal force per physiological cross-sectional area and V_{max} per muscle group, muscle, and sarcomere have been made. The relationship between the absolute force and V_{max} of four muscle groups (knee extensors, knee flexors, ankle plantarflexors, and ankle dorsiflexors) is shown in Figure 10. Peak forces of the four muscle groups varied about six-fold. As shown previously for knee extensors (Perrine & Edgerton, 1978), peak torque and force also occurred at velocities greater than zero for the KF and PF, but not the DF. Each of the four muscle groups produced a significantly lower force at zero velocity than would be expected based on Hill's equation describing the force-velocity relationship of *in vitro* maximally stimulated muscle (Hill, 1951). This unexpectedly low torque at zero velocity appears at odds with Wilkie's (1950) data on the elbow flexors of humans. At the higher velocities, the expected force-velocity relationship appears to have occurred for all four muscle groups.

Absolute maximal velocities differed among muscle groups of the human lower limb by as much as three-fold. However, there is a strong similarity of the V_{max} of pairs of agonist and antagonist muscle groups. To determine the influence of architecture on the V_{max}, angular velocities were converted to linear velocities using lever arm distances measured from cadavers, as described by Wickiewicz et al. (1984). This linear velocity then was corrected per fiber

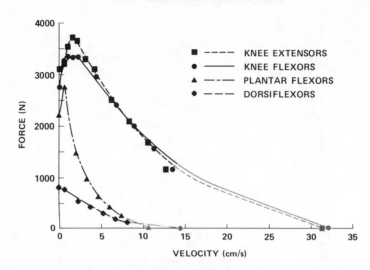

Figure 10. The force and velocity relationships of the four muscle groups noted in this figure were obtained from the subjects reported by Wickiewicz et al. (1984). The lines extended from the last two velocity points were extrapolated from the actual data points at the lower velocities. The forces and velocities were calculated from lever arms, torques, and angular velocities, as noted in Wickiewicz et al. (1984).

length, assuming a sarcomere length of 2.2 μm. The resulting calculations for the V_{max} were 90, 52, 48, and 46 mm.sec^{-1} per 1000 sarcomeres for the KE, KF, PF, and DF when it was assumed that the V_{max} was a function of the longest fibers in a muscle group.

Based on the histochemical analyses of a variety of leg muscles of humans and other mammals (Ariano, Armstrong, & Edgerton, 1973; Saltin & Gollnick, 1983) the overall intrinsic biochemical properties of the major muscle groups of the lower limb seem to vary little. Consequently, one might expect a similar V_{max} when fiber length is normalized for each muscle group. This is particularly true considering that V_{max} should be a function of the fastest muscle fibers. Three of the muscle groups had remarkably similar V_{max} values when normalized to fiber length or a constant number of sarcomeres *in series*, but the KE V_{max} remained considerably higher than the others. An explanation for this apparent discrepancy will rely on more direct measurements of the appropriate morphological features. For example, perhaps a direct measurement of lever lengths of the same subjects tested physiologically would be more desirable than estimates derived from cadavers, as we and others have done.

Based on the force-velocity measurements shown in Figure 10, power was calculated for each of the muscle groups (see Figure 11). As was true for force and velocity, the power and velocity relationships were similar for the agonist-

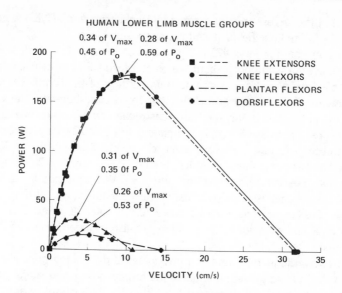

Figure 11. The power and velocity relationships shown are based on the force and velocity data shown in Figure 10. The percent of maximum velocity of shortening and of maximum tension at which peak power occurred is shown for each muscle. Note that peak power occurred at about 0.3 of V_{max} for each muscle group, whereas peak power occurred at relative values of maximum tension that were higher than 0.3.

antagonist muscle groups. However, the muscles that flex and extend the knee were much more powerful than the ankle musculature. Theoretically, peak power per unit mass of muscle should be similar for all muscle groups assuming each muscle group has similar biochemical properties and assuming all muscles in a group have similar architectural features. However, the fiber lengths do differ significantly particularly within the plantarflexors and dorsiflexors of the ankle (Wickiewicz et al., 1983). This variable makes it difficult to relate the peak power of a muscle group to a velocity of shortening because the velocity at which the maximal power occurs is a function of the length of the muscle fibers (see Figures 2,7,9). For example, when two muscles are arranged *in parallel* and have different fiber lengths, the maximal power of the two muscles stimulated simultaneously will be less than the sum of the maximal powers observed at the optimal velocity for peak power for each muscle separately. Note the velocity at which peak power occurs as well as the force at which peak power occurs.

The complication of variable fiber lengths makes any conclusion regarding power per unit of muscle weight per muscle group of limited value. However, if considerable liberty is taken with the above assumption, some calculations of power per unit weight of muscle can be made. For example, the maximum power per unit weight of knee extensors (excluding the slow vastus intermedius) of the largest cadaver studied by Wickiewicz et al. (1983) would be 536 W.Kg^{-1}. The knee flexors (semimembranosus, biceps femoris, and semitendinosus) would produce 472 W.Kg^{-1} based on the muscle weights from the same cadaver. Assumptions about the plantarflexors that actually contribute to the maximal power are more uncertain because of the complexity of the attachments of the variety of muscles that could contribute and the variety of their fiber lengths. If only the lateral gastrocnemius is included because its average fiber length was 5.9 cm in comparison to 3.5 and 2.0 cm for the medial head and the soleus, the power per muscle weight would be 405 W.Kg^{-1}. If the medial gastrocnemius is included, the calculated power is 203 W.Kg^{-1}. If all possible muscles are included, a value of 155 W.Kg^{-1} is calculated. If only the tibialis anterior is principally responsible for the power of dorsiflexion because of its longer fibers, then 470 W.Kg^{-1} is calculated. If the extensor digitorum longus and extensor hallucis longus are also included, then 125 W.Kg^{-1} is calculated (see Table 1).

Based on the architectural and physiological data noted previously, the force, velocity, and power potential of the human soleus and lateral gastrocnemius can be estimated for comparison with data on the cat soleus and medial gastrocnemius (see Figure 12). To make these calculations, the following assumptions were made:

1. Maximum force is proportional to physiological cross-sectional area.
2. The physiological cross-sectional areas of individual muscles or muscle groups in the human subjects tested were similar to that observed in the largest cadaver.
3. The maximal velocity of shortening of the plantarflexors is due principally to the lateral gastrocnemius.

Table 1. In Vivo Power of Human Lower Limb Muscles

	Wet Weight	Maximum Power (W)	(W.Kg$^-$)
KE	0.563	177	[1]536
KF	0.377	178	472
PF	0.206	32	[2]155
DF	0.128	16	[3]125

[1]Weight of heaviest cadaver quadriceps muscles (Wickiewicz et al., 1984) minus the vastus intermedius.
[2]Weight of heaviest cadaver calf muscles minus the soleus (Wickiewicz et al., 1984) and includes the gastrocnemius, plantaris, flexor hallucis longus, and flexor digitorum longus.
[3]Weight of heaviest cadaver muscles. Includes the tibialis anterior, extensor digitorum longus, and extensor hallucis longus.

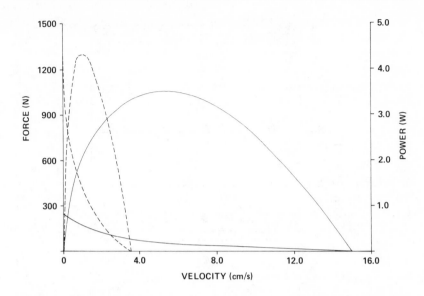

Figure 12.   Predicted force-velocity and power-velocity relationships for the soleus (---) and medial gastrocnemius (—) muscles in humans are shown. Maximum forces were based on physiological cross-sectional areas reported by Wickiewicz et al. (1983) and assuming 22.5 N.cm⁻². Maximal veloc-ities (V_{max}) were based on the findings of the plantarflexors as reported by Wickiewicz et al. (1983). It was also assumed that the V_{max} represented the lateral gastrocnemius, which has the longest fibers of the plantarflexors. It was also assumed that the intrinsic velocity of shortening for the lateral gas-trocnemius was 2.5 times greater than that of the soleus (see text for explanation).

4. The intrinsic properties of sarcomeres are such that the lateral gastroc-nemius shortens 2.5 times faster than those of the soleus.
5. Each muscle has mechanical properties that are similar to those predicted by Hill's equation.

  Given these assumptions, the maximal tension of the soleus muscle of the largest cadaver studied by Wickiewicz et al. (1983, 1984) would be 1305 N and the V_{max} would be 3.4 cm.s⁻¹. The lateral gastrocnemius maximum force would be 243 N and the V_{max} would be 14.9 cm.s⁻¹. It is estimated that the maximal force, velocity, and power curves of these two muscles in humans would ap-pear as shown in Figure 12 if they could be tested *in vitro* or *in situ* using max-imally stimulated conditions.
  A final consideration is the power output of a muscle during normal loco-motion. The most directly measured power output during normal movements and under *in situ* maximum stimulation conditions has been obtained for the cat soleus and medial gastrocnemius (Whiting, Gregor, Roy, & Edgerton, 1984). Figure 13 illustrates the *in vivo* power time curve for a cat step cycle while run-ning at relatively fast (2.2 m.s⁻¹), medium (1.5 m.s⁻¹), and slow (0.8 m.s⁻¹) speeds. The differences in the responses of the two muscles are due to the

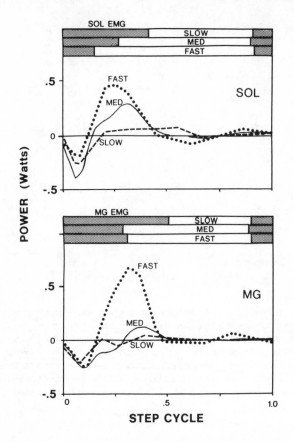

Figure 13. Mean power curves for the cat soleus and medial gastrocnemius muscles during locomotion at treadmill speeds of 0.8 (---), 1.5 (—), and 2.2 (····) m.s⁻¹. Relative EMG timing is shown
at each speed for each muscle.

net effects of their biochemical (intrinsic) properties, architectural features,
mechanical attachments, and levels of excitation by the central nervous system (Edgerton, Roy, Bodine, & Sacks, 1983). The peak power of a step cycle
during the fastest speed was 0.45 W and 0.70 W for the soleus and medial
gastrocnemius muscles, respectively (see Table 2). When expressed per unit
muscle weight, 112 and 73 W.Kg⁻¹ were produced. In comparison, when these
same muscles were tested *in situ*, a maximum of 174 and 440 W.Kg⁻¹ were measured (Spector et al., 1980). Therefore, 64% and 17% of the maximal power
potentials of the cat soleus and medial gastrocnemius muscles were produced
during a typical step cycle as shown in Figure 13.

Table 2. *In Situ* and *In Vivo* Power in the Cat Soleus and Gastrocnemius
Muscles

Muscle	In Situ Maximum Power (W)	(W·Kg⁻¹)	In Vivo Peak Power in Fast Run (W)	(W·Kg⁻¹)	Percent In Vivo In Situ
Soleus	0.7	174	0.45	112	64
Medial Gastrocnemius	6.0	440	0.70	73	17

Comparisons With Other in Situ, in Vitro, and in Vivo Measurements of Maximal Power

The power potential of a range of muscles across species can be compared
meaningfully by normalizing to the mass of the muscle as one would predict,
based on the theoretical considerations presented in Figures 1 and 2 and on
the assumptions that all fibers within a muscle have similar lengths and that
all muscles have fibers with similar intrinsic biochemical properties. The first
assumption appears to be reasonable, at least for the muscles and some muscle
groups being considered (Sacks & Roy, 1982; Wickiewicz et al., 1983). The
second assumption can be met by selecting muscles of a similar slow-fast fiber
type proportion.

Representative relative power comparisons for muscles from several species
are shown in Table 3. Two points related to comparisons within the cat are
of particular interest. First, the power per unit weight for the semitendinosus
is similar in each of the three stimulating conditions, ranging from 159 to 169
W·Kg⁻¹. Second, the medial gastrocnemius produces 2.5 times more power
than the soleus, a value equivalent to the difference in myofibrillar ATPase
activity of these two muscles (Buller et al., 1969).

How does the power per muscle mass in the cat compare to a range of
other muscles tested *in situ* or *in vitro* (see Table 3)? Rome (1983) reported a
value of 250 W·Kg⁻¹ for the frog sartorius tested at 25°C. Ritchie (1954) reported
241 and 90 W·Kg⁻¹ for strips of rat diaphragm. Faulkner, Jones, Round, and
Edwards (1980) estimated the power potential of human muscle in several ways.
Based on the peak rate of ATP utilization, they estimated human muscle with
about 50% type I and 50% type II fibers to produce 50 W·Kg⁻¹. However, this

Table 3. Maximum Power of *In Situ* or *In Vitro* Stimulated Muscles

Muscle	Maximum Power (W.Kg^{-1})	Reference
Cat Semitendinosus		
Proximal	163	Present Paper
Distal	169	Present Paper
Both	159	Present Paper
Cat Soleus	174	Present Paper
Cat Medial Gastrocnemius	440	Present Paper
Frog Sartorius	250	Rome, 1983
Rat Diaphragm	241	Ritchie, 1954
	90	
Human Diaphragm	50	Faulkner et al., 1980

method of estimating peak power probably underestimates the maximum because it is necessary to relate ATP utilized per contraction, not just peak rate
of ATP consumption.

How does the peak power of electrically stimulated muscles compare to
that achieved under voluntary conditions? Obviously, precise data regarding
this question is difficult to obtain. However, estimates can be made if some
assumptions about the mass of the muscle involved can be justified. Ralston,
Polissar, Inman, Close, and Feinstein (1949) reported about 182 W.Kg^{-1} from
the pectoralis muscle of an amputee (see Table 4). Hirano and Rome (1984)
reported 272 W.Kg^{-1} for the frog sartorius at 25°C during a maximal jump,
assuming that 14% of the body weight represented the muscle mass involved.
This assumption is the most uncertain one in light of the mechanical factors
noted in this paper, as well as the assumption that 14% of the musculature
is recruited similarly and simultaneously. The power derived from Figure 5
of Walmsley, Hodgson, and Burke (1978), using average muscle weights from
Sacks and Roy (1982) and based on a vertical jump of 120 cm is estimated to
be about 500 W.Kg^{-1} for the cat medial gastrocnemius.

As noted previously, estimates of human power per muscle mass fall within
a similar range in spite of the uncertainty of many variables in the various types
of experiments. As is the case with the frog-jumping experiments, one must
assume that there are no major differences in the mechanical properties and
architectural arrangements of muscles within a muscle group and that the
muscles actually involved in executing the movement can be identified. But,
if these uncertainties are accepted, estimates of maximum human muscle power
range from 125 to 536 W.Kg^{-1} (see Table 1).

Table 4. Maximum Power of In Vivo Stimulated Muscles

Muscle	Power (W)	Muscle Wet Weight (Kg)	Power (W·Kg⁻¹)
Human Pectoralis Voluntary activation Amputee Ralston et al., 1949)	35	0.192	182
Frog Sartorius Maximum jump at 25° (Hirano & Rome, 1984)	39	0.143	272
Cat Medial Gastrocnemius (3N × 164 mm/s) 120 cm jump (Walmsley et al., 1978)	5	0.010	500

Summary

A muscle's physiological cross-sectional area, muscle fiber length, and muscle mass are the primary morphological determinants of maximal force, velocity, and power, respectively. Angle of attachment of fibers to the tendon and the interconnections between fibers generally have a lesser influence on these parameters. Although the power potential of a muscle can be normalized in a physiologically meaningful way to muscle mass, the power potential of individual muscles will not be additive unless the net effect of fiber lengths and biochemical intrinsic properties are similar. Further, it appears that similar amounts of power but not similar levels of isometric force can be produced in voluntarily activated and maximally stimulated muscle.

Discussion

A lively discussion took place after Dr. Edgerton's paper regarding the implications of simultaneous contraction of muscles with both slow and fast twitch fibers and of fibers with differing structure. Although at first sight it might appear a physiological waste of energy to recruit slow muscle fibers during high velocity contractions, Dr. Edgerton felt that a trade-off might be involved. Taking the soleus as an example of a slow twitch muscle, he pointed out that it is very tolerant of repetitive activity and difficult to fatigue; thus if slow fibers were activated during a fast movement, their resistance to fatigue might be an advantage in maintaining force output after many repetitive contractions. As both slow and fast twitch fibers are about the same length in the same muscle, one has to conclude that the slow fibers within a fast muscle will be making a smaller contribution at the faster velocities. Dr. Edgerton concluded that if one were calculating maximum power per kilogram of muscle and the muscle in question was composed of 50% fast and 50% slow fibers, then the power per kg of muscle taking part in maximal activity would be about 50% higher than the value for the total muscle if it were composed of 100% slow fibers. Of course, the assumption being made is that the tension per cross-sectional area is the same in slow and fast muscle. Whether this assumption is true or not remains to be determined.

Mr. Herzog wanted clarification of the force velocity relationships for human muscle in concentric contractions, in which the maximal force may be higher at a slow velocity than at zero velocity. According to Mr. Herzog, this appears to be in contrast to animal muscle. Dr. Edgerton replied that the amount of tension produced at low velocities is less than that predicted from the Hill curve. Whether the force at zero velocity is actually lower than that produced at some velocity greater than zero is variable between subjects. As Mr. Perrine suggested, it seems to be related to the subject's experience in exerting high forces. Although some subjects develop torque at zero velocity that is less than at a higher velocity, others do not, and it is easy to get spuriously high values by using trick movements even without the subject realizing it. Dr. Edgerton did not think that the difference between Dr. Wilkie's findings and the data from his laboratory was related to the architectural differences between the elbow flexors and the muscles of the lower limb, as similar results had shown recently in the elbow flexors. Whether human muscle follows Hill's predictions *in vivo* at all velocities is a question that needs to be examined by other groups. However, the same phenomenon has been observed in every muscle group studied so far.

Dr. Stauber wondered what the implications were for activities that were carried out by muscles having 100% type I fibers. Could such subjects even walk up stairs? Dr. Edgerton replied that the nervous system seems to be capable of performing graduated contractions in which a relatively set recruitment order is followed even within a fiber type or unit type. This is true at least in the cat soleus. Each movement employs a certain percentage of the motor pool at any given time, and the order of recruitment appears to be rather consistent for a specific movement. However, it might be more difficult to produce a low force during fine movements in individuals that have a very high percentage of fast twitch fibers. Dr. Edgerton knew of no data that bear on this speculation.

In reply to another questioner who felt there was a difference between his findings in knee extensors generating more power than plantar flexors and the studies presented by Dr. Winter in which plantar flexors generated more power than the extensors, Dr.Edgerton pointed out that Dr. Winter's studies were carried out *in vivo* and during jogging, which was very different in design from the questions being addressed. In Dr. Edgerton's studies the muscular output from one joint was measured in maximal efforts. Dr. Winter's studies might be compared more closely to what his group had found during movement in cats in which the soleus could generate 50% more power in a fast run than a slow run. Part of the discussion dealt with the problem of fiber angulation influencing the functional length of fibers and the force velocity characteristics of the total muscle. Dr. Edgerton wanted to know what the angle of attachment of fibers was at each fiber length *in vivo* both during contraction and in relaxation, but the only fiber angle measurements that were familiar to him were ones made at a given length in which the muscle is not contracted. He found it unlikely that what is seen in formalin fixed muscle is similar to that in the *in vivo* muscle at the same length. Based on the fixed tissue, the angles that are seen in most muscles of the cat hind limb affect the tension by less than 10% and in most muscles less than 5% if the cosine of the angle is used. However, there are a number of different designs that might affect the physiological properties; for example, there are pennate muscles in which contraction is accompanied by more shortening of the common tendon than would be predicted from examining individual fiber shortening. Also, the relative number of sarcomeres in series and in parallel is a factor about which we have little information for most muscles.

On another point of clarification from a questioner who had wondered about the activity of soleus muscle relative to the gastrocnemius during walking, Dr. Edgerton replied that at the velocities reported in his paper both soleus and the gastrocnemius contributed to the force. Dr. Winter pointed out that in the human, the velocity of shortening of the gastrocnemius is about twice that of the soleus during the push off in a step when high tensions are produced in both muscles. However, the soleus is shortening through one joint and the gastrocnemius is shortening through both joints. Because the knee starts flexing at push-off, the longer muscle has to shorten to a greater extent in order to maintain tension; otherwise it would slacken. Thus, it has to contract twice as fast as the soleus in order to achieve the common tension.

Dr. Edgerton felt that this was an important point and one in which more kinematic data on two-joint muscles are required to tie the system together. These architectural features are well known, but the physiological implications have not been explored fully. In the cat the gastrocnemius has relatively short fibers compared to the soleus; when the cat jumps, for example, and extension of the knee occurs, the gastrocnemius operates closer to the isometric condition and does not experience the change in length that is observed from the soleus because the angle of the knee "compensates for" the length changes in the ankle.

Dr. McComas was interested in Dr. Edgerton's discussion of the cat semitendinosus muscle, which has two arrays of muscle fibers longitudinally and arranged end-to-end, and allowing the power of the muscle to be modulated by activation of one or both arrays at the same time. Some muscles have more than two arrays; the sartorius muscle in man, for example, has at least four. In such a muscle it might be very important to get near synchronous activation along the length of the whole muscle as opposed to having an action potential running the whole way along the muscle. He wanted to know if there was any physiological evidence that muscles were activated in a pattern that depended on the power requirements, with only one array of fibers being switched on during movements requiring little power and more being recruited if higher power generation was required. Dr. Edgerton answered that this had been studied *in situ* by stimulating muscles from both ends and recording the force generated at the tendon; cinephotography allowed calculation of the velocity of shortening under each of the circumstances. If only one end of the muscle is stimulated *in situ*, the opposite end of the muscle stretches, and it is clear that the tension generated in the muscle tendon will be less than that when both ends are stimulated. The unstimulated end of the muscle is very compliant. EMG recordings made *in vivo* during treadmill running suggested that both ends of the muscles are activated similarly. Although there is a possibility that in a muscle like the sartorius some fiber bundles may be activated while others attached in series are not, his impression, based on the results obtained in the semitendinosus, was that this would not be the usual case.

References

Ariano, M.A., Armstrong, R.B., & Edgerton, V.R. (1973). Hindlimb muscle fiber populations of five mammals. *Journal of Histochemistry and Cytochemistry*, **21**, 51-55.

Bárány, M. (1967). ATPase activity of myosin correlated with speed of muscle shortening. *Journal of General Physiology*, **50**, 197-216.

Bodine, S., Roy, R.R., Meadows, D.A., Zernicke, R.F., Sacks, R., Fournier, M., & Edgerton, V.R. (1982). Architectural, histochemical and contractile characteristics of a unique biarticular muscle: The cat semitendinosus. *Journal of Neurophysiology*, **48**, 192-201.

Buller, A.J., Mommaerts, W.F.H.M., & Seraydarian, K. (1969). Enzymic properties of myosin in fast and slow twitch muscles of the cat following cross-innervation. *Journal of Physiology*, **205**, 581-597.

Edgerton, V.R., Roy, R.R., Bodine, S.C., & Sacks, R.D. (1983). The matching of neuronal and muscular physiology. In K.T. Borer, D.W. Edington, & T.P. White (Eds.), *Frontiers of Exercise Biology* (pp. 51-70). Champaign, IL: Human Kinetics.

Faulkner, J.A., Jones, D.A., Round, J.M., & Edwards, R.H.T. (1980). Dynamics of energetic processes in human muscle. In P. Cerretelli & B.J. Whipp (Eds.), *Exercise Bioenergetics and Gas Exchange* (pp. 81-90). London: Elsevier/North Holland Biomedical Press.

Gans, C., & Bock, W.J. (1965). The functional significance of muscle architecture; a theoretical analysis. *Ergebnisse der Anatomie und entwicklungsgeschichte,* **38**, 115-142.

Hill, A.V. (1951). The mechanics of voluntary muscle. *The Lancet,* **261**, 947-951.

Hirano, M., & Rome, L.C. (1984). Jumping performance of frogs (Rana Pipiens) as a function of muscle temperature. *Journal of Experimental Biology,* **108**, 429-439.

Partridge, L.D., & Benton, L.A. (1981). Muscle, the motor. In J.M. Brookhart, V.B. Mountcastle, V.B. Brooks, & S.R. Geiger (Eds.), *Handbook of Physiology: Sec. 1. The Nervous System* (pp. 43-106). Bethesda, Maryland: American Physiological Society.

Perrine, J.J., & Edgerton, V.R. (1978). Muscle force-velocity and power-velocity relationships under isokinetic loading. *Medicine and Science in Sports and Exercise,* **10**, 159-166.

Powell, P.L., Roy, R.R., Kanim, P., Bello, M.A., & Edgerton, V.R. (1984). Predictability of skeletal muscle tension from architectural determinations in guinea pig hindlimbs. *Journal of Applied Physiology: Respiratory, Environmental and Exercise Physiology,* **57**, 1715-1721.

Ralston, H.J., Polissar, M.J., Inman, V.T., Close, J.R., & Feinstein, B. (1949). Dynamic features of human isolated voluntary muscle in isometric and free contractions. *Journal of Applied Physiology,* **1**, 526-533.

Ritchie, J.M. (1954). The relation between force and velocity of shortening in rat muscle. *Journal of Physiology,* **123**, 633-639.

Rome, L.C. (1983). The effects of long-term exposure to different temperatures on the mechanical performance of frog muscle. *Physiological Zoology,* **56**, 33-40.

Sacks, R.D., & Roy, R.R. (1982). Architecture of the hind limb muscles of cats: Functional significance. *Journal of Morphology,* **173**, 185-195.

Saltin, B., & Gollnick, P. (1983). Skeletal muscle adaptability: Significance for metabolism and performance. In L.D. Peachey (Ed.), *Handbook of Physiology: Sec. 10. Skeletal Muscle.* Baltimore: Williams and Wilkins.

Spector, S.A., Gardiner, P.F., Zernicke, R.F., Roy, R.R., & Edgerton, V.R. (1980). Muscle architecture and force-velocity characteristics of the cat soleus and medial gastrocnemius: Implications for motor control. *Journal of Neurophysiology,* **44**, 951-960.

Walmsley, B., Hodgson, J.A., & Burke, R.E. (1978). Forces produced by medial gastrocnemius and soleus muscles during locomotion in freely moving cats. *Journal of Neurophysiology, 41,* 1203-1216.

Whiting, W.C., Gregor, R.J., Roy, R.R., & Edgerton, V.R. (1984). A technique for estimating mechanical work of individual muscles in the cat during treadmill locomotion. *Journal of Biomechanics, 17,* 685-694.

Wickiewicz, T.L., Roy, R.R., Powell, P.L., & Edgerton, V.R. (1983). Muscle architecture of the human lower limb. *Clinical Orthopaedics and Related Research, 179,* 275-283.

Wickiewicz, T.L., Roy, R.R., Powell, P.L., Perrine, J.J., & Edgerton, V.R. (1984). Muscle architecture and force-velocity relationships in humans. *Journal of Applied Physiology: Respiratory, Environmental and Exercise Physiology, 57,* 435-443.

Wilkie, D.R. (1950). The relation between force and velocity in human muscle. *Journal of Physiology, 110,* 249-280.

5

Muscle Power: Fibre Type Recruitment, Metabolism and Fatigue

Howard J. Green
University of Waterloo

P ower is generated by muscles in isotonic contractions, either concentric or eccentric. The instantaneous power output may be expressed at different points through a range of motion (i.e., at different fibre lengths) by individual muscles or by groups of muscles acting over one or more joints. Also, power output may be expressed at different velocities, the output then being defined by the well-known hyperbolic relationship between force and velocity first described by Hill (1938).

Since the generation of power involves displacement associated with muscle fibre shortening or lengthening, at least two fundamentally different challenges are imposed during functional activities than in the isometric contractions that are most frequently studied in experimental settings. First, the myosin heads must cycle to successive actin sites, necessitating repeated attachment and dissociation of the actin and myosin at different interfilament distances and, depending on the load, at different rates. Secondly, since movement is involved, definite limits are imposed on the duration of the contraction (T_C). Once full extension or flexion is completed, the muscle must return to the starting position if an additional contraction cycle is to be repeated. This introduces a variable time delay depending on the velocity with which the muscle is returned to the precontraction position. This time delay represents a potential recovery period (T_R) that may allow valuable time for restoration of critical subcellular processes necessary for continued function. The concept of a duty cycle, defined as the ratio of the time of contraction to the time of relaxation plus recovery (T_C/T_{TOT}), consequently is of fundamental importance in understanding power generation that involves repetitive contraction-cycles

(Bellemare & Grassino, 1982). Indeed, the heart and respiratory muscles both depend on a duty cycle, as is the case with many activities involving the loco-motor muscles, such as those used in sprinting and cycling.

Peak power generation must be viewed as an optimal and dynamic inter-action between the muscle (excitation-contraction processes), neural recruit-ment (type of motor units, size of motor unit pool, frequency and pattern of discharge), and the metabolic source of ATP production (anaerobic and aero-bic). Any deviation from the status of optimal synchrony between these inter-acting factors would be expected to detract from the potential power capabilities of the muscle.

Specialization of Muscle Structure and Function

Evidence exists to demonstrate that mammalian skeletal muscles and mus-cle fibres assume a specialized organization and composition to function op-timally in a given set of environmental conditions (Hochachka, 1976). Although a wide mosaic in selected properties is evident between species and between muscles from the same species, the separation of motor units into two fun-damental categories, each highly adapted for the performance of certain types of contractile behavior, is well recognized (Saltin & Gollnick, 1983).

In general, slow twitch (ST) or Type I muscle fibres are specialized for pro-tracted usage at relatively low velocities. Fast twitch (FT) or Type II fibres, on the other hand, are specialized for burst work in which large power outputs and high velocities are generated for relatively brief periods of time. The phys-iologic differences between the fibre types are consistent with fundamental differences in a range of ultrastructural and metabolic properties (Pette & Heil-man, 1979). The sarcoplasmic reticulum (ATPase activity, Ca^{2+} uptake charac-teristics, phosphoprotein formation, and peptide pattern), the contractile proteins (isozymes of myosin and troponin), myosin ATPase activity, and the enzymes of energy metabolism (aerobic and anaerobic) all appear to undergo a co-ordinated expression. In the case of the FT fibres, Ca^{2+} uptake by the sar-coplasmic reticulum, actomyosin cycling rate, ATP hydrolysis, and anaerobic regeneration of ATP (high energy phosphagens, anaerobic glycolysis) are all uniformly high. Burst work muscles possess the ability to form lactate at high rates (Hochachka, 1976), but the dependence on anaerobic processes com-promises energetic efficiency. In contrast, ST fibres depend on aerobic oxida-tion of both fats and carbohydrates to produce a high degree of efficiency in energy production. Actomyosin cycling rate, ATPase activity, and calcium up-take by the sarcoplasmic reticulum are correspondingly lower than in the FT fibres.

Subdivisions of burst work muscles are also recognized. These subdivi-sions, determined largely on the basis of histochemical criteria, appear to be highly specific (Reichmann & Pette, 1982; Green, Reichmann, & Pette, 1982). The three most popular fibre-typing schema include two that are based on the pH liability of myofibrillar (myosin) ATPase reaction (Guth & Samaha, 1969; Brooke & Kaiser, 1970) and one based on the oxidative and glycolytic potential of the muscle fibre (Peter, Barnard, Edgerton, Gillespie, & Stempel, 1972). The most common fibre-typing schema employed for the human has been based on the procedure of Brooke and Kaiser (1970) with three categories (IIA, IIB, IIC) of Type II fibres recognized. It is a common error to equate the Type IIA and Type IIB fibres with the fast-oxidative glycolytic (FOG) and fast glycolytic (FG) fibres respectively, as recognized by the method of Peter et al. (1972). The Type IIA and Type IIB fibres show a substantial overlap in aerobic potential (Sjøgaard, Houston, Nygaard, & Saltin, 1978; Reichmann & Pette, 1982).

Some insight into the cellular mechanisms underlying the functional specialization exhibited by ST and FT fibres can be obtained by a more detailed comparison of the two fibre types. In this regard it is important to emphasize the differences in fibre type properties in humans as compared to nonhumans and, in particular, the laboratory rat, about which considerably more is known. In humans, both Ca^{2+} activated myosin ATPase (Essén, Jansson, Henriksson, Taylor, & Saltin, 1975) and Mg^{2+} stimulated myofibrillar ATPase (Thorstensson, Sjödin, Tesch, & Karlsson, 1977) range from twofold to threefold higher in FT as compared to ST fibres. Comparable differences in actomyosin ATPase between these fibre types have also been noted for smaller mammals such as the rat (Baldwin, Winder, & Holloszy, 1975). Although evidence is generally lacking in humans, the differences between the Type I and Type II fibres in isometric contraction time (CT) and maximal velocity of shortening (V_{max}) would be expected to parallel the differences in actin activated myosin ATPase activity (Bárány, 1967). Garnett, O'Donovan, Stephens, and Taylor (1978), using electrical stimulation of single motor units in humans, have reported contraction times ranging from 90 to 110 msec for ST motor units and from 40 to 84 msec for FT motor units. Although contraction times for rat ST and FT muscles are considerably faster, the difference between the fibre types appears to be comparable to the human (Close, 1967). For V_{max}, Faulkner, Jones, Round, and Edwards (1981) have estimated an approximately fourfold difference in the human between fibre types, a figure that is generally higher than the reported differences between muscles composed essentially of either FT or ST motor units in the rat (Fitts, Courtright, Kim, & Witzmann, 1982).

In muscles characterized by high power outputs and high rates of force development, metabolic specialization is necessary not only to provide for high rates of ATP regeneration but to satisfy the nearly instantaneous requirement for large amounts of ATP. Differentiation of anaerobic processes can occur at the level of the high energy phosphagens and in the anaerobic degradation of carbohydrates. In small mammals such as the rat, clear differences exist in the phosphagen content between the two specialized fibre types. ATP and CP concentrations are approximately 60% to 70% higher in FT muscles than in

ST muscles (Meyer & Terjung, 1979). In humans, values of ATP and CP are generally comparable between fibre types (Rehunen & Härkönen, 1980). The rat also appears to possess a higher ATP/ADP ratio in the FT fibres. This property, which is not present in the human FT fibres, has been postulated to favor a rapid increase in glycolysis and ATP production (Edström, Hultman, Sahlin, & Sjohölm, 1982). Further, the higher CP concentration in the FT fibres of the rat may be beneficial not only in offering a greater potential pool for ATP re-synthesis but also in serving as an important mechanism in buffering against the high acidosis associated with a high glycolytic rate (Edström et al., 1982).

Higher rates of ATP production in FT fibres are also facilitated on the basis of the approximately 30% higher maximal creatine kinase activity and 80% higher myokinase activity (Thorstensson et al., 1977). Compared to the rat, however, where up to fourfold differences have been reported for maximal creatine kinase activity (Staudte, Exner, & Pette, 1973), the degree of specialization between the different principal fibre types in the human is relatively modest.

In the highly specialized FT muscle of the rat, large increases in IMP formation and ammonia are found during high levels of contractile activity (Meyer & Terjung, 1979). The AMP deaminase reaction may be an important mechanism for maintaining high ratios of ATP to ADP and AMP during periods when ATP utilization exceeds supply (Lowenstein & Goodman, 1978). In humans, although increases in IMP have been found in homogenates containing a mixture of fibre types (Sahlin, Palmskog, & Hultman, 1978), the significance of the AMP deaminase reaction has not been demonstrated in the two fibre types separately. Indirect evidence has been published, however, showing a close relationship between increases in blood ammonia, blood lactate, and the percentage of FT fibres (Dudley, Staron, Murray, Hagerman, & Luginbuhl, 1983).

Metabolic differentiation between the ST and FT fibres is also evident at the level of glycogenolysis and glycolysis. Glycogenolytic and glycolytic potential as measured by maximal activities of a number of enzymes has been reported to be approximately twofold higher in the FT human fibres than in the ST fibres (Essén et al., 1975; Essén-Gustavsson & Henriksson, 1984). The twofold differences noted in the maximal activities of a number of glycolytic enzymes are also paralleled by lactate dehydrogenase (LDH), for which at least twofold differences exist between the main fibre types (Thorstensson et al., 1977). Moreover, the LDH isozyme pattern of the skeletal muscle specific subunit, (LDH-M), predominates in the FT fibres, and the heart specific subunit appears to be higher in the ST fibres (Thorstensson et al., 1977). The predominant glycogenolytic and glycolytic potential reported in the FT fibres as compared to the ST fibres of the human is not accompanied by a comparable difference in endogenous glycogen. The concentration of glycogen in FT fibres has been reported to be only 15% higher (Halkjaer-Kristensen & Ingeman-Hansen, 1979). On the average, the major human fibre types do not demonstrate as great a difference in the potential for aerobic and free fatty acid oxidation as they do in glycolytic potential. Values ranging from 30% to 40% higher have been reported for the ST fibres over the FT fibres in marker enzymes of the citric acid cycle and β-oxidation (Essén et al., 1975; Lowry et al., 1978; Essén-Gustavsson & Henriksson, 1984). However, as previously noted, FT fibres can display a wide variation in aerobic potential (Reichmann & Pette, 1982). Whether or not the FT fibres in the human with the high aerobic potential are accompanied by a lower glycolytic potential than FT fibres with a low oxidative potential is uncertain at this time.

A greater degree of differentiation between the ST and FT fibres in the rat than in the human is also evident for the metabolic pathways involved in carbohydrate metabolism. Glycogenolytic potential is approximately sixfold higher and glycolytic threefold to fourfold higher in the FT fibres in the rat as compared to the ST fibres (Baldwin, Winder, Terjung, & Holloszy, 1973). It is of interest that in the rat, where FT fibres are commonly subdivided by the Peter et al. (1972) classification into FOG and FG types, the FOG fibres display a generally lower glycolytic potential. Moreover, the FOG fibres possess an even greater oxidative potential than the ST fibres (Baldwin, Klinkerfuss, Terjung, Mole, & Holloszy, 1972). Endogenous glycogen may be up to twofold lower in the rat than in the human (Baldwin, Reitman, Terjung, Winder, & Holloszy, 1973) with the FT fibre containing on average a 25% higher concentration.

The difference in capillary supply (per unit area) and fibre size in the slow and fast contracting fibres is also less in the human than in the rat. In the rat, the area of FT fibres with a high oxidative capacity is generally similar to the area of ST fibres. The low oxidative FT fibre, however, may be up to fivefold larger, approximately the size of a human fibre (Green and Greene, 1980; Green et al., 1981). Such size discrepancies are not evident between the human FT and ST fibres (Sjøgaard, 1982). As in the rat, the number of capillaries is not different between the ST and FT fibres (Sjøgaard, 1982). However, capillary to fibre area ratios have been reported to be 40% higher for FT fibres than ST fibres in the human (Sjøgaard, 1982). In contrast, capillary to fibre area ratios may be fourfold to sixfold higher in the rat between the fibre types.

It is evident that the marked physiologic specialization between the fundamental fibre types is accompanied by a correspondingly emphasized metabolic differentiation. The metabolic differentiation is more conspicuous in the smaller mammal such as the rat than in the human. It may be speculated that the large differences between the extremes of the fibre types observed for the rat have led to the need for the development of a second FT fibre, the FOG, which differs from the FG fibre in having a highly developed capacity for both aerobic and β-oxidation (Baldwin et al., 1972). However, power output may be somewhat compromised due to the substantially smaller cross sectional area and the lower glycolytic potential than observed in FG fibres (Green & Greene, 1980).

In view of the differences between the ST and FT muscles, it is not surprising that athletes performing in specialties requiring rapid development of force and high power outputs tend to have a predominance of FT fibres (Gollnick, Armstrong, Saubert, Piehl, & Saltin, 1972; Costill et al., 1976). Evidence has also been published demonstrating a positive relationship with the percentage of FT fibres and power output (Thorstensson, Grimby, & Karlsson, 1976). This relationship seems to be most pronounced in maximal contractions involving high velocities (Coyle, Costill, & Lesme, 1979) or when the rate of force development is high (Viitasalo & Komi, 1978). This notion is consistent with the finding that no differences exist between the fibre types in the peak ability to generate isometric force (Gregor, Edgerton, Perrine, Campion, & Debus, 1979; Faulkner et al., 1981).

An additional consideration that may have some influence on the power output by a muscle relates to the accommodation that occurs during repeated stimulation in both human (Vandervoort, Quinlan, & McComas, 1983) and non-human muscle (Manning & Stull, 1982; Kushmerick & Crow, 1983). The accommodation is specific to the FT fibres, and involves a potentiation of the force developed during a supramaximal twitch. Although there is some controversy regarding the cellular mechanism involved (Butler, Siegmen, Mooers, & Barsotti, 1983; Barsotti & Butler, 1984), impressive evidence has been published demonstrating a close parallel between the increase in phosphorylation of the P light chains and the degree of potentiation (Manning & Stull, 1982). This calcium mediated event has been postulated to involve a reduction in the actomyosin cycling rate as a result of a reduced actin activated myosin ATPase activity (Kushmerick & Crow, 1983). The specific effect of the potentiation on power activities remains to be determined. Vandervoort et al. (1983) have observed a speeding up of the twitch, whereas Kushmerick and Crow (1983) observed a depression of the maximal velocity of shortening. The specific effect on the dynamic behavior of muscle must await isolation of the possible contaminating effects of fatigue induced by the tetanic tension (Kushmerick & Crow, 1983). It is evident, however, that the utilization of FT fibres for even brief periods induces an alteration in selected intracellular processes that persists for several minutes and increases the twitch output of the muscle. Whether or not the repeated utilization of FT fibres involves an obligatory reduction in power output at high velocities and whether or not such a change in mechanical behavior is mediated through similar mechanisms that lead to a potentiation of the twitch is uncertain (Butler et al., 1983; Barsotti & Butler, 1984).

Recruitment Considerations

For many muscles, expression of the maximal force output would be expected to involve maximal or near maximal recruitment of both ST and FT motoneuron pools (Belanger & McComas, 1981). Although there is some evidence to the contrary (Grimby & Hannerz, 1974), it is generally accepted that during very rapid voluntary contractions there is orderly recruitment of motor units according to the size principle (Henneman, Somjen, & Carpenter, 1965; Desmedt & Godaux, 1977a, 1977b). In mixed muscle containing both ST and FT motor units, this implies that the involvement of ST motor units is obligatory, regardless of the power and velocity being generated.

The optimization of force within each motor unit specific pool may depend on the pattern of discharge. Grimby and Hannerz (1977), while investigating the individual motor units of the short toe extensor muscle of man, identified two fundamental types of motor units based upon characteristic firing patterns believed to represent ST and FT fibres. In this scheme, the ST motor units fire continuously for long periods of time at a relatively low frequency. The FT units, on the other hand, fire intermittently at high rates for short intervals. These characteristics are consistent with what is known about the properties of ST and FT motor units. The ST, low threshold, motor units have relatively low conduction velocities and long twitch contraction times, and require low stimulus frequencies to produce a tetanic contraction. The FT high threshold motor units, in contrast, have relatively high conduction velocities and short twitch contraction times, and require high stimulus frequencies to produce a fused tetanus (Burke, 1967). Consequently, in mixed muscle with both fast and slow twitch motor units, maximal force output of the muscle is realized when both ST and FT pools of motor units are recruited at optimal rate coding to produce a fused tetanus synchronously in each of the motor units. This would suggest that given the high threshold of the FT motoneurons, relatively high firing frequencies in the FT motor nerves would be a prerequisite to attainment of maximal force. At least for the deltoid muscle and for maximal isometric force development, this appears to be the case (DeLuca, LeFever, McCue, & Xenakis, 1982). At force levels between 40% and 80% MVC in the deltoid, recruitment appeared to be the primary mechanism for increasing force development. This is in contrast to the smaller first dorsal interosseus muscle, where rate coding played the major role in development of force up to 80% of MVC. In the force range between 80% and 100% of MVC, DeLuca et al. (1982) have speculated that rate coding and, in particular, intermittent high frequency bursts of impulses may be of primary significance. How these differences relate to difference in the recruitment of specific motor unit types could not be determined from this study. In most of the experimental work where intramuscular electrodes were employed for the investigation of the discharge properties of specific motor units, isometric contraction has been employed. As previously emphasized, the expression of the power capabilities of a muscle can occur at varying velocities and, consequently, for varying durations throughout the range of motion of a joint. In these situations, it is possible that depending on the velocity, different motor units may be recruited at different points in the contraction period and display a highly unsteady firing frequency (Desmedt & Godaux, 1977a). During repetitive contractions of this nature, the characteristic pattern of frequency may change depending on the time between contractions and the time needed for specific excitation processes to recover to the pre-exercise state.

During ballistic movements or movements requiring high power output, the high frequency of activation may be of fundamental importance in capitalizing on the metabolic features of the burst work muscles. The production of ATP must be accelerated rapidly to several hundred times the resting level to support the rapid and large increase in actomyosin cycling rate and power output by the muscle. The high frequency of activation would be expected to lead to rapid increases in cytosolic calcium levels, which would provide an early stimulus to glycogenolysis through activation of phosphorylase b to a (Chasiotis, Sahlin, & Hultman, 1982). This change, in conjunction with large increases in actin-activated, myosin ATPase activity, and ATP hydrolysis, leads to rapid increases in Pi and AMP, both of which may also stimulate glycogenolysis.

Excitation-Contraction Interactions and Muscle Fatigue

It is well recognized that in bipedal activities such as cycling, maximal power output can be sustained only for a few seconds (McCartney, Heigenhauser, & Jones, 1983). Moreover, evidence has been presented demonstrating a deterioration in peak power during the course of a single maximal knee extension at 180 degrees/sec (Perrine & Edgerton, 1978), a total contraction time of approximately 0.5 sec. The failure to maintain a required or expected force has been defined as fatigue (Edwards, 1981). In recent years, a number of potential fatigue sites, both central and peripheral, that depend on the characteristics of the contractile activity and on the type of motor unit have been identified. To produce a maximal power output, a high stimulation rate and a high ATP utilization are essential, particularly in the FT motor units. Under these conditions, central inhibition, neuromuscular junction failure, and an impaired excitation of the sarcolemma have all been suggested as the cause of the early reduction in performance (Edwards, 1981). Bigland-Ritchie, Kukula, Lippold, and Woods (1982) have demonstrated the importance of central inhibition during maximal sustained voluntary contraction (MVC), and Grimby, Hannerz, and Hedman (1981) have observed the loss of intermittent, high frequency signals intramuscularly, promoting the suggestion that FT motor units are inhibited and that the inhibition is central. The concept of high frequency fatigue is consistent with the notion that the neuromuscular junction and the sarcolemma are incapable of rapidly processing high frequency stimulation except for brief periods of time (Jones, 1981). To some extent, accommodation within the muscle fibre may assist in offsetting this type of fatigue. In sustained MVC, the high frequency of impulses characteristic of the onset of activities involving maximal force is quickly reduced without an apparent further loss of force (Bigland-Ritchie, Johnsson, Lippold, Smith, & Woods, 1983). This has led to speculation that an alteration in some intracellular process assists in the maintenance of force output in the face of a lower firing frequency, thus delaying or eliminating high frequency fatigue. In this regard, both a prolongation in relaxation time and a potentiation of the motor unit twitch tension may be of significance. A sustained MVC would be expected to induce a substantial metabolic acidosis in addition to a depletion of muscle phosphocreatine. Large increases in relaxation time have been observed in such conditions (Hultman & Sjohölm, 1983). The potentiation of the twitch, a consequence of the repetitive stimulation of FT motor units (Kushmerick & Crow, 1983) could also serve to offset fatigue. It is important to note, however, that these adaptations may be specific to sustained isometric contraction. Repeated dynamic contraction, depending on the duty cycle, may minimize the occurrence of high frequency fatigue or the need to down-regulate firing frequency, providing the time between contraction cycles is sufficient to allow recovery of processes responsible for this type of impairment. Indeed, if potentiation is an obligatory event in dynamic exercise regardless of velocity, and if actomyosin cycling rate is compromised (Kushmerick & Crow, 1983), unavoidable reductions in power output would be expected and would be most notable in high velocity activities.

A phenomenon that appears to be associated with active utilization of muscle regardless of the contractile schedule is a long-lasting type of fatigue that is specific to low frequency stimulation in the range of 10 to 20 Hz and accordingly has been labelled low frequency fatigue (Edwards, Hill, Jones, & Merton, 1977). Although specific mechanisms have not been identified at this time, impairment of release of calcium from sarcoplasmic reticulum, impaired transmission in the transverse tubular system, and reduction in the binding affinity of calcium to the regulatory protein troponin may be responsible (Edwards, 1981; Faulkner, 1983). Reduction in cystolic calcium may also affect other processes involved in the mechanical output of muscle (Julian & Moss, 1981), such as activation of myosin light chain kinase and myosin light chain phosphorylation. Any resultant modification in myosin ATPase activity would be expected to reduce force output at low stimulation frequencies. Low frequency fatigue can occur independently of high frequency fatigue (Edwards et al., 1977); consequently maximal power output need not be compromised when this type of fatigue is present.

The physiologic significance of low frequency fatigue at submaximal power outputs has not been elucidated. To maintain force output in the face of low frequency fatigue, compensation must be made in the firing frequency to active motor units, in recruitment of additional motor units, or in recruitment of synergistic muscles. Increasing the firing frequency may precipitate high frequency fatigue, and increasing the pool of motor units recruited would be expected to promote a greater low frequency fatigue. Ultimately, increases in discharge rates may be the final adjustment mechanism regardless of the compensation, if fatigue is to be delayed.

The vulnerability of ST and FT muscle fibres to fatigue has been well established *in vitro* and *in situ* using varied patterns of electrical stimulation. However, little information is available regarding the fatigue patterns in these two types of motor units and the site of fatigue during voluntary activity. As has been previously noted, at least in MVC, both ST and FT fibres are extensively involved and each motor unit type appears to have a characteristic discharge pattern. The ability to resist fatigue may be intimately associated with stimulation patterns such as those experienced in vivo. Differences in subcellular composition and organization between the fibre types may make them highly specialized for translation of specific patterns of activation into force production on a repetitive basis. Further, the asynchronous nature of activation *in vivo* has added to the difficulty in trying to simulate ST and FT fibre activation using electrical stimulation protocols. It is well known that ability to sustain activities requiring large power outputs depends on the duty cycle. Relatively short contraction cycles in combination with long recovery periods can greatly enhance work output. Increasing the duty cycle by prolonging the contraction cycle or by reducing the recovery period accelerates fatigue and is accompanied by metabolic acidosis, which is known to affect excitation-contraction coupling (Hermansen, 1981). Although it is tempting to speculate that the acidosis may be indirectly associated with the primary cause of peripheral fatigue, this conclusion seems premature. It is possible that the more pronounced fatigue observed with higher duty cycles could be central in nature or may be associated with the different challenges placed on the processes involved in excitation and contraction per se and not to the acidosis. In fatigue of this nature, much emphasis has been given to the energy status of the muscle and, in particular, the ATP available for actomyosin activity. However, excitation-contraction is energy dependent, and an impairment in the energy status at any of these locations could conceivably impair performance.

The expression of maximal power output by a muscle or a muscle group depends on an intimate and optimal synchronization of neural, excitation, contractile, and energetic processes. A failure in any one of these may represent the weak link and directly contribute to fatigue. The "weak link" may be highly specific to the type of contraction, the contraction schedule, and the fibre type. It is possible that maximal isometric contraction does not represent an appropriate model for understanding the determinants of muscle power.

References

Baldwin, K.M., Klinkerfuss, G.H., Terjung, R.L., Mole, P.A., & Holloszy, J.O. (1972). Respiratory capacity of white red and intermediate muscle: Adaptive response to exercise. *American Journal of Physiology, 222, 373-378.*

Baldwin, K.M., Reitman, J.S., Terjung, R.L., Winder, W.W., & Holloszy, J.O. (1973). Substrate depletion in different types of muscle and in liver during prolonged running. *American Journal of Physiology, 225, 1045-1050.*

Baldwin, K.M., Winder, W.W., & Holloszy, J.O. (1975). Adaptation of actomyosin ATPase in different types of muscle to endurance exercise. *American Journal of Physiology, 229, 442-446.*

Baldwin, K.M., Winder, W.W., Terjung, R.L., & Holloszy, J.O. (1973). Glycolytic enzymes in different types of skeletal muscle: Adaptation to exercise. *American Journal of Physiology, 225, 962-966.*

Bárány, M. (1967). ATPase activity of myosin correlated with speed of muscle shortening. *Journal of General Physiology, 50* (Suppl., Pt. 2), 197-218.

Barsotti, R.J., & Butler, T.M. (1984). Chemical energy usage and myosin light chain phosphorylation in mammalian skeletal muscle. *Journal of Muscle Research and Cell Motility, 5,* 45-64.

Belanger, A.Y., & McComas, A.J. (1981). Extent of motor unit activation during effort. *Journal of Applied Physiology: Respiratory, Environmental and Exercise Physiology, 51,* 1131-1135.

Bellemare, F., & Grassino, A. (1982). Effect of pressure and timing of contraction on human diaphragm fatigue. *Journal of Applied Physiology: Respiratory, Environmental and Exercise Physiology, 53,* 1190-1195.

Bigland-Ritchie, B., Johnsson, R., Lippold, O.C.J., Smith, S., & Woods, J.J. (1983). Changes in motoneurone firing rates during sustained maximal voluntary contractions. *Journal of Physiology* (London), *340,* 335-346.

Bigland-Ritchie, B.R., Kukula, G.G., Lippold, O.C.J., & Woods, J.J. (1982). The absence of neuromuscular transmission failure is sustained maximal voluntary contraction. *Journal of Physiology* (London), *330,* 265-278.

Brooke, M.H., & Kaiser, K.K. (1970). Muscle fiber types: How many and what kind? *Archives of Neurology, 23,* 369-379.

Burke, R.E. (1967). Motor unit types of cat triceps surae muscle. *Journal of Physiology* (London), *193,* 141-160.

Butler, T.M., Siegmen, M.J., Mooers, S.U., & Barsotti, R.J. (1983). Myosin light chain phosphorylation does not modulate cross bridge cycling in mouse skeletal muscle. *Science, 220,* 1167-1169.

Chasiotis, D., Sahlin, K., & Hultman, E. (1982). Regulation of glycogenolysis in human muscle at rest and during exercise. *Journal of Applied Physiology: Respiratory, Environmental and Exercise Physiology, 53*, 708-715.

Close, R. (1967). Properties of motor units in fast and slow skeletal muscles of the rat. *Journal of Physiology* (London), **193**, 45-55.

Costill, D.L., Daniels, J., Evans, W., Fink, W., Krahenbuhl, G., & Saltin, B. (1976). Skeletal muscle enzymes and fiber composition in male and female track athletes. *Journal of Applied Physiology, 40*, 149-154.

Coyle, E.F., Costill, D.L., & Lesmes, G.R. (1979). Leg extension power and muscle fiber composition. *Medicine and Science in Sports, 11*, 12-15.

DeLuca, C.J., LeFever, R.S., McCue, M.P., & Xenakis, A.P. (1982). Behavior of human motor units in different muscles during linearly varying contractions. *Journal of Physiology* (London), **329**, 113-128.

Desmedt, J.E., & Godaux, E. (1977a). Ballistic contractions in man: Characteristic recruitment pattern of single motor units of the tibialis anterior muscle. *Journal of Physiology* (London), **264**, 673-693.

Desmedt, J.E., & Godaux, E. (1977b). Fast motor units are not preferentially activated in rapid voluntary contractions in man. *Nature*, **267**, 717-719.

Dudley, G.A., Staron, R.S., Murray, J.F., Hagerman, F.C., & Luginbuhl, A. (1983). Muscle fiber composition and blood ammonia levels after intense exercise in humans. *Journal of Applied Physiology: Respiratory, Environmental and Exercise Physiology, 54*, 582-586.

Edström, L., Hultman, E., Sahlin, K., & Sjohölm, H. (1982). The content of high energy phosphates in skeletal muscles from rat, guinea pig and man. *Journal of Physiology* (London), **332**, 47-58.

Edwards, R.H.T. (1981). Human muscle function and fatigue. In R. Porter & J. Whelan (Eds.), *Human muscle fatigue: Physiological mechanisms* (pp. 1-18). London: Pitman Medical.

Edwards, R.H.T., Hill, D.K., Jones, D.A., & Merton, P.A. (1977). Fatigue of long duration in human skeletal muscle after exercise. *Journal of Physiology* (London), **72**, 769-788.

Essén, B., Jansson, E., Henriksson, J., Taylor, A.W., & Saltin, B. (1975). Metabolic characteristics of fibre types in human skeletal muscle. *Acta Physiologica Scandinavica, 95*, 153-165.

Essén-Gustavsson, B., & Henriksson, J. (1984). Enzyme levels in pools of microdissected human muscle fibres of identified type. *Acta Physiologica Scandinavica, 120*, 505-515.

Faulkner, J.A. (1983). Fatigue of skeletal muscle fibers. In J. Sutton, C. Houston, & N.L. Jones (Eds.), *Hypoxia exercise and altitude* (pp. 243-253). Proceedings of the Third Banff International Hypoxia Symposium. New York: Alan R. Liss.

Faulkner, J.A., Jones, D.A., Round, J.M., & Edwards, R.H.T. (1981). Dynamics of energetic processes in human muscle. In P. Ceretelli & B.J. Whipp (Eds.), *Exercise bioenergetics and gas exchange* (pp. 75-78). Holland: Elsevier Biomedical Press.

Fitts, R.H., Courtright, J.B., Kim, D.H., & Witzmann, F.A. (1982). Muscle fatigue with prolonged exercise: Contractile and biochemical alterations. *American Journal of Physiology*, **242**, C65-C73.

Garnett, R.A.F., O'Donovan, M.J., Stephens, J.A., & Taylor, A. (1978). Motor unit organization of human medial gastrocnemius. *Journal of Physiology* (London), **287**, 33-43.

Gollnick, P.D., Armstrong, R.B., Saubert IV, C.W., Piehl, K., & Saltin, B. (1972). Enzyme activities and fiber composition in skeletal muscle of untrained and trained men. *Journal of Applied Physiology*, **33**, 312-319.

Green, H., Reichmann, H., & Pette, D. (1982). A comparison of two ATPase based schema for histochemical fibre typing in various mammals. *Histochemistry*, **76**, 21-31.

Green, H.J., Daub, B., Houston, M.E., Thomson, J.A., Fraser, I., & Ranney, D. (1981). Human vastus lateralis and gastrocnemius muscles: A comparative histochemical and biochemical analysis. *Journal of Neurological Sciences*, **52**, 201-210.

Green, H.J., & Greene, K. (1980). Histochemical characteristics of selected locomotor and respiratory muscles of the rat. In F. Nagle & H. Montague (Eds.), *Exercise in health and disease* (pp. 136-146). Springfield, IL: C.C. Thomas.

Gregor, R.J., Edgerton, V.R., Perrine, J.J., Campion, D.S., & Debus, C. (1979). Torque-velocity relationships and muscle fibre composition in elite female athletes. *Journal of Applied Physiology: Respiratory, Environmental and Exercise Physiology*, **47**, 388-392.

Grimby, L., & Hannerz, J. (1974). Differences in recruitment order and discharge pattern of motor units in the early and late reflex components in man. *Acta Physiologica Scandinavica*, **90**, 555-564.

Grimby, L., & Hannerz, J. (1977). Firing rate and recruitment order of the toe extensor units in different modes of voluntary contraction. *Journal of Physiology* (London), **264**, 865-879.

Grimby, L., Hannerz, J., & Hedman, B. (1981). The fatigue and voluntary discharge properties of single motor units in man. *Journal of Physiology* (London), **316**, 545-554.

Guth, L., & Samaha, F.J. (1969). Qualitative differences between actomyosin ATPase of slow and fast mammalian muscle. *Experimental Neurology*, **25**, 139-152.

Halkjaer-Kristensen, J., & Ingeman-Hansen, T. (1979). Microphotometric determination of glycogen in single fibres of human quadriceps muscles. *Histochemical Journal*, **11**, 629-638.

Henneman, E., Somjen, G., & Carpenter, D.O. (1965). Functional significance of cell size in spinal motoneurons. *Journal of Neurophysiology*, **28**, 560-580.

Hermansen, L. (1981). Effect of metabolic changes on force generation in skeletal muscle during maximal exercise. In R. Porter & J. Whelan (Eds.), *Human muscle fatigue: Physiologic mechanisms* (pp. 75-88). London: Pitman Medical.

Hill, A.V. (1938). The heat of shortening and the dynamic constants of muscle. *Proceedings of the Royal Society of London, Series B*, **126**, 136-195.

Hochachka, P.W. (1976). Design of metabolic and enzymatic machinery to fit lifestyle and environment. *Biochemical Society Symposium*, **41**, 3-31.

Hultman, E., & Sjohölm, H. (1983). Electromyogram, force and relaxation time during and after continuous electrical stimulation of human skeletal muscle in situ. *Journal of Physiology* (London), **339**, 33-40.

Jones, D.A. (1981). Muscle fatigue due to changes beyond the neuromuscular junction. In R. Porter & J. Whelan (Eds.), *Human muscle fatigue: Physiologic mechanisms* (pp. 178-196). London: Pitman Medical.

Julian, F.J., & Moss, R.L. (1981). Effects of calcium and ionic strength on shortening velocity and tension development in frog skinned muscle fibres. *Journal of Physiology* (London), **311**, 179-199.

Kushmerick, M.J., & Crow, M.T. (1983). Regulation of energetics and mechanics by myosin light chain phosphorylation in fast-twitch skeletal muscle. *Foundation Proceedings*, **42**, 14-20.

Lowenstein, J, & Goodman, M.N. (1978). The purine nucleotide cycle in skeletal muscle. *Federation Proceedings*, **37**, 2308-2312.

Lowry, C.V., Kimmey, J.S., Felder, S., Chi, MM-Y, Kaiser, K.K., Passoneau, P.N., Kirk, K.A., & Lowry, O.H. (1978). Enzyme patterns in single human muscle fibres. *Journal of Biological Chemistry*, **253**, 8269-8277.

Manning, D.R., & Stull, J.T. (1982). Myosin light chain phosphorylation-dephosphorylation in mammalian skeletal muscle. *American Journal of Physiology*, **242**, C234-C241.

McCartney, N., Heigenhauser, G.J.F., & Jones, N.L. (1983). Power output and fatigue of human muscle in maximal cycling exercise. *Journal of Applied Physiology: Respiratory, Environmental and Exercise Physiology*, **55**, 218-224.

Meyer, R.A., & Terjung, R.L. (1979). Differences in ammonia and adenylate metabolism in contracting fast and slow muscle. *American Journal of Physiology*, **237**, C111-C118.

Perrine, J.J., & Edgerton, V.R. (1978). Muscle force-velocity and power-velocity relationships under isokinetic loading. *Medicine and Science in Sports*, **10**, 159-166.

Peter, J.B., Barnard, R.J., Edgerton, V.R., Gillespie, C.A., & Stempel, K.E. (1972). Metabolic profiles of three fiber types of skeletal muscle in guinea pigs and rabbits. *Biochemistry*, **11**, 2627-2633.

Pette, D., & Heilman, C. (1979). Some characteristics of sarcoplasmic reticulum in fast and slow-twitch muscles. *Biochemical Society Transactions*, **7**, 765-767.

Rehunen, S., & Härkönen, M. (1980). High-energy phosphate compounds in human slow-twitch and fast-twitch muscle fibres. *Scandinavian Journal of Clinical Laboratory Investigation*, **40**, 45-54.

Reichmann, H., & Pette, D. (1982). A comparative microphotometric study of succinic dehydrogenase activity levels in Type I, IIA and IIB fibres of mammalian and human muscles. *Histochemistry*, **74**, 27-41.

Sahlin, K., Palmskog, G., & Hultman, E. (1978). Adenine nucleotide and IMP contents of the quadriceps muscles in man after exercise. *Pflugers Archives*, **374**, 193-198.

Saltin, B., & Gollnick, P.D. (1983). Skeletal muscle adaptability: Significance of metabolism and performance. In L. Peachey (Ed.), *Handbook of physiology* (pp. 555-631). Maryland: American Physiological Society.

Sjøgaard, G. (1982). Capillary supply and cross-sectional area of slow and fast twitch muscle fibres in man. *European Journal of Applied Physiology*, **50**, 136-146.

Sjøgaard, G., Houston, M.E., Nygaard, E., & Saltin, B. (1978). Subgroupings of fast twitch fibres in skeletal muscles of man. *Histochemistry*, **58**, 79-87.

Staudte, H.W., Exner, G.U., & Pette, D. (1973). Effect of short term, high intensity (sprint) training on some contractile and metabolic characteristics of fast and slow muscle of the rat. *Pflügers Archives*, **344**, 159-168.

Thorstensson, A., Grimby, G., & Karlsson, J. (1976). Force-velocity relations and fibre composition in human knee extensor muscles. *Journal of Applied Physiology*, **40**, 12-16.

Thorstensson, A., Sjödin, B., Tesch, P., & Karlsson, J. (1977). Actomyosin ATPase, myokinase, CPK and LDH in human fast and slow twitch muscle fibres. *Acta Physiologica Scandinavica*, **99**, 225-229.

Vandervoort, A.A., Quinlan, J., & McComas, A.J. (1983). Twitch potentiation after voluntary contraction. *Experimental Neurology*, **81**, 141-152.

Viitasalo, J.T., & Komi, P.V. (1978). Force-time characteristics and fiber composition in human leg extensor muscles. *European Journal of Applied Physiology*, **40**, 7-15.

6

Power Output of Fast and Slow Fibers From Human Skeletal Muscles

John A. Faulkner, Dennis R. Claflin, and
Kevin K. McCully
University of Michigan Medical School

Muscle physiologists measure force development and shortening velocity of skeletal muscles of small animals but rarely discuss power output (Hill, 1950). Conversely, investigators of human performance have had a long and continued interest in maximum, short-term power output (Margaria, Aghemo, & Rovelli, 1966; McCartney, Heigenhauser, & Jones, 1983) and sustained, long-term power output (Wilkie, 1959; Wilkie, 1960).

Skeletal muscle fibers may be classified fast or slow on the basis of contractile properties (Close, 1972). Most of our knowledge of the properties of fast and slow skeletal muscle fibers is based on studies of whole extensor digitorum longus and soleus muscles of rats (Close, 1964) and cats (Murphy & Beardsley, 1974; Faulkner, Niemeyer, Maxwell, & White, 1980). This knowledge has been supplemented by more limited data on the contractile properties of single motor units in fast and slow muscles of mice (Lewis, Parry, & Rowlerson, 1982), rats (Close, 1967), and cats (Burke, Levine, Tsairis, & Zajac, 1973). Data have been collected by less direct techniques on fast and slow motor units in the extensor hallucis brevis (Sica & McComas, 1971) and the medial gastrocnemius (Garnett, O'Donovan, Stephens, & Taylor, 1979) muscles of humans.

Controversy exists as to whether fast and slow skeletal muscles develop the same maximum isometric force per unit cross-sectional area (Close, 1972). If a difference does exist for whole skeletal muscles, it is small with slow muscles having lower values (Close, 1964). While the force development per unit area of fast and slow fibers is similar, the shortening velocity of fast fibers is threefold greater than that of slow fibers at zero load and up to fourfold greater at other loads (Close, 1964; Ranatunga, 1983). The fatigability of fast and slow muscles (Witzmann, Kim, & Fitts, 1983) or fast and slow motor units (Edstrom & Kugelberg, 1968) has been based exclusively on their ability to sustain isometric force development. Under these circumstances, slow compared to fast muscles or motor units show a much greater resistance to fatigue.

Our purpose was to collect data on the force-velocity characteristics of small bundles of fast and slow fibers from human skeletal muscles, calculate the power curves, and model the contribution of fast and slow fibers to the composite power curve for a mixed muscle. We postulated that within a muscle composed of both fast and slow fibers, the fast fibers would make a significantly greater contribution to peak and sustained high power output.

Methods

Contractile properties were measured on bundles of fiber segments from human skeletal muscles (Faulkner, Jones, Round, & Edwards, 1980). The validity of measuring contractile properties on segments of fibers was verified through comparisons with data on bundles of intact fibers (Faulkner, Claflin, McCully, & Jones, 1982). The bundles of fiber segments were 10 to 25 mm long, 0.5 to 2.0 mm^2 in cross-sectional area, and each contained 200 to 800 fibers. Bundles were suspended in a muscle bath containing buffered mammalian Ringer's solution at 37°C. Stimulus pulses were unidirectional square waves, 0.2 ms in duration and of supramaximal intensity. Measurements of contractile properties were made at optimal length for force development. Measurements included contraction time, maximum isometric tetanic force development (F_m), and velocity of shortening (V) at 12 to 15 different afterloads. A hyperbola described by the Hill equation (Hill, 1938) was fit to the shortening velocities by computing the Hill constants, a/F_m and b, which minimized the sum of the squared errors in the velocity dimension (Claflin, 1984). The maximum velocity of shortening (V_m) was determined by extrapolation along the hyperbola to zero load.

Following measurement of contractile properties, the fibers in bundles were classified Type I and Type II based on histochemical demonstration of myofibrillar ATPase activity (Brooke & Kaiser, 1970). The contraction times for bundles of fibers containing 100% Type II fibers and bundles containing 85% Type I fibers were 55 and 160 ms, respectively. These times are in agreement with data reported for the fastest and slowest motor units from human muscles (Sica & McComas, 1971; Garnett et al., 1979). Therefore, data on these bundles of fiber segments were taken as representative of pure fast and slow muscle fibers.

Force development of bundles of fast and slow fiber segments was normalized by maximum isometric tetanic force on the assumption that both types of fibers develop similar forces per cross-sectional area. Shortening velocities (fiber-lengths/s) were normalized by the maximum velocity of shortening of the fast fibers (Vm_{fast}). The power developed by fast and slow fibers was calculated from the force-velocity data and normalized by maximum power output of the fast fibers (Pm_{fast}).

To make realistic comparisons of the relative contributions of fast and slow fibers to the power development of a mixed muscle, a model representative of human mixed muscles was required. In an autopsy study of 36 human muscles, the mean for Type I fibers in 15 different limb muscles was 51 $\pm$ 2% (Johnson, Polgar, Weightman, & Appleton, 1973). No difference was observed between the percentages of Type I fibers in muscles from the upper limbs and those from the lower limbs for these untrained control subjects. Data on limb muscles of different species indicate a good correlation between the histochemical classification of Type I and Type II fibers and the identification of slow and fast fibers through measurements of contractile properties (Burke et al., 1973; Garnett et al., 1979). Based on these data, a muscle composed of 50% fast fibers and 50% slow fibers was chosen as representative of human limb muscles. A composite power curve was constructed for this mixed muscle.

Results

The maximum velocities of shortening of fast and slow fibers from human skeletal muscles were 6 and 2 fiber-lengths/s, respectively. The force-velocity relationships for bundles of fast and slow fiber segments from human skeletal muscles are presented in Figure 1A. The a/F_m ratios were 0.25 and 0.15 for fast and slow fibers, respectively. The difference in the a/F_m ratios indicates greater curvature of the force-velocity curve of slow fibers than that of fast fibers (see Figure 1A, inset). The power outputs for fast and slow fibers are shown as a function of afterload in Figure 1B. The power developed by fast fibers is greater than that developed by slow fibers at all velocities of shortening. The peak power output of the fast fibers is fourfold that of the slow fibers.

In Figure 2A, the power curves for a muscle composed of 100% fast fibers and a muscle of equal fiber length and cross-sectional area composed of 100% slow fibers are plotted against normalized velocity of shortening (V/Vm_{fast}). Each muscle achieves its peak power at approximately one-third of its maximum velocity of shortening. The power contributed by slow and fast fibers in a muscle composed of 50% of each fiber type is illustrated as a function of the shortening velocity of the mixed muscle in Figure 2B. The composite power curve for the mixed muscle indicates how little the slow fibers contribute to

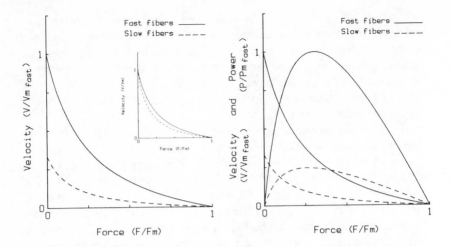

Figure 1. Velocity of shortening and power output as a function of force for fast and slow muscle fibers of humans. Force is normalized by maximum isometric tetanic force. A. Velocity of shortening as a function of force for fast and slow fibers. Velocities are normalized by the maximum velocity of shortening of the fast fibers. Insert illustrates the difference in curvature of the force-velocity curves of the fast and slow fibers (velocities are normalized by their respective maximum velocities of shortening). B. Power output as a function of force added to A. Power is normalized by maximum power output of the fast fibers.

the maximum power of the mixed muscle (see Figure 2B, shaded area). Even at the velocity of shortening at which peak power is achieved by the slow fibers, the fast fibers contribute 2.5 times more than the slow fibers to the total power. At velocities of shortening greater than those attainable by the slow fibers, the power developed by mixed muscle is due exclusively to that contributed by the fast fibers. The muscle with 50% fast and 50% slow fibers has a peak power that is 55% of the peak power for a muscle composed exclusively of fast fibers.

Discussion

The ratio between the maximum velocity of shortening of slow and fast muscles varies from twofold to threefold for mice (Close, 1965), rats (Close, 1964; Ranatunga, 1983), and cats (Murphy & Beardsley, 1974; Faulkner et al., 1980). Our data on the maximum velocity of shortening of small bundles of fast and slow fiber segments from human muscles are in good agreement with data on whole muscles from smaller mammals. Therefore, the force-velocity and power relationships between fast and slow muscle fibers from different mammalian species, including humans, can be discussed in a general sense.

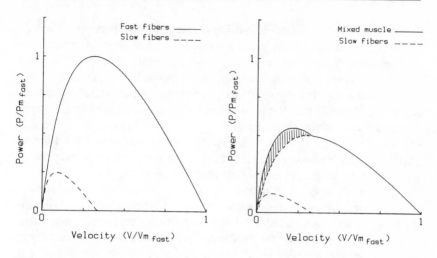

Figure 2. Power output as a function of velocity for fast, slow, and mixed muscle. A. Power curves for pure fast and pure slow muscle fibers. Power and velocity are normalized by peak power output and maximum velocity of shortening of the fast fibers. B. Power output of a mixed muscle (50% fast and 50% slow fibers) and of the slow fibers of the mixed muscle. The shaded portion of the curve represents the contribution of the slow fibers to power output of the mixed muscle. Velocities are normalized by the maximum shortening velocity of the fast fibers, and power is normalized by the maximum power output of a muscle composed of fast fibers.

Fast and slow fibers have similar capacities to generate isometric force, but fast fibers are much more effective than slow fibers in producing power. Compared to a pure fast muscle, a mixed muscle composed of approximately 50% slow fibers is at a considerable disadvantage in performing tasks requiring substantial power development. When all fibers in a mixed muscle are contracting, the slow fibers contribute almost as much power as the fast fibers at very low velocities, only slightly to power at moderate velocities, and not at all at high velocities. However, slow fibers are more efficient in performing both isometric contractions and isotonic contractions at very low velocities (Wendt & Gibbs, 1974).

The difference between the power output of fast and slow fibers can be applied to the analysis of maximum power produced by humans. McCartney, Heigenhauser, and Jones (1983) observed a 33% difference between the maximum power output of their best and worst cyclists. The performance of the poorest cyclist was attributed to a low percentage of Type II fibers and a small active muscle mass. The subject with a peak power of 2539 watts had 72% Type II fibers, and the subject with a peak power of 1708 watts had 53% Type II fibers (McCartney et al., 1983). If the distribution of fiber types observed in the vastus lateralis muscle is representative of all muscles active in cycling, the difference in muscle composition alone could account for 85% of the difference in maximum power.

Most comparisons of the fatigability of fast and slow fibers have involved isometric contractions. Slow fibers are superior to fast fibers in maintaining force with time (Edstrom & Kugelberg, 1968). The greater capacity of fast fibers to generate power makes the comparison of fatigability quite different when the criterion is the ability to sustain a given power output. The ability to sustain power depends on whether the fibers in a motor unit are fast-glycolytic, fast-oxidative, or slow (see Figure 3). Fast-glycolytic fibers lose power rapidly, whereas slow fibers can sustain a high percentage of their peak power for long periods of time. Fast-oxidative fibers can sustain much higher proportions of peak power for longer periods of time than fast-glycolytic fibers can. Because of their capacity to develop greater peak power, fast-oxidative fibers sustain higher power outputs than slow fibers during short-term exercise. With endurance training, fast-oxidative fibers have oxidative capacities greater than slow fibers. Consequently, fast-oxidative fibers may be capable of sustaining higher power outputs than slow fibers even during activities lasting several hours.

The soleus muscle in all species is composed predominantly of Type I fibers and has a relatively long contraction time and low maximum velocity of shortening (Close, 1972; Murphy & Beardsley, 1974). For six different human cadavers, the composition of the soleus muscle varied from 70% to 100% Type I fibers (Johnson et al., 1973). Of the more than 600 other muscles in the human body, almost all have a significant proportion of Type I fibers (Johnson et al., 1973). Untrained control subjects rarely initiate contractions that require high or even moderate power. Many of the leg and trunk muscles are involved in the maintenance of posture during standing and in the very low power move-

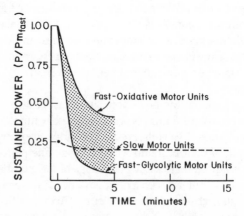

Figure 3. The maximum power output that can be sustained with time for fast and slow motor units. Sustained power is normalized by the peak power of the fast motor units. Fast motor units are shown with a range of sustained power outputs depending on their oxidative capacity. Compared to slow motor units, the ability of fast motor units to sustain power for periods of time greater than five minutes is not known.

ments of walking. Because of the frequency of such activities, the presence of slow fibers in these muscles results in a significant gain in economy. Conversely, the fast fibers in mixed muscles provide a potential for more rapid movements and substantially higher power outputs than would be possible for a purely slow muscle.

In contrast to untrained control subjects, the presence of high percentages of slow fibers in the leg muscles of weight lifters (Gollnick, Armstrong, Saubert, Piehl, & Saltin, 1972), world champion sprint cyclists (Burke, Cerny, Costill, & Fink, 1977), and sprint runners (Costill et al., 1976), and in the arm muscles of canoeists and competitive swimmers (Gollnick et al., 1972) is unexpected. The muscles of these athletes are trained for high power contractions. The presence of a high proportion of slow fibers suggests either that their presence is genetically determined and the fiber type is immutable, or that the slow fibers are not adapting to the training stimulus.

An alternative explanation for human skeletal muscles containing high percentages of apparently slow fibers is that some of the fibers that demonstrate Type I fiber characteristics histochemically might have contractile properties that are representative of fast fibers. The adductor pollicis muscle of humans is composed of 80% Type I fibers (Johnson et al., 1973) yet has a contraction time of 55 ms (Merton, 1954). A contraction time of 55 ms is similar to that of the fast fibers reported in this study. There is not sufficient data on the histochemistry, biochemistry, and contractile properties of the same biopsy samples of human muscles to differentiate among these alternative explanations.

Interest is focused currently on eccentric contractions of skeletal muscle because of their apparent role in exercise-induced injury to the skeletal muscle fibers of humans (Newham, Jones, & Edwards, 1983; Hikida, Staron, Hagerman, Sherman, & Costill, 1983) and other animals (Armstrong, Ogilvie, & Schwane, 1983; Vihko, Salminen, & Rantamaki, 1979). During an active contraction, skeletal muscle fibers appear to be much more susceptible to injury when the fibers are lengthening than when they are shortening (Newham et al., 1983).

The force-velocity and power relationships during eccentric contractions provide insights into the possible mechanisms of the injury. Data available on the soleus muscles of cats (Joyce & Rack, 1969; Joyce, Rack, & Westbury, 1969) suggest that at low velocities of lengthening small changes in velocity result in large changes in force. At higher velocities of lengthening, changes in velocity result in little change in force. The point in the relationship where this transition occurs remains to be documented clearly. The power absorbed by the muscle fibers increases rapidly with increasing velocities of lengthening and can reach magnitudes that equal or exceed the peak power output attainable during concentric contractions. The high power eccentric contractions that occur during the braking of high velocity ballistic movements (Marsden, Obeso, & Rothwell, 1983), downward stepping (Newham et al., 1983), and downward jumping (Dyhre-Poulsen & Laursen, 1984) are the most likely to produce injury.

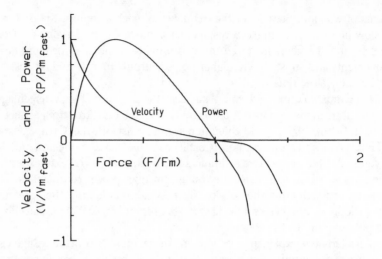

Figure 4. Velocity and power as a function of force for concentric and eccentric contractions of fast muscle. Velocity and power are normalized by the maximum velocity of shortening and maximum power output, respectively. Force is normalized by maximum isometric tetanic force.

In summary, the peak power output of fast fibers is fourfold that of slow fibers due to a greater shortening velocity for a given afterload. Slow fibers are more economical than fast fibers in generating a sustained force. Consequently, slow fibers are ideally suited for the maintenance of posture. Because of their high peak power and resistance to fatigue, fast-oxidative fibers may sustain moderate power better than slow fibers even during long-term contractions. Most human muscles are composed of a mixture of approximately 50% fast and 50% slow fibers. This mixture of fiber types appears to provide adequate power for both short-term peak demands and for low power sustained activities. A better understanding of the capacity of fast and slow fibers to produce and sustain power is needed. Little is known about power absorption by fast and slow fibers during eccentric contractions. The absorption of power during eccentric contractions may be responsible for exercise-induced injury.

Acknowledgements

We acknowledge the assistance and support of our colleagues whose names appear as co-authors on our references. The research on which this paper is based was supported by a National Institutes of Health Program Project Grant, NS 17017 and Grant HL-34164.

References

Armstrong, R.B., Ogilvie, R.W., & Schwane, J.A. (1983). Eccentric exercise-induced injury to rat skeletal muscle. *Journal of Applied Physiology: Respiratory, Environmental and Exercise Physiology*, **54**, 80-93.

Brooke, M.H., & Kaiser, K.K. (1970). Muscle fiber types: How many and what kind? *Archives of Neurology*, **23**, 369-379.

Burke, R.E., Cerny, F., Costill, D., & Fink, W. (1977). Characteristics of skeletal muscle in competitive cyclists. *Medicine and Science in Sports*, **9**, 109-112.

Burke, R.E., Levine, D.N., Tsairis, P., & Zajac, F.E. (1973). Physiological types and histochemical profiles in motor units of the cat gastrocnemius. *Journal of Physiology* (London), **234**, 723-748.

Claflin, D.R. (1984). Least-squares fit of the Hill equation to force-velocity data from muscle preparations. *Federation Proceedings*, **43**, 533.

Close, R.I. (1964). Dynamic properties of fast and slow skeletal muscles of the rat during development. *Journal of Physiology* (London), **173**, 74-95.

Close, R.I. (1965). Force: velocity properties of mouse muscles. *Nature*, **206**, 717-718.

Close, R.I. (1967). Properties of motor units in fast and slow skeletal muscles the rat. *Journal of Physiology* (London), **193**, 45-55.

Close, R.I. (1972). Dynamic properties of mammalian skeletal muscles. *Physiological Reviews*, **52**, 129-197.

Costill, D.L., Daniels, J., Evans, W., Fink, W., Krahenbuhl, G., & Saltin, B. (1976). Skeletal muscle enzymes and fiber composition in male and female track athletes. *Journal of Applied Physiology*, **40**, 149-154.

Dyhre-Poulsen, P., & Laursen, A.M. (1984). Programmed electromyographic activity and negative incremental muscle stiffness in monkeys jumping downward. *Journal of Physiology* (London), **350**, 121-136.

Edstrom, L., & Kugelberg, E. (1968). Histochemical composition, distribution of fibres and fatigability of single motor units. *Journal of Neurology, Neurosurgery, and Psychiatry*, **31**, 424-433.

Faulkner, J.A., Claflin, D.R., McCully, K.K., & Jones, D.A. (1982). Contractile properties of bundles of fiber segments from skeletal muscles. *American Journal of Physiology*, **242**, *(Cell Physiology*, **12**), C66-C73.

Faulkner, J.A., Jones, D.A., Round, J.M., & Edwards, R.H.T. (1980). Dynamics of energetic processes in human muscle. In P. Cerretelli & B.J. Whipp (Eds.), *Proceedings of the International Symposium on Exercise, Bioenergetics, and Gas Exchange* (pp. 81-90). Milan.

Faulkner, J.A., Niemeyer, J.H., Maxwell, L.C., & White, T.P. (1980). Contractile properties of transplanted extensor digitorum longus muscles of cats. *American Journal of Physiology*, **238**, *(Cell Physiology*, **7**), C120-C126.

Garnett, R.A.F., O'Donovan, M.J., Stephens, J.A., & Taylor, A. (1979). Motor unit organization of human medial gastrocnemius. *Journal of Physiology* (London), **287**, 33-43.

Gollnick, P.D., Armstrong, C.W., Saubert IV, C.W., Piehl, K., & Saltin, B. (1972). Enzyme activity and fiber composition in skeletal muscle of untrained and trained men. *Journal of Applied Physiology*, **33**, 312-319.

Hikida, R.S., Staron, R.S., Hagerman, F.C., Sherman, W.M., & Costill, D.L. (1983). Muscle fiber necrosis associated with human marathon runners. *Journal of Neurological Science*, **59**, 185-203.

Hill, A.V. (1938). The heat of shortening and the dynamic constants of muscle. *Proceedings of the Royal Society of London, Series B*, **126**, 136-195.

Hill, A.V. (1950). The dimensions of animals and their muscular dynamics. *Royal Institution of Great Britain Proceedings*, **34**, (Pt. III, 156), 450-471.

Johnson, M.A., Polgar, J., Weightman, D., & Appleton, D. (1973). Data on the distribution of fibre types in thirty-six human muscles: An autopsy study. *Journal of the Neurological Sciences*, **18**, 111-129.

Joyce, G.C., & Rack, P.M.H. (1969). Isotonic lengthening and shortening movements of cat soleus muscle. *Journal of Physiology* (London), **204**, 475-591.

Joyce, G.C., Rack, P.M.H., & Westbury, D.R. (1969). The mechanical properties of cat soleus muscle during controlled lengthening and shortening movements. *Journal of Physiology* (London), **204**, 461-474.

Lewis, D.M., Parry, D.J., & Rowlerson, A. (1982). Isometric contractions of motor units and immunohistochemistry of mouse soleus muscle. *Journal of Physiology* (London), **325**, 393-401.

Margaria, R., Aghemo, P., & Rovelli, E. (1966). Measurements of muscular power (anaerobic) in man. *Journal of Applied Physiology*, **21**, 1661-1669.

Marsden, C.D., Obeso, J.A., & Rothwell, J.C. (1983). The function of the antagonist muscle during fast limb movements in man. *Journal of Physiology* (London), **335**, 1-13.

McCartney, N., Heigenhauser, G.J.F., & Jones, N.L. (1983). Power output and fatigue of human muscle in maximal cycling exercise. *Journal of Applied Physiology: Respiratory, Environmental and Exercise Physiology*, **55**, 218-224.

Merton, P.A. (1954). Interaction between muscle fibers in a twitch. *Journal of Physiology* (London), **124**, 311-324.

Murphy, R.A., & Beardsley, A.C. (1974). Mechanical properties of the cat soleus muscle *in situ*. *American Journal of Physiology*, **227**, 1008-1013.

Newham, D.J., Jones, D.A., & Edwards, R.H.T. (1983). Large delayed plasma creatine kinase changes after stepping exercise. *Muscle and Nerve*, **6**, 380-385.

Ranatunga, K.W. (1983). Temperature-dependence of shortening velocity and rate of isometric tension development in rat skeletal muscle. *Journal of Physiology* (London), **329**, 465-483.

Sica, R.E.P., & McComas, A.J. (1971). Fast and slow twitch units in a human muscle. *Journal of Neurology, Neurosurgery, and Psychiatry*, **34**, 113-120.

Vihko, V., Salminen, A., & Rantamaki, J. (1979). Exhaustive exercise, endurance training, and acid hydrolase activity in skeletal muscle. *Journal of Applied Physiology, 47,* 43-50.

Wendt, I.R., & Gibbs, C.L. (1974). Energy production of mammalian fast- and slow-twitch muscles during development. *American Journal of Physiology, 226,* 642-647.

Wilkie, D.R. (1959). The work output of animals: Flight by birds, and by man-power. *Nature, 183,* 1515-1516.

Wilkie, D.R. (1960). Man as a source of mechanical power. *Ergonomics, 3,* 1-8.

Witzmann, F.A., Kim, D.H., & Fitts, R.H. (1983). Effect of hindlimb immobilization on fatigability of skeletal muscle. *Journal of Applied Physiology: Respiratory, Environmental and Exercise Physiology, 54,* 1242-1248.

Discussion

Following Dr. Faulkner's paper there was a long discussion regarding the differential recruitment patterns of slow and fast twitch muscle fibers, muscle injury in eccentric contractions, and the effects of training on both.

Dr. Ianuzzo felt that if we were using fast twitch fibers at their full capacity for only a very short time every day, we paid for it by carrying them around; the 15 kg of fast twitch fibers extract a cost in terms of protein and ATP synthesis. Dr. Faulkner replied that the answer might be that in the evolution of man fast twitch fibers were once critical for survival and the balance between slow and fast fibers was established then. This particularly applies to the fast twitch oxidative fibers that enable us to sustain power output over several hours. Man has an astounding capacity for long distance running, which may have been very important to survival. Skeletal muscle fibers have only partially adapted to the inactivity of modern day life styles.

Dr. Komi was interested in the power velocity curves of fast and slow fibers; it seemed a waste of energy to use slow fibers at high velocities in concentric contractions when slow fibers are unlikely to contribute much. Dr. Faulkner replied that if the size principle prevails, as it appears to for most types of recruitment, slow fibers are apparently recruited even at high velocities of shortening. Under these circumstances, they may not contribute much to power, being essentially unloaded. If slow fibers are unloaded, the energetic cost of their shortening is not very costly. Dr. Bigland-Ritchie wondered whether, in fact, even in the fastest movements, muscle ever acted in the part of the force velocity relationship that was beyond the range of the slow fibers. She had calculated that in bicycle pedalling one probably never went beyond about 0.2 of V_{max}. Perhaps the discussion of the relative contributions made to power by fast and slow muscles is a little misleading, if considered in the context of velocities that are only possible in isolated muscle strips. Dr. Faulkner agreed that undoubtedly much of human movement is performed at power outputs within the velocity range of the slow fibers.

Mr. Perrine felt that one point being forgotten in the discussion was that the so-called fast or high power fibers have to function both in the velocity and the time domain. For convenience, power is measured because without knowing the capacity of the series elastic component it is impossible to tell how quickly muscle is generating energy by monitoring its rate of force development. However, a high power fiber would generate force initially at a greater rate than a slow fiber. Even if a person spends most of his or her time in sedentary activity, there are many occasions during the day where bursts of energy are needed for safety purposes (for example, in correcting a stumble). Such circumstances are associated with very explosive contractions; force velocity curves are fine, but we must also consider the force:time domain.

Dr. Edgerton questioned whether slow muscles should be described as postural muscles; most are obviously capable of working as flexors and extensors, and they are present in fish, in which posture is irrelevant. Should the concept be continued? Dr. Winter took up this point and asked that muscle function be examined in voluntary acts like walking and running. In walking and jogging he had found only one major muscle group on the positive part of the force-velocity curve: the plantarflexor of the ankle. Other muscles were mainly involved with eccentric contractions at weight acceptance and push-off. This type of activity does not activate a large proportion of the total motor units and the level of recruitment is low except for the plantarflexors, which generate 80% to 90% of what is needed during walking.

Dr. Gollnick pointed out that there are large differences between fibers in mixed population muscles, even though they are typed as being slow; as long ago as 1938 Brown and von Euler showed differences between the slow fibers in gastrocnemius and in the soleus. Schmalbruch (1977) showed that slow fibers in mixed muscle may have a sarcoplasmic reticulum that is very similar to that of a fast muscle and quite different from that of the soleus. Thus, there are differences within both slow and fast muscles that are generally overlooked, and a fast muscle in one limb may have a completely different contractile speed than that in another part of the body. Also, the whole concept falls apart when different animals are being considered; a fast muscle may behave like a fast muscle in one animal yet be on the slow end of the range in another. Dr. Gollnick also pointed out that even when muscles are typed according to their myosin ATPase activity, there is a huge overlap in the oxidative capacity. Stephens and Usherwood (1977) showed that some so-called fast glycolytic motor units could contract at a high level for 20 to 30 minutes. Dr. Faulkner agreed that there was no question that slow fibers in soleus are quite different from those in the medial gastrocnemius or in extensor digitorum longus muscles. Differences are evident through measurements made on small bundles of fibers and on single motor units. The characterization of human muscle power output was presented in a simple model to demonstrate contributions of slow and fast fibers individually and when combined in the contractions of a mixed muscle. At the present time one cannot elaborate human power output further.

Dr. Faulkner was asked by Dr. Howald to explain how the high forces associated with eccentric contraction lead to injury through power absorption. He replied that cross bridges and other parts of the muscle absorb the power in some way, and specifically how power is dissipated during eccentric contractions is not known. Dr. Howald asked whether power might be stored in some elastic element or dissipated as heat. Perhaps there might even be a local hot spot. Dr. Knuttgen doubted that muscle soreness could be explained on the basis of power absorption; if someone cycles concentrically at a power output of 20% to 25% of peak force for that velocity, and the same exercise is carried out eccentrically, the muscles are now only at about 10% of peak force. Dr. Faulkner felt that we had very limited information with regard to the magnitude of power during the braking of movements such as in stepping down. Dr. Komi agreed that eccentric contractions could be used as a model to induce muscle soreness but pointed out that adaptation can occur even to this type of movement. He felt that it was not so much the eccentric contraction that causes muscle soreness but a high tension related to the capacity of the muscle that was activated. Any tension, if high enough, would cause soreness. Dr. Faulkner added that even world class marathon runners sustain injury to skeletal muscle that may be just as severe as those that occur in the untrained person. Dr. Gollnick wondered whether this was because in the course of a marathon some motor units are activated that are not trained. Consequently, training may still exert some degree of protection. Dr. Faulkner agreed that the injury to fibers was related to the relative stress.

Dr. Morrison asked what Dr. Faulkner's definition of injury was, in view of the fact that this is usually defined as an abnormality resulting in a lessening or stopping of performance. Dr. Faulkner was not defining it functionally but morphologically. The fibers are actually damaged, with disruption of the Z-line, disruption of sarcomeres, and sarcoplasmic streaming; there is also an inflammatory response with invasion of the injured area with macrophages. Dr. Morrison wondered how these findings could be compatible with a runner going out and doing 20 miles the next day. Dr. Faulkner responded that the runners probably did not use injured motor units in that situation. Dr. Ianuzzo quoted the work of Armstrong, Ogilvie, and Schwane (1983), who found 5% of fibers injured in running rats. His own work carried out in human knee extension showed that if a level of power was achieved at which leakage of CPK occurred, the individual was unable to generate a maximal voluntary contraction on the next day. Dr. Faulkner pointed out that marathon runners do not recruit a large proportion of their motor units, and thus if only 5% of the fibers are injured, they are capable of recruiting others. Newham, Mills, Quigley, and Edwards (1983) found that 24 hours following eccentric contractions, only about 80% of maximal force was obtained in a muscle myogram.

Dr. Faulkner commented that 80% of maximal force was much more than that required to run at a reasonable velocity.

Dr. Stauber wished to suggest that a reason for human muscle having an average of 50% slow and 50% fast twitch fibers might be related to the muscle acting as a protein store. During long-term starvation we could lose much of the functional capacity for high power output work with loss of Type II fibers, but there would still be a large percentage of fibers that could still maintain a repertoire of fine movements necessary for survival. Under these circumstances, power output would be significantly decreased. Dr. Faulkner agreed that the phenomenon of Type II fiber atrophy is also seen with aging. Muscle biopsies in very elderly bedridden patients show almost no Type II fibers.

References

Armstrong, R.B., Ogilvie, R.W., & Schwane, J.A. (1983). Eccentric exercise-induced injury to rat skeletal muscle. *Journal of Applied Physiology: Respiratory, Environmental and Exercise Physiology, 54*, 80-93.

Brown, G.L., & von Euler, U.S. (1938). The after effects of a tetanus on mammalian muscle. *Journal of Physiology* (London), *93*, 39-60.

Newham, D.J., Mills, K.R., Quigley, B.M., & Edwards, R.H.T. (1983). Pain and fatigue after concentric and eccentric muscle contractions. *Clinical Science, 64*, 55-62.

Schmalbruch, H. (1977). Regeneration of soleus muscles of rat autografted in toto as studied by electron microscopy. *Cell Tissue Research, 177*, 159-180.

Stephens, J.A., & Usherwood, T.P. (1977). The mechanical properties of human motor units with special reference to their fatigability and recruitment threshold. *Brain Research, 125*, 91-97.

Section **3**

Neural

7

The Control of Muscle Force: Motor Unit Recruitment and Firing Patterns

R.E. Burke
National Institute of Neurological and
Communicative Disorders and Stroke,
National Institute of Health

More than a half century ago, the basic concepts about the control of muscle force were developed by two pioneering neurophysiologists, Sherrington and Adrian. Sherrington defined the "motor unit" as the quantum of motor system output and formulated the notion of "recruitment" to describe the gradation of total muscle force by addition and subtraction of active motor units (Liddell & Sherrington, 1925; Eccles & Sherrington, 1930). At about the same time, Adrian and Bronk (1929) demonstrated the action currents of individual motor axons and showed that their discharge frequency could vary over a considerable range. The notions of motor unit recruitment and frequency modulation of motor unit firing are now ingrained in the thinking of motor systems physiologists as the primary mechanisms for the control of muscle force. This brief essay will focus on recruitment and some possible functional consequences of recruitment flexibility.

Recruitment

Denny-Brown, Sherrington's illustrious student, furthered our understanding of recruitment when he showed in 1919 that it was important to consider the *identities* of active motor units as well as their numbers. He showed that, under some conditions such as the stretch reflex, motor units in slow, red muscles are recruited more readily than those in fast, white muscles. It is less often remembered that he also demonstrated preferential recruitment of fast, white muscles under other conditions (Denny-Brown, 1929). Denny-Brown introduced the notion of "threshold grades" among the motoneurons innervating a given muscle and suggested that these were scaled according to relative intensities of excitatory and inhibitory synaptic input. In his subsequent work on electromyography in human subjects, he went on to demonstrate that orderly patterns of recruitment also occur in voluntary contractions, with the lowest threshold units ordinarily showing the smallest EMG potential amplitudes (Denny-Brown & Pennybacker, 1938; Denny-Brown, 1949).

In this connection, it is important to recall that recruitment orders are defined within a *functional* pool of motor units, which is not necessarily identical to the pool belonging to an anatomically-defined muscle. Denny-Brown (1949), in fact, pointed this out when he described separate recruitment sequences within three different sets of motor units within the complex, multi-articular flexor digitorum profundus of man. These appeared to function independently in wrist flexion versus ulnar deviation versus grasp. Loeb (1984) has recently discussed this phenomenon using the notion of "task groups" to describe sets of motor units, whether within a single muscle or different muscles, that subserve a given action, or "task."

These early ideas and observations have been confirmed and elaborated upon considerably in the past 25 years. A major advance was made in 1965 when Henneman and his co-workers at Harvard surveyed the mechanical properties of large samples of individual motor units in the nominally "white" gastrocnemius and the "red " soleus muscles of the cat hindlimb. They demonstrated a much wider range of physiological properties in the former than in the latter. They also demonstrated systematic interrelations between force outputs, isometric contraction times, and motor axon conduction velocities in these motor unit populations (Wuerker, McPhedran, & Henneman, 1965; McPhedran, Wuerker, & Henneman, 1965; Henneman & Olson, 1965). At the same time, Henneman and colleagues demonstrated quite precise patterns of orderly recruitment among gastrocnemius motoneurons, using the spike amplitudes to "label" their motor axons and to infer the size of the parent motoneurons (Henneman, Somjen, & Carpenter, 1965a, 1965b). Since extracellular spike amplitude was expected to vary according to axonal conduction velocity (Clamann & Henneman, 1976), Henneman's "size principle" of motor pool organization suggested (1) that small force, slow twitch muscle units are innervated by small alpha motoneurons while larger, faster muscle units are innervated by correspondingly larger motoneurons; and (2) that functional thresholds vary along the same continuum, starting with the lowest thresholds among the smallest motoneurons. In the original size principle formulation (Henneman et al., 1965a, 1965b), motoneuron size was viewed as an anatomically "built-in" mechanism for controlling the orderly patterns of recruitment that had been observed by Denny-Brown and others.

A voluminous literature documents the fact that, under many conditions, the recruitment of motor units in animal and human muscles occurs in an orderly sequence, consonant with the predictions of the size principle (see reviews in Burke, 1981; Henneman & Mendell, 1981; Buchthal & Schmalbruch, 1980). There is a great deal of inferential, and some direct, evidence that slow twitch, small force units ordinarily are recruited first in many actions, and demands for larger forces are met by recruitment of increasingly forceful, faster contracting units. Although the factors that produce such recruitment sequences are highly complex and involve motoneuron size only tangentially (Burke, 1981), the net result is essentially consonant with the predictions of the size principle.

In the face of this evidence, it may seem odd to question the generality of the size principle and its predictions. However, despite its attractive simplicity, the original formulation of the size principle cannot account for the early observation of Denny-Brown (1929) that, under some conditions, the usually high threshold units of "white" muscles can be activated before, or even without, activation of the usually low threshold units of red muscle. Such apparent "violations" of the size principle could not be explained if all of the factors controlling recruitment were intrinsic to the motoneurons themselves.

More recent observations have confirmed Denny-Brown's early observations. For example, stimulation of distal skin regions can produce significant reversals of the usual recruitment sequence, both in animals (Kanda, Burke, & Walmsley, 1977) and man (Garnett & Stephens, 1981; Datta & Stephens, 1981). Preferential activation of very high threshold units has been described during extremely rapid voluntary shortening in the human extensor digitorum brevis (Grimby & Hannerz, 1977). EMG patterns recorded from the heterogeneous, but largely fast twitch, lateral gastrocnemius and the slow, red soleus in the cat show that though the former is intensely activated during the rapid alternating movements in the paw shake reflex, the soleus participation is suppressed (Smith, Betts, Edgerton, & Zernicke, 1980). Such major shifts in recruitment patterns, even under specialized conditions, indicate that the organization of synaptic inputs to motoneurons must also play a role in controlling recruitment sequences (Burke, 1973, 1981; Kanda et al., 1977). Some synaptic input systems must be differentially distributed to motoneuron pools so as to reorder the sequence of functional thresholds under particular conditions.

One such system has been demonstrated experimentally in the cat lumbosacral spinal cord. Electrical stimulation of low threshold afferents in the sural nerve produces polysynaptic (minimum trisynaptic) excitation in medial gastrocnemius motoneurons that innervate fast twitch muscle units. The short latency, polysynaptic EPSPs in slow twitch motoneurons are generally much smaller than in the cells that innervate fast twitch muscle units and are, in fact, undetectable in many slow motoneurons (Burke, Jankowska, & Bruggencate, 1970; Burke, Rymer, & Walsh, 1973). Transmission in this excitatory pathway is facilitated by the rubrospinal and corticospinal tracts (Pinter, Burke,

O'Donovan, & Dum, 1982), implying that descending motor command systems have access to the same interneuronal pathway. With this organization, both supraspinal and reflex systems could, in principle, produce preferential excitation of fast twitch motor units.

The organization of this cutaneous pathway in the cat has certain features that suggest a useful degree of functional flexibility. In the diagram in Figure 1, when the motoneurons A through D are excited by the left pathway, one might expect a gradation of function threshold rising for A to D (upper recruitment pattern). Excitation coming exclusively from the right hand pathway, organized in a reverse sequence of synaptic efficacy, would presumably produce the reverse pattern of recruitment. However, input from both pathways, especially if excitatory and inhibitory effects were admixed, might produce complex recruitment sequences, such as shown in the lower recruitment pattern. One may also envision that pure excitation arriving over both pathways would generate simultaneous activation of all the motoneurons.

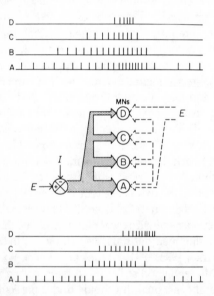

Figure 1. Alternative synaptic organizations (central diagram) that may explain different patterns of motor unit recruitment. The thickness of the arrows denotes synaptic efficacy in four motoneurons (MNs; circles labeled A through D). Many excitatory (E) and inhibitory (I) input systems are organized to produce parallel grades of synaptic efficacy, as denoted by the shaded arrows on the left. Activation of the motoneurons by these pathways would produce recruitment sequences such as shown in the upper diagram. The addition of an excitatory input with the reverse gradation of efficacy (dashed arrows on the right) would generate more complex recruitment patterns, including preferential activity among normally high threshold cells such as shown in the lower recruitment diagram (see text for further discussion). Figure reproduced from Kanda, Burke and Walmsley, 1977.

Thus, the addition of a pathway with a pattern of distribution different from that of all other input pathways can confer a measure of flexibility in motor unit usage. This does not imply chaos but simply that alternative recruitment sequences are available to the CNS.

Such flexibility appears to be used in actual movement. "Ballistic" contractions, as studied, for example, by Desmedt and Godaux (1977, 1978), are produced by more or less synchronous activation of large fractions of the motor unit pool. To achieve such simultaneity with a single pattern of input organization would presumably require an inordinate amount of "surplus excitation" in the lowest threshold units. It would seem both more economical and more effective to use a dual input organization, such as that suggested in Figure 1. The results of Stephens and coworkers (Stephens, Garnett, & Buller, 1978; Garnett & Stephens, 1981; Datta & Stephens, 1981) suggest that alternative input organizations such as those shown in Figure 1 may exist in man. These investigators have shown that electrical stimulation of the finger-tip can dramatically alter the sequence of functional thresholds among motor units in the first dorsal interosseous muscle and thus produce large reversals among units of originally high versus low functional threshold. When fully developed, there was preferential voluntary recruitment of high threshold motor units. At intermediate levels of effect, there was simply a narrowing of the range of functional thresholds.

One may question whether there are functional advantages in preferential recruitment of usually high threshold units under some conditions. Recent studies of the paw shake reflex in cats are of interest on this point. The paw shake involves very rapid (up to 10 Hz) alternate flexions and extensions of the hindfoot when stimulated by a mild irritant, such as water or tape (Smith et al., 1980). The rapid movement is designed to shake off the irritant. As noted above, the slow twitch soleus muscle often exhibits minimal participation in this reflex, even though it is usually fully activated over a wide range of other hindlimb actions (Walmsley, Hodgson, & Burke, 1978). Spector, Gardiner, Zernicke, Roy, and Edgerton (1980) have argued that the slow contraction and particularly the slow relaxation of the cat soleus would be mechanically disadvantageous in a movement that requires maximally rapid alternating movements of a limb in order to be effective.

Adaptability

The neuromuscular apparatus of the limb must be effective over a very wide dynamic range. It therefore seems logical to consider the option that alternative neural control organizations exist to subserve different regions within this range. These considerations are of obvious importance to understanding the basis of athletic performance, which often entails usage of the motor system well beyond the range encountered in everyday life. The ability to perform at the limit of physical capacity is the essence of competitive sport. This must involve training not only the muscles, which are marvelously adaptable, but also the nervous system, which is no less so. Optimum usage of muscles may well require strategies of usage for which the "usual" sequence of recruitment is poorly adapted.

The slow to fast, small force to large force, fatigue resistant to fatigable sequence that is the usual rule appears to be optimized for minimizing the energy cost of motor activities within the normal range of an animal's activities. This cost must reflect not only the energy consumed during activity but also that required to maintain muscle while inactive. It seems likely that the maintenance cost of glycolytic, fatigable muscle units is much lower than that of fibers more heavily dependent on oxidative systems. For example, there is evidence that the resting blood flow in red muscles is higher than that in white, whereas the increase with exercise is much more dramatic in white (Laughlin & Armstrong, 1982).

The Design of Motor Unit Populations

The existing data about the organization of motor unit populations is most extensive for those present in the hindlimb of the domestic cat. For example, about half of the motor unit population in the medial gastrocnemius (MG) of this sedentary predator is made up of large force but highly fatigable type FF motor units, which have muscle units that are highly dependent on glycolytic enzyme systems and have little aerobic capacity (Burke, Levine, Tsairis, & Zajac, 1973). The fibers of FF muscle units, based on estimates of fiber number and average area, make up about 72% of the MG volume (Burke, 1981) and produce, in aggregate, about 80% of the maximum tetanic force that the fully tetanized MG can generate (Walmsley et al., 1978). The slow twitch, fatigue resistant type S units, which comprise about 25% of the MG pool, make up about 14% of MG volume because of their small fiber size but produce, in aggregate, only about 5% of MG tetanic force. The remaining 25% of the MG motor unit population consists of type FR motor units, which are fast contracting, fatigue resistant, and produce moderate force outputs. In aggregate, they also make up about 14% of MG volume and produce, in aggregate, about 15% of MG tetanic force.

Why does the cat carry around over two-thirds of its MG muscle volume in type FF muscle units that can deliver only a few thousand contractions before losing their ability to contract? The answer lies perhaps in a trade-off between the mechanical demands placed on the muscle by the most frequent motor behaviors and the metabolic cost of different types of muscle units, evaluated at rest as well as when active.

The MG muscle of the cat needs to generate only about 20% of its peak theoretical force output to subserve the full range of normal postural and loco-motor activities, from quiet standing to fast running. Only galloping and jumping require recruitment into the force range that must involve activation of significant numbers of type FF muscle units (Walmsley et al., 1978). Although the life-style of the domestic cat does involve galloping and jumping, these actions tend to occur only in short and intermittent bursts. The same is true of its larger relative, the lion, which exhibits a rather extreme degree of glycolytic dependence (Armstrong, Marum, Saubert, Seeherman, & Taylor, 1977). The cat MG appears to be designed to provide all of the force required for "usual" activities from fatigue resistant muscle units that have high capacity for oxida-tive metabolism. As noted above, it seems likely that such muscle units require significant energy expenditure while inactive as well as active. On the other hand, the large bulk of glycolytic fibers probably incurs a small metabolic cost, on a volume basis, when inactive and is therefore economical to maintain in reserve for short bursts of intense activity.

The striped skunk provides an interesting contrast to the cat. The MG and other locomotor muscles of this animal contain no type IIB fibers (the fiber type associated with FF units) and no motor units with the fatigability of type FF (Van de Graaf, Frederick, Williamson, & Goslow, 1977). Rather, they are made up exclusively of fatigue resistant fast (type FR) and slow (type S) twitch motor units. The life-style of the skunk, a scavenger, involves foraging for food over extensive territories. The animal thus requires endurance but has no need to run or jump to escape from predators or to obtain food. As is the case with the cat, the skunk's MG appears well suited to the motor demands imposed by its life-style, although one may infer that the maintenance cost of its muscles may be higher than that of the cat.

A Synthesis

The available evidence suggests that the design of motor unit populations and the usual ordering of motor unit recruitment are well suited to the de-mands placed on the motor system by the normal, predictable modes of a given animal's existence. The motor apparatus appears to be optimized not only for mechanical action but also for minimizing total metabolic cost, including the cost of maintenance. Both goals have survival value and probably shape the motor unit composition found in different muscles or in disparate species of animals (e.g., see Burke, 1981). It seems likely that recruitment patterns that fit the size principle predictions also fit the functional demands placed by the normal and predictable dynamic range that operates most of the time. However, most of the time is not all the time.

Because life for most animals, including man, is not always normal or predictable, it seems likely that certain demands for mechanical action may require patterns of motor unit activity that are inconsistent with minimal metabolic cost. Examples could include the rapid paw shaking reflex in the cat or rapid, forceful throwing movements in a human athlete. In such actions, metabolic economy is presumably sacrificed in favor of mechanical performance. Obviously, such actions occur only intermittently, but they are nevertheless within the dynamic range that the motor system must accommodate. The existence of "alternative" or "reversed" patterns of motor unit recruitment suggests that the mammalian central nervous system is equipped to deal with such demands. A search in this direction may well increase our understanding of athletic performance.

References

Adrian, E.D., & Bronk, D.W. (1929). The discharge of impulses in motor nerve fibers, Part II. The frequency of discharge in reflex and voluntary contractions. *Journal of Physiology* (London), **67**, 119-151.

Armstrong, R.B., Marum, P., Saubert, C.W., Seeherman, H.J., & Taylor, C.R. (1977). Muscle fiber activity as a function of speed and gait. *Journal of Applied Physiology: Respiratory, Environmental and Exercise Physiology*, **43**, 672-677.

Buchthal, F., & Schmalbruch, H. (1980). Motor unit of mammalian muscle. *Physiological Reviews*, **60**, 90-142.

Burke, R.E. (1973). On the central nervous system control of fast and slow twitch motor units. In J.E. Desmedt (Ed.), *New developments in electromyography and clinical neurophysiology* (pp. 69-94). Basel: Karger.

Burke, R.E. (1981). Motor units: Anatomy, physiology and functional organization. In V.B. Brooks (Ed.), *Handbook of physiology: Sec. 1. The nervous system: Vol. 3. Motor systems* (pp. 345-422). Bethesda, MD: American Physiological Society.

Burke, R.E., Jankowska, E., & Bruggencate, G. (1970). A comparison of peripheral and rubrospinal synaptic input to slow and fast twitch motor units of triceps surae. *Journal of Physiology* (London), **207**, 709-732.

Burke, R.E., Levine, D.N., Tsairis, P., & Zajac, F.E. (1973). Physiological types of histochemical profiles in motor units of the cat gastrocnemius. *Journal of Physiology* (London), **234**, 723-748.

Burke, R.E., Rymer, W.Z., & Walsh, J.V. (1973). Functional specialization in the motor unit population of cat medial gastrocnemius muscle. In R.B. Stein, K.B. Pearson, R.S. Smith, & J.B. Redford (Eds.), *Control of posture and locomotion* (pp. 29-44). New York: Plenum.

Clamann, H.P., & Henneman, E. (1976). Electrical measurement of axon diameter and its use in relating motoneuron size to critical firing level. *Journal of Neurophysiology*, **39**, 844-851.

Datta, A.K., & Stephens, J.A. (1981). The effects of digital nerve stimulation on the firing of motor units in human first dorsal interosseous muscle. *Journal of Physiology* (London), **318**, 501-510.

Denny-Brown, D. (1929). On the nature of postural reflexes. *Proceedings of the Royal Society of London, Series B,* **104**, 252-301.

Denny-Brown, D. (1949). Interpretation of the electromyogram. *Archives of Neurology and Psychiatry,* **61**, 99-128.

Denny-Brown, D., & Pennybacker, J.B. (1938). Fibrillation and fasciculation in voluntary muscle. *Brain,* **61**, 311-344.

Desmedt, J.E., & Godaux, E. (1977). Ballistic contractions in man: Characteristic recruitment pattern of single motor units of the tibialis anterior muscle. *Journal of Physiology* (London), **264**, 673-694.

Desmedt, J.E., & Godaux, E. (1978). Ballistic contractions in fast or slow human muscles: Discharge patterns of single motor units. *Journal of Physiology* (London), **285**, 185-196.

Eccles, J.C., & Sherrington, C.S. (1930). Numbers and contraction values of individual motor units examined in some muscles of the limb. *Proceedings of the Royal Society of London, Series, B,* **106**, 326-357.

Garnett, R., & Stephens, J.A. (1981). Changes in the recruitment threshold of motor units produced by cutaneous stimulation in man. *Journal of Physiology* (London), **311**, 463-473.

Grimby, L., & Hannerz, J. (1977). Firing rate and recruitment order of toe extensor motor units in different modes of voluntary contraction. *Journal of Physiology* (London), **264**, 865-879.

Henneman, E., & Mendell, L.M. (1981). Functional organization of motoneuron pool and its inputs. In V.B. Brooks (Ed.), *Handbook of physiology: Sec. 2. The nervous system: Vol. 2. Motor control. Part 2* (pp. 423-507). Bethesda, MD: American Physiological Society.

Henneman, E., & Olson, C.B. (1965). Relations between structure and function in the design of skeletal muscles. *Journal of Neurophysiology,* **28**, 581-598.

Henneman, E., Somjen, G., & Carpenter, D.O. (1965a). Functional significance of cell size in spinal motoneurons. *Journal of Neurophysiology,* **28**, 560-580.

Henneman, E., Somjen, G., & Carpenter, D.O. (1965b). Excitability and inhibitability of motoneurons of different sizes. *Journal of Neurophysiology,* **28**, 599-620.

Kanda, K., Burke, R.E., & Walmsley, B. (1977). Differential control of fast and slow twitch motor units in the decerebrate cat. *Experimental Brain Research,* **29**, 57-74.

Laughlin, M.H., & Armstrong, R.B. (1982). Muscular blood flow distribution patterns as a function of running speed in rats. *American Journal of Physiology,* **243**, H296-H306.

Liddell, E.G.T., & Sherrington, C.S. (1925). Recruitment and some other factors of reflex inhibition. *Proceedings of the Royal Society of London, Series B,* **97**, 488-518.

Loeb, G.E. (1984). The control and responses of mammalian muscle spindles during normally executed motor tasks. *Exercise and Sport Sciences Review*, **12**, 157-204.

McPhedran, A.M., Wuerker, R.B., & Henneman, E. (1965). Properties of motor units in a homogeneous red muscle (soleus) of the cat. *Journal of Neurophysiology*, **28**, 71-84.

Pinter, M.J., Burke, R.E., O'Donovan, M.J., & Dum, R.P. (1982). Supraspinal facilitation of cutaneous polysynaptic EPSPs in cat medial gastrocnemius motoneurons. *Experimental Brain Research*, **45**, 133-143.

Smith, J.L., Betts, B., Edgerton, V.R., & Zernicke, R.F. (1980). Rapid ankle extension during paw shakes: Selective recruitment of fast ankle extensors. *Journal of Neurophysiology*, **43**, 612-620.

Spector, S.A., Gardiner, P.F., Zernicke, R.F., Roy, R.R., & Edgerton, V.R. (1980). Muscle architecture and force-velocity characteristics of cat soleus and medial gastrocnemius: Implications for motor control. *Journal of Neurophysiology*, **44**, 951-960.

Stephens, J.A., Garnett, R., & Buller, N.P. (1978). Reversal of recruitment order of single motor units produced by cutaneous stimulation during voluntary muscle contraction in man. *Nature*, **272**, 362-364.

Van de Graaff, K.M., Frederick, E.C., Williamson, R.G., & Goslow, G.E., Jr. (1977). Motor units and fiber types of primary ankle extensors of the skunk *(mephitis mephitis)*. *Journal of Neurophysiology*, **40**, 1424-1431.

Walmsley, B., Hodgson, J.A., & Burke, R.E. (1978). Forces produced by medial gastrocnemius and soleus during locomotion in freely moving cats. *Journal of Neurophysiology*, **41**, 1203-1216.

Wuerker, R.B., McPhedran, A.M., & Henneman, E. (1965). Properties of motor units in a heterogeneous pale muscle (M. gastrocnemius) of the cat. *Journal of Neurophysiology*, **28**, 85-99.

Discussion

Dr. McComas opened the discussion by considering the relevance of Dr. Burke's animal studies to humans. So far as human motor units were concerned, there was good evidence that twitch speeds varied considerably. In the extensor digitorum brevis muscle, Sica and McComas (1971) had found the motor unit contraction times to range from 35 to 96 ms, and similar values had been reported subsequently by others using different muscles. The work of Milner-Brown, Stein, and Yemm (1973) was of particular importance in demonstrating orderly recruitment of progressively larger motor units in the first dorsal interosseus muscle as the force of voluntary abduction of the index finger was increased. However, the correlation between contraction time and twitch tension was not as high as in animal studies. Information was also available concerning different synaptic inputs to human motor neurons. Caccia, McComas, Upton, and Blogg (1973) have shown that some motor neurons innervating the intrinsic muscles of the hand were very sensitive to mechanical stimulation of the fingertip or to weak electrical stimulation of the digital nerve fibers. In an extension of this work, Garnett and Stephens (1981) found that digital nerve stimulation could alter the thresholds of motor units to voluntary activation so that the larger fast twitch units were recruited early. In considering the question of efficacy of synaptic input to motor neurons, the function of the muscle had to be taken into account. Thus, those motor neurons which supply muscles participating in the flexor withdrawal response would be expected to receive a powerful input from the skin; a good example of this was the innervation to the posterior part of the human deltoid muscle (McComas & Robinson, 1983).

Dr. Stein enquired how the recruitment model presented by Dr. Burke would be affected by the modulation of individual unit forces through impulse rate-coding. Dr. Burke explained that this factor had for simplicity been ignored as part of the assumptions in the model; also the model assumed that all type S units in the available motor pool were recruited before type FR, and that all FR units were recruited before any type FF. He noted that both assumptions were clearly oversimplifications, but that both had sufficient basis in experimental evidence as to provide useful results. However, Dr. Burke also noted that rapid ballistic movements involved more or less synchronous activation of large numbers of motor units, probably including all of the available types in the muscle, and that the "recruitment model" under discussion represented only a caricature of the situation in slower graded contractions. He mentioned that the paw shaking reflex in cats, studied particularly by Judith Smith, Betts, Edgerton, and Zernicke (1980), was an interesting example of the possible reversal of functional thresholds in which the slow twitch soleus muscle exhibits less recruitment during rapid alternating shakes than does the "faster" lateral gastrocnemius, even though the reverse is true in standing or walking. The reason for this observation could be that the slowly contracting and slowly relaxing soleus may be mechanically disadvantageous during rapid alternating shaking movements.

Dr. Edgerton asked if there were situations in which the soleus was unloaded even though an EMG signal was obtained, thus indicating dissociation between the EMG and force production. In his laboratory this had been seen often in movements in which both muscles contributed; because the gastrocnemius was fast contracting, it unloaded the soleus. Dr. Burke tended to discount the notion of unloading because in the locomotion and postural activity studied in his own laboratory, the ankle extensor soleus and gastrocnemii are active mainly during eccentric lengthening, when they act as stiff springs and generate considerable tendon force. Both muscles participate through a wide range of postural and locomotor actions, with the soleus usually fully activated, whereas the gastrocnemius showed much wider modulation of peak force output that depended on locomotion speed. He noted that tendon force records are difficult to interpret when muscle contractions are unopposed, such as when the limb is in the air, unless accurate length records are also available.

Dr. Stein felt that there were good arguments for the reverse order of recruitment in rapidly alternating movements, but he did not see the need for this in ballistic movements per se. Even if all motor units were recruited together temporally, there were still advantages in recruiting the soleus before the gastrocnemius because of the different contraction times; this order of recruitment would lead to all units reaching their peak force at the same time, as shown by Desmedt and Godaux (1977).

Dr. Burke emphasized the importance of eccentric contractions in ballistic movements, particularly in jumping. Force traces obtained from the soleus and medial gastrocnemius during locomotion could usually be superimposed. In some recordings the soleus appeared to peak before the gastrocnemius. The reason for this was that contraction was occurring during a time that the muscle was being stretched and the recorder was really measuring stiffness of the muscle rather than the isometric contraction. Similarly in jumping, the cat always lengthens the muscle first. Dr. Burke felt further that the concept of a dichotomy between "tonic" or "postural" muscles versus "phasic" muscles was misleading; the soleus, for example, acts throughout the whole range of movement, except perhaps in very rapidly alternating movements.

Dr. Bigland-Ritchie wondered whether it was appropriate to compare the activities of two such dissimilar muscles as the soleus and gastrocnemius. Perhaps the same factors needed to be taken into account in comparing slow and fast twitch units within a single muscle, such as the gastrocnemius. Dr. Bigland-Ritchie asked if Dr. Burke would extend his speculation regarding the recruitment pattern that occurred in a coordinated movement as being one functional entity. Dr. Burke replied that studies were only just beginning to look at this topic. However, in many movements contributions from the synergistic muscles might be viewed as the output from one vast motor unit pool. There are also some muscles with several distinct motor unit pools that can act more or less independently. An example of this is the cat sartorius, in which different parts of the muscle are active at different phases of the step cycle.

Dr. Green referred to Dr. Burke's graph of the percentage of tetanic force achieved by different motor units and the hierarchy he had established related to the twitch characteristics. This suggested that the oxidative potential of a muscle would also be a good indicator of the recruitment patterns. Dr. Burke considered that this was another valid way to look at the scheme, but he pointed out that the interrelationships between the various observations that had been made on motor units with different characteristics showed a linkage throughout the system extending from the motor axon through to the mitochondrion. All these characteristics were very tightly coupled.

References

Caccia, M.R., McComas, A.J., Upton, A.R.M., & Blogg, T. (1973). Cutaneous reflexes in small muscles of the hand. *Journal of Neurology, Neurosurgery and Psychiatry*, **36**, 960-977.

Desmedt, J.E., & Godaux, E. (1977). Ballistic contractions in man: Characteristic recruitment pattern of single motor units of the tibialis anterior muscle. *Journal of Physiology* (London), **264**, 673-694.

Garnett, R., & Stephens, J.A. (1981). Changes in the recruitment threshold of motor units produced by cutaneous stimulation in man. *Journal of Physiology* (London), **311**, 463-473.

McComas, A.J., & Robinson, K.R. (1983). Identification of a low-threshold cutaneous reflex in the human arm. *Journal of Physiology* (London), **343**, 111 P.

Milner-Brown, H.S., Stein, R.B., & Yemm, R. (1973). The orderly recruitment of human motor units during voluntary isometric contractions. *Journal of Physiology* (London), **230**, 359-370.

Sica, R.E.P., & McComas, A.J. (1971). Fast and slow twitch units in a human muscle. *Journal of Neurology, Neurosurgery and Psychiatry*, **34**, 113-120.

Smith, J.L., Betts, B., Edgerton, V.R., & Zernicke, R.F. (1980). Rapid ankle extension during paw shakes: Selective recruitment of fast ankle extensors. *Journal of Neurophysiology*, **43**, 612-620.

8

Single Motor Unit Discharge During Voluntary Contraction and Locomotion

Lennart Grimby
Karolinska Hospital

T he aim of the studies presented here is to determine the use of the main motor unit in normal activities of man. Our knowledge about its uses has been limited by technical difficulties. Electromyographic studies have been performed mainly under isometric conditions (Freund, 1983), although movements are far more important in normal daily activities. Glycogen depletion studies have a limited value because only prolonged motor functions can be studied and because the resistance of the fibre types differs greatly (Kugelberg & Edstrom, 1968). Microneurographic techniques also pose a problem; they are simply too difficult to apply to man (Freyschuss & Knutsson, 1971).

In conformance with the symposium's title the presentation below will concentrate on maximal voluntary performance. Special attention will also be paid to locomotion because the use of a motor unit during locomotion plays a major role in its long-term use and thus also for its contractile properties (Salmons & Henriksson, 1981).

Methods

Electromyographic (EMG) techniques were used to study single motor units in the extensor digitorum brevis (EDB) and tibialis anterior (TA) muscles. Sufficient selectivity for identification of single motor unit potentials during sustained isometric maximal contraction was achieved by means of microelectrodes (Hannerz, 1974a; Bigland-Ritchie, Johansson, Lippold, Smith, & Woods, 1983). However, the more selective a recording was, the more sensitive was the electrode to being dislocated; the latter was unavoidable when shortening muscle fibres were studied. Thus, single motor unit recordings during movements were possible only under certain conditions.

Technique I.

In the lower leg muscles, clusters of muscle fibres innervated by one motoneurone were found in some normal subjects, particularly athletes. The clusters may be the result of denervation-reinnervation processes that occur in normal muscles (Stalberg & Trontelj, 1979).

When a recording electrode made up of two 20-100 μm wires was inserted into such a cluster and retained by means of a hook, recordings of the single motor unit could be achieved even during movements. However, clusters of a sufficient number of fibres were scarce in the normal EDB and TA, and only a few motor units could be studied in each subject (Hannerz, 1974a; Grimby, 1984).

Technique II.

A representative number of low as well as high threshold motor units could be measured in the EDB in three members of the research group who had taken part earlier in several electromyographic studies requiring the use of needle electrodes. The latter had caused repeated lesions to the terminal nerve twigs and muscle fibres; consequently, collateral sprouting and an increase in muscle fibre density within the units took place (Grimby & Hannerz, 1976).

Technique III.

Fifteen subjects with an accessory innervation of just a few motor units in the EDB were studied (Lambert, 1969). These units could easily be studied during lidocaine blocking of the main innervation (Marsden, Meadows, & Merton, 1971; Borg, Grimby, & Hannerz, 1977).

Locomotion was studied by using a small pre-amplifier that was strapped to the leg and connected to the main amplifier with a cable that permitted 40 m of movement (Grimby, 1984). Methodological details are given in the legends and the original papers cited above.

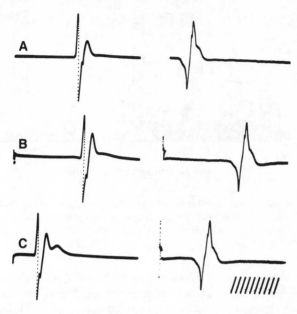

Figure 1. Calculation of axonal conduction velocity of single extensor digitorum brevis motor units. Left and right columns are two different experiments from the same muscle. (A) the only spike potential recorded during maximal voluntary effort, (B) distal, and (C) proximal, peroneal nerve stimulation. Time divisions were 1 ms. The latency differences B–C in the two experiments were 10 ms and 7.5 ms, respectively. The distance between distal and proximal stimulation points was 38 cm. The axonal conduction velocities were 38 m/s and 51 m/s, respectively. Reprinted from Borg, Grimby, and Hannerz 1978, with permission.

Results

Axonal Conduction Velocity

Axonal conduction velocities were calculated for 135 EDB units (Borg et al., 1977) using Techniques II and III. The calculations were based on the latency differences between the single motor unit potentials evoked by proximal and distal peroneal nerve stimulation, as illustrated in Figure 1.

Figure 2 shows that the conduction velocities ranged between 30 and 58 m/s. There was a unimodal distribution, and about half of the units had conduction velocities between 40 and 45 m/s. There was no significant difference between units studied after reinnervation (Technique II) and those examined after blocking the main innervation (Technique III).

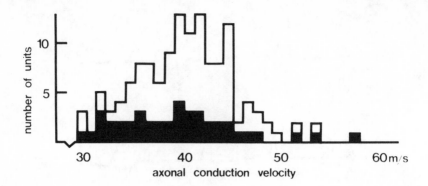

Figure 2. Axonal conduction velocities of 135 single extensor digitorum hallucis brevis motor units calculated as illustrated in Figure 1. Open squares denote reinnervated units (Technique II), filled squares denote accessorily innervated units (Technique III).

During slow voluntary increase of tension under isometric conditions, single motor units were recruited between 0% and 80% of maximal tension (defined as the tension evoked by supramaximal tetanization). However, such a broad range of threshold tensions probably does not exist in all muscles. In the small hand muscles the role of recruitment was mainly confined to the generation of force at low levels of voluntary contraction (Milner-Brown, Stein, & Yemm, 1973). The threshold tensions of low threshold units remained stable or decreased on prolonged contraction in parallel with the decrease of maximal tension. The threshold tensions of high threshold units, on the other hand, increased relative to the maximal tension and sometimes also in absolute terms during prolonged contraction (Figure 3).

There was a close relationship between the recruitment thresholds and axonal conduction velocities as implied by the "size principle" (see Figure 4)

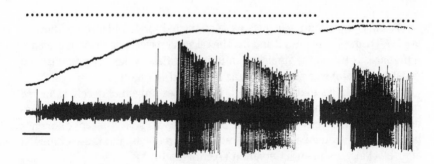

Figure 3. Threshold tension of a high threshold unit from the extensor hallucis brevis at recruitment (left) and upon prolonged contraction (right). The dotted lines denote the tension evoked by supramaximal electrical tetanization at rest (left) and immediately after the prolonged voluntary contraction (right). Time bar=1 s.

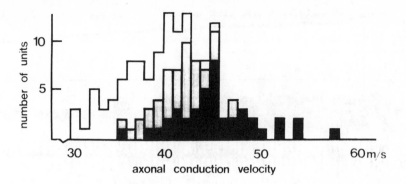

Figure 4.   The relationship between axonal conduction velocities and thresholds of 135 single extensor digitorum hallucis brevis motor units. Filled squares denote motor units with such high thresholds that they mainly operate phasically in ordinarily motivated and untrained subjects. Open squares denote motor units with such low thresholds that they could be driven tonically for apparently unlimited periods of time. Hatched squares denote intermediate motor units.

(Henneman, Somjen, & Carpenter, 1965a, 1965b). Units with such high thresholds that they could not be driven continuously had axonal conduction velocities between 40 and 55 m/s. Units that could be driven for apparently unlimited periods of time had conduction velocities between 30 and 45 m/s. The overlapping between high and low threshold units was less for individual subjects than for the whole group.

Maximal Voluntary Tension

The firing properties during maximal voluntary effort were studied under isometric conditions in 100 EDB and TA units with Techniques I, II, or III (Hannerz, 1974b: Grimby, Hannerz, & Hedman, 1981).

Maximal tension was obtained by supramaximal electrical stimulation of the peroneal nerve at 50 Hz because the units with the shortest contraction times did not fuse completely at lower rates. During fatigue the stimulation rate required for maximal tension decreased because of prolongation of the relaxation times; the rate tolerated by the peripheral electrical propagation decreased in parallel so that the stimulation rate had to be carefully adjusted to maintain maximal tension (Bigland-Ritchie, Jones, & Woods, 1979).

Maximal voluntary tension could be maintained for a few seconds without difficulty. The motor units with the highest thresholds then fired at 50-60 Hz, whereas the ones with lower thresholds, longer contraction times, and lower fusion rates fired at only 30-50 Hz. During prolonged maximal effort the firing rates decreased progressively. In ordinarily motivated and untrained subjects, the voluntary firing rates decreased more rapidly than the rates required for full excitation of the contractile mechanisms (i.e., there was "cen-

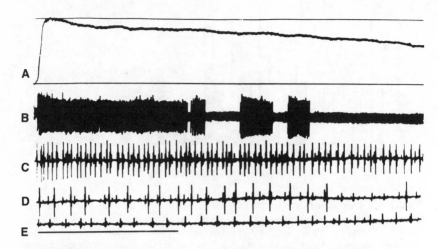

Figure 5.   Firing properties of one high threshold unit (large amplitude potential) and one low threshold unit (small potential) from the extensor hallucis brevis during prolonged maximal voluntary effort. (A) toe dorsiflexion tension (lower and upper thin lines denote 0% and 100% tension, respectively). (B) EMG at the same film speed as the tension curve. (C) EMG at maximal tension at fast film speed. (D) EMG after about 10 s. (E) EMG after about 25 s at fast film speed. Time bar: A–B=10 s; C–F=0, 5 s. Reprinted from Grimby, Hannerz, Borg, & Hedman, 1981, with permission.

tral" fatigue). Ordinary subjects did not drive their units with the highest thresholds for more than a few seconds, even though they claimed to have done their utmost and appeared very exhausted. Low threshold units, on the other hand, continued tonic firing at 20-10 Hz for apparently unlimited periods of time (see Figure 5).

Central fatigue could, however, be overcome by extraordinary motivation and training (Merton, 1964). Highly motivated and trained subjects could drive high threshold units tonically for up to a minute. The safety margin between the voluntary firing intervals and the shortest intervals tolerated by the peripheral electrical propagation was usually broad. Only in high threshold units driven continuously for extraordinarily long periods of time did the shortest tolerated intervals approach the voluntary ones so that blocking occurred (Borg, Grimby, & Hannerz, 1983).

Ballistic Voluntary Movements

Ballistic voluntary movements were studied in 35 units using Techniques II and III (Grimby & Hannerz, 1977). High threshold units fired at higher rates and with the appearance of less effort than during prolonged tension. They might attain discharge intervals corresponding to 100 Hz in twitches evoked with very little effort (see Figure 6A), whereas during prolonged maximal contraction they fired at no more than 30 Hz (see Figure 6B). Figure 7 compares

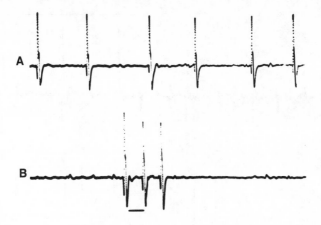

Figure 6. Firing of a high threshold unit from the extensor digitorum brevis during prolonged maximal voluntary effort (A) and a tiny voluntary twitch (B). Time bar = 10 ms.

the simultaneous recording of high and low threshold units during both movement and prolonged tension. It can be seen that during voluntary movement the high threshold unit played a much greater role than during prolonged tension. Upon acceleration, firing rates increased more rapidly in the high threshold unit than in the low threshold unit. This higher "gain" of high threshold units was most significant after a period of rest.

When the subject was instructed to dorsiflex toes and foot with maximal rapidity under isotonic conditions, high threshold units attained 100 Hz (see Figure 8), but their firing intervals were irregular and there was a tendency for a short interval to be followed by a relatively long one. Even the potentials of reinnervated units, consisting of many components, behaved in an all-or-none manner; thus, the irregularity of the interdischarge intervals was not due to failure of peripheral electrical propagation. The units with lower thresholds fired at 60-80 Hz and with greater regularity. The high frequency discharge lasted for about 200 ms, and there was a pause separating the discharge into two bursts of about 100 ms each. The pause is compatible with the three phase organization of ballistic contractions, agonist - antagonist - agonist (Hallett, Shahani, & Young, 1975).

It was possible to wave the toes at regular rates up to 3-4 Hz. At such high rates, the single units fired in short high frequency bursts of 2-5 discharges with interdischarge intervals of 10-50 ms. When one high and one low threshold unit were recorded simultaneously, it was found that in almost all bursts both units fired as illustrated in Figure 9B. Occasionally the low threshold unit might fire once or twice without the high threshold unit firing. In the average burst, however, the number of discharges of high and low threshold units were similar. The differences in threshold were compensated by differences in gain (cf. above). When the rate of toe waving decreased to below 2 Hz, the low

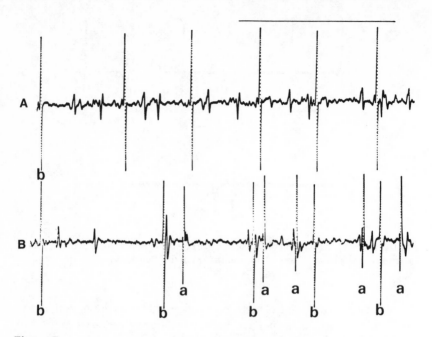

Figure 7. Firing of one high threshold unit from the extensor hallucis brevis (marked a) and one low threshold unit from the same muscle (marked b) during prolonged maximal isometric contraction (A) and during a voluntary movement (B). Time bar = 100 ms.

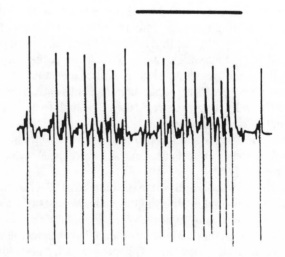

Figure 8. Firing of a high threshold unit from the extensor digitorum brevis during a maximal ballistic voluntary movement. Time bar = 100 ms. (Adapted with permission from Grimby, Hannerz, & Hedman, 1980.)

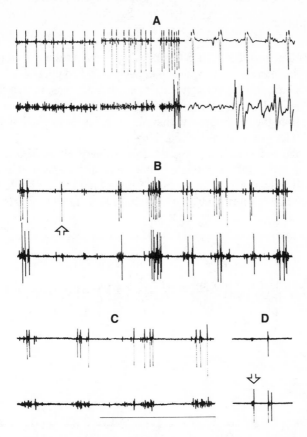

Figure 9. Firing of one low threshold unit from the extensor hallucis brevis (upper trace) and one high threshold unit from the same muscle (lower trace) recorded simultaneously. (A) slowly increasing isometric voluntary contraction (on the right recruitment of the high threshold unit at 10 times faster film speed). The low threshold unit is used selectively within a large tension range. (B) alternating voluntary movements at 3-4 Hz. The low threshold units fire selectively (↑) when the voluntary drive is so weak that none of the units respond in the next burst. (C) alternating voluntary movements at 2 Hz. The low threshold unit is used selectively. (D) attempt of alternating voluntary movement at 6 Hz. Only the high threshold unit fires occasionally (↓). Time bar = 100 ms.

threshold unit was selectively used when the amplitude of the movement was small (see Figure 9C). The high threshold unit was only recruited when the amplitude was high. When the contractions were repeated as rapidly as possible, the high threshold unit might fire selectively (see Figure 9D). Unfortunately, extremely rapid toe waving could not be studied systematically because the subjects had to make many attempts to achieve more than 4 Hz even temporarily; also, the recording electrodes were dislocated during prolonged experiments. A systematic correlation between recruitment and rate of cyclic movements is, however, demonstrable in the cat as discussed below.

Locomotion

Locomotion was studied in 50 units using Techniques II and III (Grimby, 1984). The single motor units were successively recruited upon slowly increasing the walking speed in the same order as voluntary tension was slowly increased; that is, the motor units with low axonal conduction velocities were recruited before the motor units with high velocities, as implied by the "size principle" (Henneman et al., 1965a, 1965b).

When allowed to *walk at free speed*, most subjects chose 55-60 cycles per minute. The use of different single motor units at this speed of locomotion is illustrated in Figure 10. Low threshold units fired in each stride for most of the cycle and with relatively long mean interdischarge intervals (see Figure

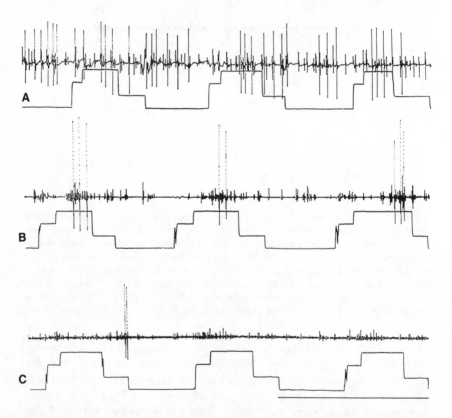

Figure 10.   Firing properties during ordinary walking (50 cycles/min) of one low threshold unit, (A) one intermediate threshold unit, (B) and one high threshold unit, (C) from the extensor digitorum brevis. The lower recordings in A, B and C show signals from foot-switches. Upward deflexions indicate pressure on the sole of the tested foot. The small amplitude indicates pressure only on the anterior part of the sole. Intermediate amplitude indicates pressure only on the heel. High amplitude indicates pressure on both of these sites. Time bar=1s.

10A). Intermediate threshold units fired also in each stride but only during the peak activation and with relatively short interdischarge intervals (see Figure 10B). Finally, high threshold units did not participate in the ordinary cycle but fired when the speed or direction of locomotion was changed, when obstacles were to be avoided, or when the subject stumbled. They then fired in high frequency bursts of 2-5 discharges with short interdischarge intervals (10-25 ms). These findings agree with observations made in the cat during treadmill locomotion (Hoffer, O'Donovan, Pratt, & Loeb, 1981) and in the freely moving rat (Henning & Lomo, 1982).

The corrective movements could appear during any part of the cycle and not just during the peak activation of the ordinary stride. They were seldom noted during a straight 40 m walk on a smooth laboratory floor but were frequently seen during a walk in the hospital park.

During *running* the proportion of motor units active in each stride was greater than in walking, and the proportion of units active only in corrective movements was correspondingly smaller. Certain high threshold units were recruited during each stride when the speed of locomotion was increased (see Figure 11A). Other high threshold units appeared to have only corrective roles

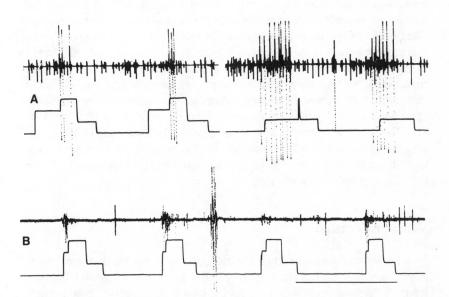

Figure 11. Firing properties during rapid locomotion of two high threshold units from the extensor digitorum brevis (A and B). The lower recordings show signals from foot-switches as in Figure 10. The unit in A fired a few times per step cycle during walking at 75 cycles/min and several times per cycle when the subject was running at 80 cycles/min. The unit in B, on the other hand, did not participate in the ordinary cycle even during running at 85 cycles/min. After the second stance phase the subject jumped over the cable connecting the preamplifier and the oscilloscope, and the test unit fired. Time bar=1 s. (Adapted with permission from Grimby, 1984.)

during the most rapid running that was possible under our laboratory conditions (see Figure 11B).

Discussion

Techniques

Satisfactory single motor unit recordings during movements could be achieved only with units having high muscle fibre densities or with units forming part of an accessory innervation (see Methods).

It is known from animal experiments that lesions to the axon of a motoneuron can change its firing properties (Eccles, Libet, & Young, 1958), but cross-reinnervation experiments indicate that the original firing properties reappear (Buller, Eccles, & Eccles, 1960). In man, motoneurons with newly regenerated axons had abnormal firing properties, but the abnormalities rapidly disappeared (Hannerz & Grimby, 1979). Some months after having made distal nerve lesions, the voluntary firing properties, the axonal conduction velocities in proximal segments, the contraction times, and the relationships between these parameters for reinnervated muscles were the same as those in normal muscles (Borg et al., 1977; Grimby, Hannerz, & Hedman, 1979). There is no evidence that making lesions in the distal axon causes permanent abnormalities in the discharge of motoneurons. Blocking of a muscle nerve reduces the feedback from muscle receptors that is known to play an important part in regulating motoneuron firing properties during voluntary contractions. However, the lidocaine blocking used in the present studies reduced the feedback from the short extensors only, whereas the long muscles were the main source of the proprioceptive control for all toe muscles. Finally, because the sources of error were different in the two techniques discussed, findings reproduced by both techniques should be conclusive.

Voluntary Tension

The findings during steady isometric contraction indicate that recruitment according to the "size principle" plays a major role in force regulation. In lower leg muscles small motoneurons were selectively used over a broad tension range, but large motoneurons were not readily available.

The firing rates decreased more rapidly under isometric conditions than during movement, suggesting that inhibitory impulses from tension receptors play a role. During prolonged maximal voluntary effort there was an increase in the threshold tension of some large motoneurons indicating that a fatigue mechanism was selectively affecting these motoneurons (Grimby et al., 1981).

The time course and its relationship to the firing rates were compatible with the late adaption of large motoneurons described in animal studies (Kernell & Monster, 1982a, 1982b). After a short period of rest the firing rates became normal. The muscle ischemia produced by a prolonged voluntary contraction was preserved, however, by occluding the circulation, and so the firing rates remained low (Bigland-Ritchie in this symposium). Thus, there seems to be some feedback from ischemic muscle that inhibits motoneurons.

The disfavoring of large, lower leg motoneurons during prolonged contraction must make their tonic firing exceedingly rare in everyday life. The term "phasic motoneurons" seems to be applicable to man. It must be emphasized, however, that large motoneurons in other muscles might have a better tonic capacity.

Voluntary Movement

The findings during rapid movements indicated that large and small motoneurons were readily available. Each motor unit fired with high frequency bursts and force was regulated by the number of discharges in the bursts rather than by recruitment. Four or five discharges of each unit were required for maximal force, and one discharge of each unit caused no more than one fifth of maximal force (for example, see review by Burke, 1981).

The firing rates were much higher in all units during rapid movements than during sustained maximal tensions, indicating a higher level of facilitation in the motoneuron pool. However, the greater role of the large motoneurons during such movements was only partly explained in terms of maximal activation of the whole pool. There must also have been a more favorable distribution of the synaptic input because selective activation of large motoneurons occurred. Perhaps synchronous activation of the whole muscle may be more easily achieved if large threshold steps within the motoneuron pool are eliminated.

Selective use of the large motoneurons innervating fast twitch muscle fibres is an advantage only for those movements that are so rapidly reversed that slow twitch muscle fibres would be counteractive. In the cat, fast gastrocnemius units are active and slow soleus units inactive when the paw is wet and the animal shakes it dry (Smith, Betts, Edgerton, & Zernicke, 1980). During slower cyclical movements, however, both muscles are active, and in even slower movements only the slow soleus participates (Smith, Edgerton, Betts, & Collatos, 1977).

In man, no systematic use of only the large motoneurons has been observed, but it proved impossible for subjects to perform toe waving at a rate requiring use of just the fast twitch muscle fibres. Occasionally, selective activation of the large motoneurons was, however, found during extremely rapid reversal of a movement. The reason why so many investigators have overlooked these deviations from orderly recruitment may be the technical difficulties encountered in studying such movements. It is not known whether the deviations from an orderly recruitment reflect just the elimination of large threshold steps discussed above or whether man also is capable of using only large motoneurons systematically under certain conditions. Unfortunately, there are no techniques available that permit the study of athletes on the sports field.

In any event, the transition from sustained tension to rapid movement causes great changes in the relative number of discharges of the various motor unit types.

Locomotion

Leg muscles are predominantly used for locomotion, and the use of a single leg motor unit during ordinary walking should reflect its long-term use. It has been shown in animal experiments that long-term electrical tetanization of a muscle nerve changes all the contractile properties of the muscle (Salmons & Henriksson, 1981). The tonic use of low threshold units in each step cycle, the phasic use of intermediates in each step cycle, and the merely corrective role of high threshold units might contribute to the differentiation of muscle fibres into S, FR and FF types, respectively.

References

Bigland-Ritchie, B., Jones, D.A., & Woods, J.J. (1979). Excitation frequency and muscle fatigue: Electrical responses during human voluntary and stimulated contractions. *Experimental Neurology, 64*, 415-427.

Bigland-Ritchie, B., Johansson, R., Lippold, O.C.J., Smith, S., & Woods, J.J. (1983). Changes in motoneuron firing rates during sustained maximal voluntary contractions. *Journal of Physiology* (London), **340**, 335-345.

Borg, J., Grimby, L., & Hannerz, J. (1977). Axonal conduction velocity and voluntary discharge properties of individual short toe extensor motor units in man. *Journal of Physiology* (London), **277**, 143-152.

Borg, J., Grimby, L., & Hannerz, J. (1983). The fatigue of voluntary contraction and the peripheral electrical propagation of single motor units in man. *Journal of Physiology* (London), **340**, 435-455.

Buller, A., Eccles, J.C., & Eccles, R.M. (1960). Interactions between motoneurons and muscles in respect of their characteristic speeds of their responses. *Journal of Physiology* (London), **150**, 417-439.

Burke, R.E. (1981). Motorunits: Anatomy, physiology and functional organization. In V.B. Brooks (Ed.), *Handbook of physiology: Sec. 1, Vol. II* (pp. 345-422). Bethesda, MD: American Physiological Society.

Eccles, J.C., Libet, B., & Young, R.R. (1958). The behavior of chromatolysed motoneurons studied by intracellular recording. *Journal of Physiology* (London), **143**, 11-40.

Freund, H.J. (1983). Motor unit and muscle activity in voluntary motor control. *Physiological Reviews*, **63**, 387-436.

Freyschuss, U., & Knutsson, E. (1971). Discharge patterns in motor nerve fibres during voluntary effort in man. *Acta Physiologica Scandinavica*, **83**, 278-279.

Grimby, L. (1984). Firing properties of single human motor units during locomotion. *Journal of Physiology* (London), **346**, 195-202.

Grimby, L., & Hannerz, J. (1977). Firing rate and recruitment order of toe extensor motor units in different modes of voluntary contraction. *Journal of Physiology* (London), **264**, 865-879.

Grimby, L., Hannerz, J., & Hedman, B. (1979). Contraction time and voluntary discharge properties of individual short toe extensor motor units in man. *Journal of Physiology* (London), **289**, 191-201.

Grimby, L., Hannerz, J., & Hedman, B. (1981). Fatigue and voluntary discharge properties of single motor units in man. *Journal of Physiology* (London), **316**, 545-554.

Hallett, M., Shahani, B.T., & Young, R.R. (1975). EMG analysis of stereotyped voluntary movements in man. *Journal of Neurology, Neurosurgery and Psychiatry*, **38**, 1154-1162.

Hannerz, J. (1974a). An electrode for recording single motor unit activity during strong muscle contractions. *Electroencephalography and Clinical Neurophysiology*, **37**, 179-181.

Hannerz, J. (1974b). Discharge properties of motor units in relation to recruitment order in voluntary contraction. *Acta Physiologica Scandinavica*, **91**, 374-384.

Hannerz, J., & Grimby, L. (1979). The afferent influence on the voluntary firing range of individual motor units in man. *Muscle and Nerve*, **2**, 414-422.

Henneman, E., Somjen, G., & Carpenter, D.O. (1965a). Functional significance of cell size in spinal motoneurons. *Journal of Neurophysiology*, **28**, 560-580.

Henneman, E., Somjen, G., & Carpenter, D.O. (1965b). Excitability and inhibitability of motoneurons of different sizes. *Journal of Neurophysiology*, **28**, 599-620.

Henning, R., & Lomo, T. (1982). Motor unit discharge patterns in rat fast and slow skeletal muscle. *Abstract*, 5th International Congress on Neuromuscular Diseases. Marseilles.

Hoffer, J.A., O'Donovan, M.J., Pratt, C.A., & Loeb, G.E. (1981). Discharge patterns of hindlimb motoneurons during normal cat locomotion. *Science*, **213**, 466-468.

Kernell, D., & Monster, A.W. (1982a). Time course and properties of late adaptation in spinal motoneurons of the cat. *Experimental Brain Research*, **46**, 191-196.

Kernell, D., & Monster, A.W. (1982b). Motoneuron properties of motor fatigue. *Experimental Brain Research*, **46**, 197-204.

Kugelberg, E., & Edstrom, L. (1968). Differential histochemical effects of muscle contractions on phosphorylase and glycogen in various types of fibres: Relation to fatigue. *Journal of Neurology, Neurosurgery and Psychiatry*, **31**, 415-423.

Lambert, E.H. (1969). The accessory deep peroneal nerve: A common variation in innervation of extensor digitorum brevis. *Neurology* (Minneapolis), **19**, 1169-1176.

Marsden, C.D., Meadows, J.C., & Merton, P.A. (1971). Isolated single motor units in human muscles and their rates of discharge during maximal voluntary effort. *Journal of Physiology* (London), **217**, 12-13.

Merton, P.A. (1954). Voluntary strength and fatigue. *Journal of Physiology* (London), **123**, 553-564.

Milner-Brown, H.S., Stein, R.B., & Yemm, R. (1973). Changes in firing rate of human motor units during linearly changing voluntary contractions. *Journal of Physiology* (London), **230**, 371-390.

Salmons, S., & Henriksson, J. (1981). The adaptive response of skeletal muscle to increased use. *Muscle & Nerve*, **4**, 94-105.

Stalberg, E., & Trontelj, J.V. (1979). *Single fibre electromyography*. Old Woking, Surrey, Misvalle Press Ltd.

Smith, J.L., Edgerton, V.R., Betts, B., & Collatos, T.C. (1977). Recruitment of slow and fast muscles of the ankle and elbow during locomotion and rapid non-support movements. *Proceedings of the International Union of Physiological Sciences: 27th Congress International des Science Physiologique*, **13**, 704.

Smith, J.L., Betts, B., Edgerton, V.R., & Zernicke, R.F. (1980). Rapid ankle extension during paw shakes: Selective recruitment of fast ankle extensors. *Journal of Neurophysiology*, **43**, 612-620.

Discussion

Dr. Grimby was congratulated by Dr. McComas and Dr. Burke for the quality of the records that he had obtained during activity. Dr. Grimby warned that each record was not of long duration; he was delighted to obtain records during 50 meters walking in a given subject.

Dr. McComas was interested in Dr. Grimby's observations that perhaps in man, as in animals, it was possible to alter the physiological and biochemical properties of motor units by changing the firing pattern. Dr. McComas presented the results of a study (Corley, Kowalchuk, & McComas, 1984) in which young hamsters were suspended for a month by their hind quarters, thus restricting activity to the forelimbs. The twitches evoked from the soleus became smaller and briefer, the tetanic tension diminished, and the rate of rise of tetanic tension increased. Histochemical studies suggested that the changes were due, in part, to conversion of 10% of the slow twitch motor units to fast twitch. Another experimental preparation used by Dr. McComas and his colleagues involved the placing of a ligature over the hind limb of a rat so as to compress the sciatic nerve and thereby induce blocking of impulse conduction (neurapraxia). After only one week, the contractile properties of the plantaris and soleus were altered, showing that these muscles were very sensitive to brief periods of disuse. These findings were in contrast to those in humans. After five weeks of immobilization of the elbow and wrist, Sale, McComas, MacDougall, and Upton (1982) found no changes in the contraction and half relaxation times of the thenar muscles. Although the firing pattern of motor units in some humans might be dominant in determining their properties, this was unlikely to be the case in muscles that were little used in the course of everyday activity. Other factors, notably axoplasmic transport, might be more important.

Dr. Grimby was questioned regarding the apparent contradictions between his results and those of Desmedt and Godaux (1977). Dr. Grimby replied that the main difference was that these authors studied graded ramp movements, whereas in his own experiments there was a rapid development of maximal effort that was quickly reversed by an antagonistic movement. The two experimental conditions were dissimilar; Dr. Grimby agreed with their results but not with their generalization.

Dr. Winter thought that the pattern of activity obtained by Dr. Grimby with single motor unit recordings was different than that obtained in his own laboratory with surface electromyography. During slow walking and jogging there were two bursts of activity in the tibialis anterior, one as the heel made contact and the other as the toe was lifted. Dr. Grimby pointed out that the examples he had shown were from the extensor digitorum brevis and not the tibialis anterior. The findings in the two muscles were qualitatively similar, but the distributions of activity within the step cycle were different; in the extensor digitorum brevis there was weak activity during the swing phase of walking and strong activity during the stance phase. In the tibialis anterior there was a small burst of EMG activity during the early swing phase and a larger burst just before heel strike (see Figure 1).

Dr. Edgerton was interested in knowing whether it was possible for subjects to activate one motor unit voluntarily rather than another, particularly if the two units had similar threshold. Dr. Grimby replied that although his group has not systematically studied changes in the order of recruitment during sustained voluntary contractions, some motor units could be made to discharge before others with similar thresholds by small changes in the activity of agonist or antagonist muscles.

In reply to a question from Dr. Faulkner, Dr. Grimby pointed out that the amplitude of motor unit potentials changes with the shortening and length-

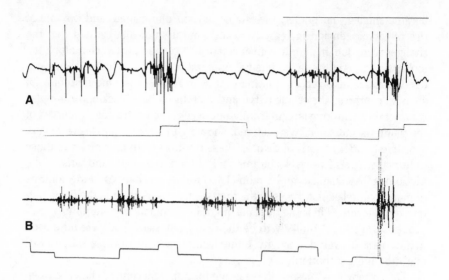

Figure 1. Firing properties during walking of one low threshold unit (A) and one high threshold unit (B) from the tibialis anterior muscle. The lower recordings in A and B show signals from foot switches: Upward deflexions indicate pressure on the sole of the tested foot, small amplitude indicates pressure only on the anterior part, intermediate amplitude only on the posterior part, and high amplitude indicates pressure on both these sites. The low threshold unit fires at about 10 Hz during the swing phase and at about 20 Hz during the heel strike. The high threshold unit, on the other hand, does not participate in the ordinary step cycle (left) but fires when the subject stumbles (right). Time bar 1 s.

ening of muscle fibers. This problem could not be avoided, but by recording from only one motor unit any confusion due to changes in amplitude was eliminated. In jumping movements the maximal activation of motor units was obtained with a burst of about four discharges at relatively short intervals. Dr. Faulkner felt that the recordings obtained from single motor units indicated that the motor units were not heavily loaded during rapid activity but that they were probably contracting at high shortening velocities, in this way generating almost maximum power. Dr. Grimby added that this type of activity may play an important role in corrective movements that occur often during ordinary walking on uneven ground.

Dr. McComas provided some information on the number of impulses required to generate maximal tension; in unpublished experiments from his laboratory, Quinlan and Vandervoort had shown that if stimuli to the dorsiflexors of the ankle were separated by as short a time as 4 msec, tension still increased from the fourth to fifth stimulus. Unless a burst of activity was associated with at least this number of impulses, maximum tension for the motor unit might not be developed. He asked Dr. Stein to comment in view of his studies on this topic carried out on the cat, and Dr. Stein replied that with five stimuli 85% to 90% of tetanic tension was generated. However, he cautioned that when muscle physiologists talk about maximum shortening velocity, they usually assume that this occurs during unloaded contractions, whereas in walking movements the load of the skeleton prevents generation of maximum shortening velocity. This topic had been discussed earlier in the meeting when differences between slow and fast twitch muscles were considered in terms of their recruitment in movements of different velocities. Dr. Faulkner agreed that slow units could contract at their highest velocity at the same time as fast units were contracting; some of the fast units, however, might contract beyond the maximum velocity of the slow twitch units, thus leading to unloading of the slow twitch units in a mixed muscle.

Dr. Green mentioned the work of Gollnick, Piehl, and Saltin (1974), who showed in cycling a progressive recruitment of fast twitch motor units. He wondered whether this was achieved through a low frequency stable type of recruitment pattern or whether an intermittent pattern might be employed. The distinction might be important because of the contrasting fatigue characteristics of different motor units. Dr. Grimby suggested that during increasing speed of locomotion, the motor units were recruited according to the size principle, and when motor units fatigued new ones were recruited. Unfortunately, it was difficult to study this phenomenon with single fiber recordings, which seldom last for 40 or 50 m of running. With surface electrode recordings the amount of EMG activity increased, and he speculated that in a trained subject all the motor units might fire during rapid running, particularly as fatigue ensued.

At Dr. McComas's invitation, Dr. Basmajian described studies of single motor unit activity carried out some years ago, which indicated that activation patterns may be modified by training. A motor unit that was normally recruited "late" could be trained to fire in an isolated manner without the activation of surrounding motor units; this observation indicated that the size principle might be overcome voluntarily in some situations. However, he pointed out that it was much easier to train units that were normally recruited later than those with low thresholds. The interest in these findings was not that they challenged the size principle but that voluntary mechanisms might be used to reverse it. There was some indication that the findings might be applied to the management of patients with neurological diseases.

Dr. Howell wondered whether Dr. Grimby might divulge the secrets of his success in obtaining motor unit recordings of such high quality. Dr. Grimby replied that the main difficulty was not in obtaining selectivity but in ensuring that the electrode remained in position. The more selective an electrode, the more sensitive was it to movement; thus, it was often possible to record selectively from a muscle fiber during isometric conditions, but as soon as the fiber was allowed to shorten, the recording became lost or blurred. This effect could reduce by recording from a part of the muscle where there were very few active motor units. With these techniques records had been obtained from about 40 or 50 units in ordinary walking and for 15 to 20 units during running.

Dr. Burke emphasized a point made earlier by Dr. Bigland-Ritchie that the order of recruitment of motor units might be altered in muscles having a number of functions if the direction of action of the muscle was changed; thus, different motor unit pools might be recruited, even though they remained within a functional grouping and within the same muscle. Dr. Grimby said that the muscle studied most often by his group, the extensor digitorum brevis, had two portions, one acting on the big toe and the other on the small toes. However, the recruitment studies had been made on low and high threshold units acting on the big toe.

In summarizing Dr. Grimby's paper and the discussion, Dr. McComas pointed out that the results complemented those recently obtained in animals and reported by Dr. Burke earlier in the meeting and that demonstrated an important function role for those motor units with very high thresholds during isometric voluntary contractions.

References

Corley, K., Kowalchuk, N., & McComas, A.J. (1984). The contrasting effects of suspension on hindlimb muscles in the hamster. *Experimental Neurology*, **85**, 30-40.

Desmedt, J.E., & Godaux, E. (1977). Fast motor units are not preferentially activated in rapid voluntary contractions in man. *Nature* (London), **267**, 717-719.

Gollnick, P.D., Piehl, K., & Saltin, B. (1974). Selective glycogen depletion in human muscle fibers after exercise of varying intensity and at varying pedalling rates. *Journal of Physiology* (London), **241**, 45-57.

Sale, D.G., McComas, A.J., MacDougall, J.D., & Upton, A.R.M. (1982). Neuromuscular adaptation in human thenar muscles following strength training and immobilization. *Journal of Applied Physiology: Respiratory, Environmental and Exercise Physiology*, **53**, 419-424.

9

What is Optimized in Muscular Movements?

R.B. Stein, M.N. Oğuztöreli, and C. Capaday
University of Alberta

At a symposium on muscle power and performance, most of the papers will report the latest details of muscle mechanics and neural control mechanisms. However, at least initially, this paper will approach the problem from quite a different perspective. In making movements, humans share common physical constraints with other animals and with artificial systems, including robots. The pattern of movement produced against these constraints will depend on the strategies used by man and machines (Nelson, 1983).

The choice of a strategy depends on the goals of the movement; that is, what variable or variables are being optimized. In a robot this optimization may be explicitly programmed or it may follow implicitly from the properties of the motors used and their limitations (Brady, Hollerbach, Johnson, Lozano-Perez, & Mason, 1982). Similarly, human movements may be consciously optimized or they may be determined at a mechanical level by muscle properties or neural circuitry. By considering the predictions of various simple optimization strategies and comparing these predictions with human movements, some insight may be gained about the question raised in the title of this paper.

Optimization of Kinematic Variables

Muscles and motors work against physical loads, which may consist, as shown in Figure 1, of a mass M, a dashpot with viscosity D, and a spring of

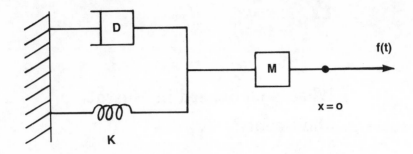

Figure 1. A load consisting of a mass M, a dashpot of viscosity D, and a spring of stiffness K is moved by a force f(t) from an initial position x = 0 at time t = 0.

stiffness K. In order to move the load from a point $x = 0$ to $x = X$ in a time T, some force must be imparted to the load. The force f(t) as a function of time will obviously depend on the way in which the movement is carried out. The power being imparted to the load at any time t will simply be the product of the force and the velocity dx/dt. The total energy required in moving the load from $x = 0$ at $t = 0$ to $x = X$ at $t = T$ will be given from basic Newtonian mechanics by the integral

$$\int_0^T f(t) \, x' \, dt = \int_0^T [Mx'' + Dx' + Kx]x' \, dt \tag{1}$$

in which $x' = dx/dt$ and $x'' = d^2x/dt^2$. However,

$$\int_0^T Mx''x' \, dt = 1/2 \, M[x'^2]_0^T = 0 \tag{2}$$

if the mass is initially at rest $(x' = 0)$ and is brought to rest again at time T. Also,

$$\int_0^T Kxx' \, dt = 1/2 \, K[x^2]_0^T = KX^2/2 \tag{3}$$

independently of the pathway taken from $x = 0$ to $x = X$. Finally, since D is a constant, minimization of energy dissipation by the load requires minimization of the integral

$$I_1 = \int_0^T [x']^2 dt. \tag{4}$$

Note that minimization of energy dissipation by the load does *not* imply minimizing the energy consumption of the muscle (or motor) producing the force to move the load. This is a separate problem that will be further considered below. From the calculus of variation (Akhieser, 1962), the integral I_1 will be minimized if

$$\partial Y/\partial x - d(\partial Y/\partial x')/dt = 0 \tag{5}$$

in which $Y = (x')^2$ in our example. The Euler-Lagrange equation (5) implies that $d(2x')/dt = 0$, and hence that

$$x' = c_1; \; x = c_1 t + c_0 \tag{6}$$

subject to the boundary conditions. If $x = 0$ at $t = 0$, $c_0 = 0$, and if $x = X$ at $t = T$, $c_1 = X/T$. Thus, to minimize energy dissipation, the load should be moved at constant velocity between the two points, as shown in Figure 2A. Note that this requires that the mass be accelerated instantaneously at $t = 0$

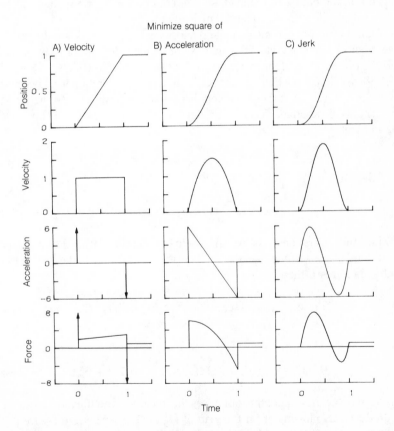

Figure 2. To minimize the mean square velocity in moving from a position $x = 0$ to $x = 1$ in time $t = 1$, the movement should take place linearly with a square velocity profile and pulses of acceleration and deceleration. For a load such as shown in Figure 1 with $M = K = 1$, $D = 2$, the force required is shown at the bottom. (B) To minimize mean square acceleration, the form of the movement becomes sigmoid with corresponding changes in the other parameters. (C) To minimize mean square jerk (jerk is the derivative of acceleration), parameters of the movement and the force required become smoother. Further discussion in text.

and decelerated instantaneously at $t = T$ if it is to remain at $x = X$ for $t \geqslant T$. We have set $X = T = 1$ in Figure 2A, but the movement could obviously be scaled to any value of X or T required. The force required to obtain the optimal trajectory is

$$f(t) = Mx'' + Dx' + Kx = \{M[\delta(t) - \delta(t-T)] + D + Kt\}(X/T) \qquad (7)$$

in which $\delta(t)$ is the Dirac delta function or unit impulse. A real force generator would not be able to produce the infinite force for instantaneous acceleration. The effect of constraints on movements will be considered later. The form of the force (without limiting its maximum value) is also shown in Figure 2A, assuming $M = K = 1$, $D = 2$. Calculation of the optimal trajectory did not depend on the nature of the load, so the required force for any load can be easily calculated with an equation analogous to Equation 7.

Optimization of the mean square velocity for Equation 4 is only one of a number of kinematic variables that might be considered. For example, in robotics optimization of mean square acceleration is often considered (Chaudet & O'Shea, 1983). Note that one cannot "optimize" acceleration itself because $\int_0^T x'' \, dt = x' |_0^T = 0$, if the movement begins and ends at rest. Again, using the calculus of variations, it can be shown that the trajectory that will optimize the integral

$$I_2 = \int_0^T [x'']^2 dt \qquad (8)$$

is of the form

$$x = c_0 + c_1 t + c_2 t^2 + c_3 t^3 \qquad (9)$$

in which the c_i's are constants, which have to be determined from the boundary conditions. If we assume that $x'(0) = 0$ at times 0 and T (i.e., the load starts and ends at rest), then

$$c_0 = c_1 = 0; \; c_2 = 3X/T^2; \; c_3 = -2X/T^3 \qquad (10)$$

so

$$x = c_2 t^2 + c_3 t^3; \; x' = 2c_2 t + 3c_3 t^2; \; x'' = 2c_2 + 6c_3 t. \qquad (11)$$

The form of the movement that optimizes the integral I_2 and the force required to produce this movement for the load of Figure 1 are shown in Figure 2B, again assuming $X = T = M = K = 1$, $D = 2$. The position follows a sigmoid curve. The velocity follows a parabolic curve, which is symmetric about the time $T/2$. The acceleration decreases linearly, passing through 0 at $T/2$. The force is more complex in form, being the sum of the three curves above, but is bounded (as is the acceleration) for all values of T.

If the mean square values of still higher order derivatives are minimized, increasingly smooth curves of position, velocity and acceleration are obtained. For example, Flash and Hogan (1982) suggested that the integral

$$I_3 = \int_0^T [x''']^2 \, dt \tag{12}$$

might be minimized in arm movements, in which x''' is the third derivative of position and is referred to as jerk. In this case, position is a fifth order polynomial

$$x = \sum_{i=0}^{5} c_i t^i \tag{13}$$

in which the constants are again calculable from the boundary conditions (Nelson, 1983). If it is also assumed that $x''(0) = x''(T) = 0$, then

$$c_0 = c_1 = c_2 = 0; \; c_3 = 10X/T^3; \; c_4 = -15x/T^4; \; c_5 = 6X/T^5 \tag{14}$$

The form of the motion is shown in Figure 2C. Position again increases in a sigmoid fashion. The velocity profile is smoother and still shows a symmetry about time $T/2$, as in Figures 2A and 2B. The acceleration now increases and decreases smoothly according to a cubic equation and shows a negative symmetry about the time $T/2$. These results can be generalized to higher order derivatives. The integral I_n that minimizes the square of the n-th order derivative subject to the boundary conditions $x^{(k)}(0) = 0$, $(k = 0,1,...,n-1)$ and $x(T) = X$, $x^{(k)}(T) = 0$ $(K = 1,2,...,n-1)$ will have a polynomial solution of order $2n-1$. The velocity will show an even symmetry with a polynomial of order $2n-2$, and the acceleration an odd symmetry with a polynomial of order $2n-3$.

Minimization of Energy Consumption

In Figure 2 the force required to move the load also becomes increasingly smooth as higher order derivatives are optimized. The force produced by a motor is proportional to the current I in the motor windings. To produce more current a larger voltage must be applied, and the power consumption is the product $IV = I^2/R$, in which R is the resistance of windings; that is, power varies as current or force squared. Thus, another possible strategy is to minimize the energy consumed by the motor (rather than that dissipated by the load), which is proportional to the integral J in which

$$J = \int_0^T [f(t)^2] dt. \tag{15}$$

Again, using the calculus of variations, it follows that minimization of energy consumption requires that

$$Mf''(t) - Df'(t) + Kf(t) = 0. \tag{16}$$

This equation can be solved by the use of Laplace transforms (Sokolnikoff & Redheffer, 1958), which give

$$[Ms^2 - Ds + K]f^*(s) = M[sf(0) + f'(0)] - Df(0), \tag{17}$$

in which $f^*(s) = \int_0^\infty f(t)e^{-st}dt$, and $f^*(s)$ denotes the Laplace transform of $f(t)$, which is a function of the Laplace variable s. From the relation between force and the parameters of movement, an equation for the Laplace transform of $x(t)$ can be obtained, namely

$$x^*(s) = \frac{M[sf(0) + f'(0)] - Df(0)}{[Ms^2 + Ds + K][Ms^2 - Ds + K]}. \tag{18}$$

The form of the movement will depend on the load and will be different if the system is underdamped, overdamped, or critically damped.* If M = K = 1, D = 2, the system is critically damped (see Figure 3B) and the form of the movement is similar to that obtained for minimizing acceleration (see Figure 2B). For a pure inertial load M, the position and its derivatives will also be identical to that given by Equations 9 and 10 for minimizing acceleration. If D = K = 0, the force will not be the same as that shown in Figure 3 because the load is different. The similarity of Figures 2B and 3B implies that, with numerically comparable values of the parameters, the inertial term dominates the force requirements to move the load a unit distance in a unit time.

If the damping is increased by increasing D, the position changes more linearly, the velocity becomes more square and the change in acceleration sharper (see Figure 3A, in which D = 10, M = K = 1). The form of the movement approaches that found for minimizing the velocity (see Figure 2A). Indeed, for a pure viscous load D the motion will be identical to that shown in Figure 2A. The forces required to produce these movements will, of course, depend on the load.

Finally, the load can be made underdamped by various means. If D is decreased, it has little effect because the inertial term already is the dominant one, as mentioned above. However, in Figure 3C the stiffness K has been increased to 10 (M = 1, D = 2) and the movement becomes assymmetrical (i.e., the load does not reach the halfway point in distance until t > 0.5). This assymmetry becomes increasingly large if K is increased relative to M and D. The reason is that with a pure spring load, force is only required to maintain

---

*Solutions of Equation 18 for different values of damping have not been derived here in the interest of space, but are shown in Figure 3.

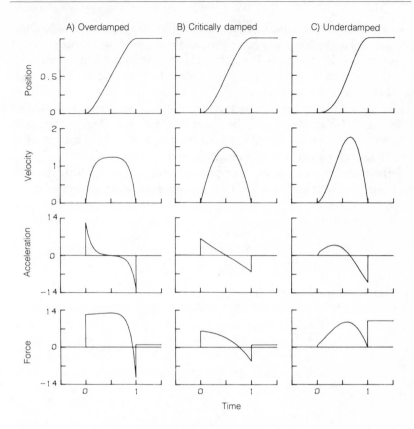

Figure 3. Increasing the viscosity D from the critically damped value of 2 (B) to 10 (A), while keeping M = K = 1, produces an overdamped load. Increasing K to 10 (C), while keeping M = 1 and D = 2, produces an underdamped load. The form of the movement required to minimize the mean square force, which corresponds to minimizing energy consumption for an electrical motor, varies with the degree of damping. Further discussion in text.

a nonzero position. Thus, the way to minimize force or its square under these conditions is to move the load to the position X at the last possible moment before t = T.

Constrained Movements

Up to this point we have considered the optimal movement without regard to the constraints that will be imposed by any physical or biological force generating system. For example, in Figure 2A an infinite force would be required to accelerate or decelerate the mass instantaneously. Similarly, the forces required for other optimal conditions may exceed the force-generating capability of a muscle or electrical motor. Constraints of this sort can be dealt with mathematically using Pontryagin's Principle (Pontryagin, Bottyanskii, Camkendze, & Mischenko, 1962; Fan, 1966) and form the basis of this section.*

Control of the movement in Figure 2A has a "bang-coast-bang" form; that is, the maximum force should be used initially to accelerate the load, which can then coast at constant velocity until it is decelerated by the maximum force (Hollerbach, 1980). Figure 4A compares the form of the optimal movement with infinite (solid lines) and finite (diamonds) forces available. For ease of calculation a pure inertial load has been used with M = 1, so the values of force and acceleration will be numerically equal.

The acceleration and deceleration phases will then be identical in form with symmetry about the midpoint (t = T/2). With an elastic load some of the limited

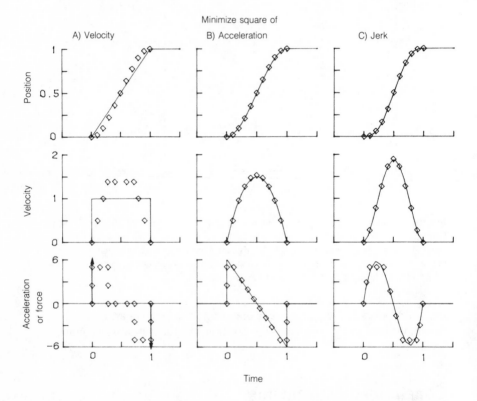

Figure 4. The effect of a limited force range ($-5 < F < 5$) on the form of movements produced so as to minimize the square of (A) velocity, (B) acceleration, or (C) jerk. The solid lines are the values without constraints on force (see also Figure 2), whereas the diamonds show the corresponding values with force limitation. Pure inertial load (M = 1; D = K = 0).

---

*An Appendix explaining the application of Pontryagin's principle to these problems is available on request.

force available would be required to stretch the spring and the symmetry would be lost. The problem is to determine the times t_1 and t_2 when switching from one mode to the other should occur. (This is a simple example of a two-point boundary value problem, which occurs frequently in optimal control with constraints.) From the physical symmetry we know that $t_2 = T - t_1$. Clearly, if there is a maximum force F available

$$x'' = F/M, \quad x' = Ft/M, \quad x = Ft^2/(2M) \tag{19}$$

in the region $0 < t < t_1$. For $t_1 < t < T - t_1$ the inertial load will move at a constant velocity Ft_1/M. To satisfy the boundary conditions this velocity must be such that it covers the distance required, $X - (Ft_1^2/M)$, in the time available, $T - 2t_1$. Thus,

$$Ft_1 = \frac{MX - Ft_1^2}{T - 2t_1}$$

which requires that

$$t_1 = [T \pm (T^2 - 4XM/F)^{\frac{1}{2}}]/2 \tag{21}$$

Equation 21 will have a real solution only if $F \geqslant 4XM/T^2$. (The force must be above a minimum value to move the mass M the distance X in time T.)

Similar considerations apply to optimal control of acceleration and jerk in Figures 4B and 4C. For minimizing acceleration the movement starts identically to Figure 4A up to a time t_1. Then, for $t_1 < t < T - t_1$,

$$x'' = c_1t + c_2; \quad x' = c_1t^2/2 + c_2 t + c_3' \tag{22}$$

$$x = c_1t^3/6 + c_2t^2/2 + c_3t + c_4$$

in which $c_1 = \dfrac{-2F}{M(T-2t_1)}$, $c_2 = \dfrac{FT}{M(T-2t_1)}$, $c_3 = Ft_1/M - c_1 t_1^2/2 - c_2 t_1$

$c_4 = Ft_1^2/(2M) - c_1t_1^3/6 - c_2t_1^2/2 - c_3t_1$.

The constants are obtained from the boundary conditions when $t = t_1$. Because of the symmetry of the movement, the correct value of t_1 will produce a movement that covers a distance $X/2$ when $t = T/2$. Equation 22 could be solved explicitly for the value of t_1, which satisfies this requirement, but it is easier to use a method of successive approximations. Similar considerations apply to minimizing jerk, but the details have been omitted. Although the forms of the acceleration remain distinct in Figures 4A-C, the velocity and particularly the position records become more similar as the force is limited. Thus, to distinguish experimentally which mode, if any, was being used, measurements should be done under conditions in which the maximum force output of the system is used briefly, if at all.

Limits apply in a real system not only to the maximum force but to its rate of change. Thus, rather than having the force (and hence the acceleration) in Figure 4 change instantaneously, there will be a maximum positive or negative slope, which will affect the acceleration records of Figures 4A and 4B in particular and make them even closer to those in Figure 4C. In fact, the limits on rates in both physical and biological systems are often due to exponential processes that affect the behavior of the system at all levels, not only near maximum values. When an electric motor is turned on, a back EMF is created, which prevents the current from building up immediately. Similarly, even when a muscle is stimulated tetanically, the force builds up to its final level gradually

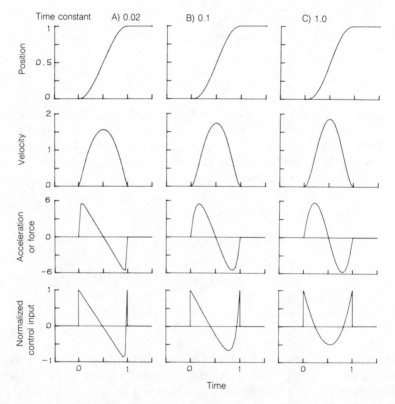

Figure 5. Effect of exponential lags in force production on the form of movement produced. The time constants used were (A) 0.02, (B) 0.1, and (C) 1. As the time constant increases, the movement changes from the form typical of minimizing acceleration (see Figure 2A) to that typical of minimizing jerk (see Figure 2C). The control inputs needed to produce the required forces are also shown and have been normalized to their maximum values.

with an approximately exponential time course (see Figure 5). As the time constant is increased from $\tau = 0.02$ to $\tau = 1$, the form of the acceleration is smoothed and shows a transition from the form obtained for minimizing acceleration (see Figure 2B) to that obtained for minimizing jerk (see Figure 2C). Mathematically, the form of the movement must agree with that for minimization of jerk if $t \ll \tau$, but good agreement was found even when $t = \tau$ (compare Figures 2C and 5C). Also shown in Figure 5 are the control inputs required to generate the forces with an exponential lag. The control input changes from a mainly biphasic shape (see Figure 5A) to a triphasic shape (see Figure 5C). The shape in Figure 5A is similar to the force, except for a brief pulse at the end, which is required for the boundary conditions. The shape of the control input in Figure 5C approaches the derivative of force. No limits were put on the control inputs in Figure 5, but the effects of a limit would be similar to that illustrated in Figure 4.

Optimization of Muscle Function

In previous sections, examples were chosen to be general enough so that the results might apply to electrical motors or muscles. Now we turn more specifically to muscle movements that will minimize energy consumption by the muscle. From the early work of Hill (1965), the rate of energy expended by a muscle and can be expressed as a sum

$$E = E_0 + E_1 g(t) + E_2 g(t)y' + f(t)x'. \tag{23}$$

E_0 is the rate of heat expended at rest. E_1 is the coefficient for the extra rate of energy expenditure needed to maintain force generation. Maintenance heat is assumed to be proportional to the activation $g(t)$ of force generating elements (i.e., cross-bridges) within the muscle, in contrast to the situation discussed earlier of a second power relation for electric motors. E_2 is the coefficient for the extra rate of heat production during shortening. Shortening heat is assumed to be proportional to the degree of activation and the velocity of shortening y' of the force generators (Oğuztöreli & Stein, 1983). A term has also been included for the rate of doing work on the load, which is the product of the external force being generated and the velocity x' at which the load is moving.

These various components are illustrated in Figure 6. Shortening heat is not exactly proportional to the speed of shortening (Hill, 1964), and it is largely unknown whether maintenance heat is proportional to the degree of activation, particularly under time-varying conditions. Nonetheless, these relatively simple assumptions will be adequate for the present purpose. To minimize energy consumption, we must minimize the integral J, in which

$$J = \int_0^T E dt = \sum_{i=0}^{3} J_i. \tag{24}$$

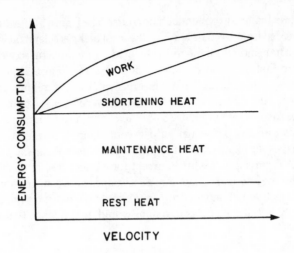

Figure 6. The rate of energy consumption increases with the velocity of shortening. The total can be divided into various components, as described in the test (see also Huxley, 1957; Oğuztöreli & Stein, 1983).

From Equation 23, $J_0 = \int_0^T E_0 dt = E_0 T$ (a constant), $J_1 = \int_0^T E_1 g(t) dt$,

$J_2 = \int_0^T E_2 g(t) y' dt$, and $J_3 = \int_0^T f(t) x' dt$. We showed earlier that minimization

of energy dissipation (integral J_3) in moving a load from one point to another required minimization of the velocity squared, a purely kinematic variable, during the period of the movement.

Determining the contribution of integrals J_1 and J_2 requires assumptions about force generation within the muscle. For this purpose we need a model that is sufficiently simple that analytical and computational results can be obtained for comparison with the previous sections. Figure 7A shows such a model coupled to the load from Figure 1. The model contains a force generator with time course $g(t)$ that interacts with internal series and parallel elastic components having stiffness K_i and K_p, respectively. Also included is a dashpot of viscosity B, which provides the force-velocity properties of the model.

All the elements are initially assumed to be linear, although this assumption will be relaxed later. Even in its linear form, the model has been widely used and agrees remarkably well with data from a number of muscles (Bawa, Mannard, & Stein, 1976; Cannon & Zahalak, 1982). The equations of motion for the model can be immediately written from the balance of forces at the two nodes x and y, namely

$$f(t) = Mx'' + Dx' + K_e x = K_i (y-x) \tag{25}$$

$$g(t) = By' + K_p y + K_1 (y-x) \tag{26}$$

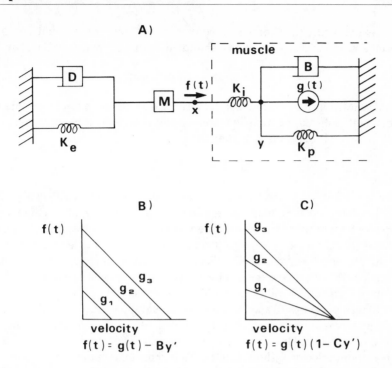

Figure 7.   The load in Figure 1 has been connected to a simple muscle model (A) with internal series (K_i) and parallel (K_p) elastic elements, a force generator (g), and a viscosity (B) that determines its force-velocity properties. The external spring has been denoted K_e to distinguish it from the internal elastic elements. A series of force-velocity curves will be obtained at increasing levels of muscle activation (g_1, g_2, and g_3) that will be parallel (B) if the viscosity is independent of force generation or convergent (C) at a point if the viscosity varies proportionally with activation. The point of convergence in (C) is the maximum unloaded shortening velocity.

Equation 25 can be solved for y and this value substituted into Equation 26, which gives

$$g(t) = a_3 x''' + a_2 x'' + a_1 x' + a_0 x \tag{27}$$

in which $a_0 = [K_e K_i + K_e K_p + K_i K_p]/K_i$, $a_1 = [D(K_i + K_p) + B(K_i + K_e)]/K_i$, $a_2 = [M(K_i + K_p) + DB]/K_i$, and $a_3 = MB/K_i$. Using Equation 27 we have

$$J_1 = E_1[a_1 X + a_0 \int_0^T x\, dt] \tag{28}$$

if we assume as before that $x = x' = x'' = 0$ at $t=0$, while $x = X$ and $x' = x'' = 0$ at $t = T$. Interestingly, only terms dependent on position (and not its derivatives) contribute to integral J_1.

In considering integral J_2, we will ignore the term involving K_p in Equation 26 because K_p is often small compared to K_i experimentally. If this assumption is not made, the expressions become rather more complex but do not change in form. Using Equations 25 and 26, J_2 can be written in the form

$$J_2 = \int_0^T [E_2/B]g(t)[g(t) - f(t)]dt. \tag{29}$$

As discussed in relation to Figure 3, terms involving the mass M are often dominant. Substituting from Equations 25 and 27 and ignoring terms that do not involve M, Equation 29 becomes

$$J_2 = \int_0^T (MB/K_i)(x'')^2 dt. \tag{30}$$

Hence, minimizing J_2 (and energy consumption) involves minimization of jerk.

Up to this point no nonlinearities have been considered, although many types of nonlinearities have been observed for muscle. For example, the series elasticity is not a simple constant but depends on the force being generated (Ford, Huxley, & Simmons, 1977). Equation 30 can generally be derived from Equations 26 & 27, independent of the type of nonlinearity for K_i, but the evaluation of Equation 30 will obviously depend on the form of K_i.

Similarly, Figures 7B and 7C show two simple approximations to the force-velocity curve of muscle (Hill, 1965). Figure 7B illustrates the form used in which the slope and hence the viscosity B are constants. The form in Figure 7C has a maximum velocity of shortening that is independent of the level of activation, as has been found experimentally in most, but not all, studies (Edman, 1979). If we had used the alternative form (see Figure 7C), Equation 29 would become

$$J_2 = \int_0^T [E_2/C][g(t) - f(t)]dt \tag{31}$$

in which C is a constant. There would now be no dependence on jerk or other derivatives, but only on x (see analysis of integral J_1 above). Various other nonlinearities could be considered, but it may be more helpful at this point to discuss some of the results already obtained in relation to experimental data and their implications for the control of movement.

Comparison With Experiments

In the previous sections, the forms of movements predicted by various control schemes have been calculated. Figure 8 shows experimental data from Cooke (1980) for a human subject holding a handle and moving the elbow from one angle to another. Similar data have been obtained by others (e.g., Abend, Bizzi, & Morasso, 1982). The data seem to be of the form expected for minimizing jerk (see Equations 12 and 14). Flash and Hogan (1982) suggested that jerk might normally be minimized in human arm movements.

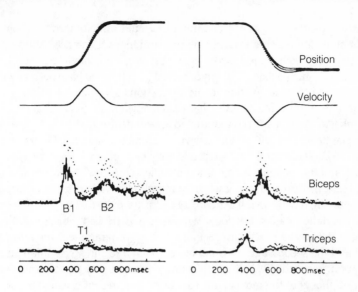

Figure 8. Average position and velocity records for flexion (left) and extension (right) movements of the human elbow joint are shown. Below are the corresponding rectified and integrated EMG records from an elbow flexor (biceps) and an elbow extensor (triceps) muscle. Note the triphasic pattern (B1, T1, B2) associated particularly with the flexion movement. Standard deviations are given by the dotted lines on each part of the Figure (Cooke, 1980).

However, it should be noted that the handle was connected to a torque motor, so that movement was probably limited by the inertia of the arm and the assembly to which it was attached. There was no spring to act as a restoring force, and care is usually taken to minimize the viscosity in this sort of apparatus. Under such conditions, we have shown that exponential lags in the muscle, minimization of energy, or even the limits on muscle power can lead to an identical form of movement to that obtained by minimizing jerk. One way to distinguish these possibilities is to vary the conditions. For example, if movement time is increased, force limitations become less important, but the movement should simply be scaled up in time if jerk is being minimized. It is well known that slow movements are often segmented (Brooks & Thach, 1981), instead of remaining continuous in form. Having accelerations and decelerations in each segment would clearly not minimize jerk but would be reasonably efficient energetically because the muscle need only be activated occasionally and the movement could coast in between.

Another interesting condition would be to have the handle attached to a spring load with a substantial restoring force and low inertia. The predictions for minimum jerk would remain unchanged, but for minimum energy consumption the movement would be delayed so that energy would not be wasted to maintain the spring in an extended state (see Figure 3C). If no compensation were made by the brain at all, the movement would become asymetric in the opposite direction because the arm would initially move rapidly and would slow down as it encountered more and more resistance. Although experiments in which subjects work against spring loads have been conducted from time to time (Wilkie, 1950; Joyce & Rack, 1974), none have been analysed, to our knowledge, in relation to the predictions given above.

Another interesting point is that all the acceleration records shown here are biphasic. Positive force is required to accelerate the load and negative force to decelerate it. This will require pairs of antagonistic muscles (Oğuztöreli and Stein, 1982). The control inputs will generally be triphasic if there are exponential lags and the movement time is comparable to the exponential time constant (see Figure 5). The electrical signals from muscles (EMGs) are generally triphasic (see Figure 8), having an initial period of agonist activity followed by antagonist activity and then a second period of agonist activity (Hallett, Shahani, & Young, 1975). Whereas the initial burst seems to be preprogrammed, the antagonist burst and the second agonist burst are correlated to the acceleration and deceleration, respectively (Ghez & Martin, 1982) and may be reflex responses to those phases of the movement. However, the present calculations specify the optimal form of a movement under prescribed conditions, irrespective of whether the signals are preprogrammed or produced by feedback.

Muscles show a tremendous array of nonlinearities that have also been ignored here for the most part. For example, the two types of force-velocity curves considered are quite crude approximations of Hill's characteristic equation (Hill, 1965). However, any curve can be approximated by a straight line and a linearized force-velocity curve works surprisingly well under many conditions (Bawa et al., 1976; Cannon & Zahalak, 1982). We have purposely used simple models of muscle for the most part so that the form of the movement could be determined analytically under many conditions. Previous work on energy minimization has often involved more complex models with so many parameters that it has been difficult to know which ones had important effects on the overall results (Hatze & Buys, 1977; Oğuztöreli & Stein, 1983). Computation of results from such complex models remains a formidable task, even for the largest digital computers.

Over the past few years the progress in understanding the molecular basis of muscular contraction has been exciting. Clearly, there is a need to begin to integrate this information into theories that adequately explain the form of the complex, elegant, and beautiful movements of which all animals including man are capable. The work presented here represents a preliminary attempt toward such theories.

Conclusions

The strategy for making a movement will clearly influence the form of the movement. By analysing various potential strategies, we may suggest what variables could be optimized in human and animal movements. Optimizing kinematic variables such as the mean square velocity, acceleration, or jerk produces quite distinct movement patterns. Minimizing the mean square force produces patterns that depend on the nature of the load. Similarly, minimizing energy consumption by a muscle will depend on muscle properties. Constraints of the maximum force or time lags in force production tend to blur the differences between alternative strategies. Many natural movements are consistent with minimization of jerk. This form could arise from limitations of force output and time lags associated with muscular force production than from any computation carried out in the brain. Experiments to distinguish these possibilities are discussed. Minimum jerk movements will also minimize energy consumption by the muscle over a range of conditions.

Discussion

Dr. Winter opened the discussion by congratulating Dr. Stein on his development of the topic, beginning with a simple ballistic movement without gravity and building up a picture of more complex movements involving different types of muscles and several joints, such as those involved in walking and running. Dr. Stein had shown that certain strategies were not functionally effective and that the variability of the load on the system and the characteristics of the muscle had to be considered. Dr. Winter pointed out that the situation that Dr. Stein had resolved by increasing the value of K could also be treated by increasing V. Dr. Stein agreed that one could make the system work in more than one way, but when this was carried out by increasing $\dot{V}$ it produced a very asymmetric movement that was limited by mass and inertia; the physiological implications were thus difficult to define. Dr. Winter wondered whether the model allowed for co-contraction, particularly if this might minimize energy. Dr. Stein answered that there were many ways in which the model might be improved and the effects of contraction of antagonistic muscles would be extremely important. Hogan had shown that if one wished to carry out a movement with extreme accuracy against the variable background, co-contraction was of great importance but would involve an energy cost. On the other hand, if the movement did not involve accuracy, co-contraction was less necessary and energy would be saved. This type of factor had not yet been built into the model.

Mr. Perrine wondered about the importance of isometric contractions; if no movement occurred, there was no power output, but in movements such as walking, isometric contractions might still be important. Dr. Faulkner had asked earlier whether a muscle might be totally activated in the gait cycle, but EMG evidence suggested that this was unlikely because the forces generated were not sufficiently large. Even in sprinting the joint velocities were not high, so single muscles might not be operating at full power. These considerations were relevant to situations in which muscles of different contraction characteristics might be activated at the same time. One synergist might operate with another of quite different force velocity characteristics, and thus might not be capable of generating much power because the movement might be outside its optimal velocity range. On the other hand, if power was defined as the rate at which energy was produced and one considered events at the sarcomere level, then a muscle might operate powerfully even when it was generating energy that was absorbed by the elastic component without any associated shortening. This behavior might become very important in a movement associated with a large acceleration. An explosive isometric contraction in which energy was generated at the highest possible rate could start the movement, but then the muscle might be inhibited so as not to exceed structural limitations. At this point power might be generated but at a very submaximal level. Dr. Stein commented that although the muscle operated to dissipate a lot of energy, the external work under isometric conditions was still zero; in such a situation there was no output in the face of very high input and thus an efficiency of zero. Mr. Perrine was unhappy about the efficiency concept and felt we should be more concerned about the ability of muscles to generate energy at the sarcomere level, even though it may not be released externally.

Dr. Wilkie felt that much of the discussion had centered around concepts that were obvious 30 to 40 years ago, such as the nonlinearity in both the internal viscosity of muscle and in the force length curve of the series' elastic component (Wilkie, 1950). These factors had to be taken into account if one was going to model a muscle operating against an external load. One might summarize the laws of motion by saying that an object did not move until a certain force (i.e., the limiting frictional force) was exceeded. The harder one pulled, the faster the object moved; that was viscosity. The harder one pulled, the more rapidly it accelerated, and that was inertia. In presenting a picture of the performance of an external task, Dr. Stein did not appear to have taken friction into account, which even Galileo realized was inherent in the relationship between force and motion.

References

Abend, W., Bizzi, E., & Morasso, P. (1982). Human arm trajectory formation. *Brain, 105*, 331-348.

Akhiezer, N.I. (1962). *The calculus of variations* (A.H. Frink, Trans.). New York: Blaisdell.

Bawa, P., Mannard, A., & Stein, R.B. (1976). Predictions and experimental tests of a visco-elastic muscle model using elastic and intertial loads. *Biological Cybernetics, 22*, 139-145.

Brady, M., Hollerbach, J., Johnson, T., Lozano-Perez, T., & Mason, M. (Eds.). (1982). *Robot motion: Planning and control.* Cambridge, MA: MIT Press.

Brooks, V.B., & Thach, W.T. (1981). Cerebellar control of posture and movement. In *Handbook of physiology* (Secs. I-II, pp. 877-946). Bethesda, MD: American Physiology Society.

Cannon, S.C., & Zahalak, G.I. (1982). The mechanical behavior of active human skeletal muscle in small oscillations. *Journal of Biomechanics,* **15,** 111-121.

Chaudet, R., & O'Shea, J. (1983). Validation of an adaptive robot control structure by means of simulation. In J. Bruger & Y. Jarny (Eds.), *Simulation in engineering sciences* (pp. 411-416). Amsterdam: Elsevier-North Holland.

Cooke, J.D. (1980). The organization of simple skilled movements. In G.E. Stelmach & J. Requin (Eds.), *Tutorials in motor behavior* (pp. 199-212). Amsterdam: Elsevier-North Holland.

Edman, K.A.P. (1979). The velocity of unloaded shortening and its relation to sarcomere length and isometric force in vertebrate muscle fibres. *Journal of Physiology* (London), **290,** 143-159.

Fan, L.-T. (1966). *The continuous maximum principle.* New York: John Wiley and Sons.

Flash, T., & Hogan, N. (1982). Evidence for optimization strategy in arm trajectory formation. *Society for Neuroscience Abstracts,* **8,** 282.

Ford, L.E., Huxley, A.F., & Simmons, R.M. (1977). Tension responses to sudden length change in stimulated frog muscle fibres near slack length. *Journal of Physiology* (London), **269,** 441-515.

Ghez, C., & Martin, J.H. (1982). The control of rapid limb movement in the cat: III. Agonist-antagonist coupling. *Experimental Brain Research,* **45,** 115-125.

Hallett, M., Shahani, B.T., & Young, R.R. (1975). EMG analysis of stereotyped voluntary movements in man. *Journal of Neurology, Neurosurgery and Psychiatry,* **38,** 1154-1162.

Hatze, H., & Buys, J.D. (1977). Energy-optimal controls in the mammalian neuromuscular system. *Biological Cybernetics,* **27,** 9-20.

Hill, A.V. (1964). The effect of load on the heat of shortening of muscle. *Proceedings of the Royal Society, London,* **159,** 297-318.

Hill, A.V. (1965). *Trails and trials in physiology.* London: Arnold.

Hollerbach, J.M. (1980). *An oscillation theory of handwriting.* Unpublished doctoral dissertation, Massachusetts Institute of Technology, Cambridge, MA.

Joyce, G.C., & Rack, P.M.H. (1974). The effects of load and force on tremor at the normal human elbow joint. *Journal of Physiology* (London), **240,** 375-396.

Nelson, W.L. (1983). Physical principles for economies of skilled movements. *Biological Cybernetics,* **46,** 135-147.

Oğuztöreli, M.N., & Stein, R.B. (1982). Analysis of a model for antagonistic muscles. *Biological Cybernetics,* **45,** 177-186.

Oğuztöreli, M.N., & Stein, R.B. (1983). Optimal control of antagonistic muscles. *Biological Cybernetics,* **48,** 91-99.

Pontryagin, L., Bottyanskii, V., Gamkendze, R., & Mischenko, E. (1962). *The mathematical theory of optimal processes* (K.N. Trigoroff, Trans.). New York: Wiley Interscience.

Sokolnikoff, I.S., & Redheffer, R.M. (1958). *Mathematics of physics and modern engineering*. New York: McGraw-Hill.

Wilkie, D.R. (1950). The relation between force and velocity in human muscle. *Journal of Physiology* (London), **110**, 249-280.

Section **4**

Energy Metabolism

10

Lactic Acid Production in Intact Muscle, as Followed by ^{13}C and ^{1}H Nuclear Magnetic Resonance

Michael Bárány and Carlos Arús
University of Illinois

Since Berzelius's discovery of lactic acid in muscles of hunted deers in 1807 (for history, see Needham, 1971), the search for this compound in tissues has continued. Lactic acid is the end product of glycolysis, one of the energy yielding processes of living cells; thus, changes in the lactic acid concentration may be related to tissue energy requirements under physiological conditions. Accumulation of lactic acid leads to acidification of intracellular pH, which may alter the rate of cellular reactions or may result in pain and muscular fatigue.

Several biochemical assays exist for detection and quantification of lactic acid in tissues, all of which require disruption of cells and measurement of lactic acid in the extracts. With such a procedure, changes in lactic acid concentration cannot be followed within a single cell population, but a series of tissue extracts must be prepared for a comparison of lactic acid levels. Naturally, this introduces the error of specimen variation into the kinetics of the lactic acid production. The application of nuclear magnetic resonance (NMR) to intact tissues opened a new avenue for monitoring intracellular lactic acid in a nondestructive way. Dawson, Gadian, and Wilkie (1978) used ^{31}P NMR for estimation of lactic acid in frog muscle under anaerobic conditions, based on the chemical shift of the cytoplasmic inorganic phosphate due to the protons generated from lactic acid in the fatigued muscle. In contrast to this indirect determination of lactic acid, Doyle and Bárány (1982) introduced the direct quantitation of muscle lactic acid by natural abundance ¹³C NMR from the integral of its hydroxyl carbon resonance. Recently, Arús, Bárány, Westler, and Markley (1984b) succeeded in quantifying lactic acid by ¹H NMR from the integral of its methyl proton resonance in muscle.

In this paper we summarize our results on lactic acid determination by both ¹³C and ¹H NMR in human muscle samples obtained at surgery, in frog gastrocnemius and other muscles of rats and chickens. ¹³C and ¹H NMR spectra of muscles were recorded as described by Bárány, Doyle, Graff, Westler, and Markley (1984) and Arús, Bárány, Westler, and Markley (1984a), respectively.

Studies with ¹³C NMR

Lactate production in resting frog muscle may be followed by the appearance of the characteristic resonances due to the methyl and alcoholic carbons at 21.0 and 69.3 ppm, respectively (see Figure 1) (Doyle & Bárány, 1982). In

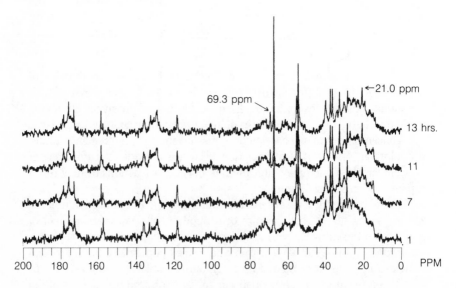

Figure 1. Natural abundance ¹³C NMR spectra (90.5 MHz) of resting frog gastrocnemius muscles at 24°C. Before sacrifice, the frogs were chilled in ice, the muscles dissected, loaded into an NMR tube on ice, and equilibrated in the spectrometer at 24°C for 10 min. Spectra of 6000 transients each (2 h) were collected, and the hours shown on the spectra refer to the midpoint of the data collection. The peaks at 21.0 and 69.3 ppm are due to lactate methyl and hydroxyl carbons. The large peak at 67.4 ppm is from the dioxane external standard. (Reproduced with permission from Doyle & Bárány, 1982.)

the freshly dissected muscle, the lactic acid concentration is so low that it is not observable by ¹³C NMR and it takes about 11 hrs incubation of the gastrocnemius muscle at room temperature to demonstrate the lactic acid peaks. These data agree with the low lactate content of resting frog muscle, 1.4 μmol lactic acid per g of muscle, determined chemically (Nassar-Gentina, Passonneau, Vergara, & Rapoport, 1978) and with the slow metabolic rate of resting frog muscle (Kushmerick, 1983).

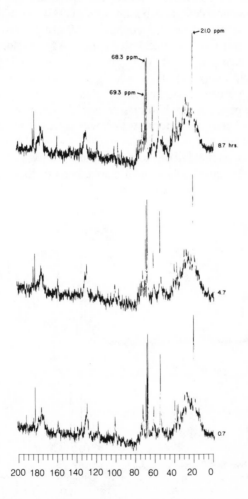

Figure 2. Natural abundance ¹³C NMR spectra of caffeine-treated frog gastrocnemius muscles. The muscles were treated with 10 mM caffeine in frog Ringer's solution for 10 min, then blotted, and transferred into NMR tubes. The time course of lactate production was measured at 1.33 h intervals (4000 scans) for 9 h at 31°C. The lower, middle, and upper spectra were obtained in the first, third, and fifth interval, respectively. A coaxial capillary containing 4.4% dioxane and 1.68 M lactate (pD 3.8) was inserted into the NMR tube to give reference signals at 67.4 and 68.3 ppm, respectively. (Reproduced with permission from Doyle & Bárány, 1982.)

In contrast, if frog muscle is stimulated by caffeine at 31°C, the production of lactic acid is already maximal after 42 min (first observation time) and decreases slightly after 4.7 and 8.7 hrs of caffeine treatment (see Figure 2). The lactate content of caffeine-treated muscles, 72-82 μmol/g, as determined by ^{13}C NMR, agrees with the chemically determined value of 79μmol/g in frog muscles treated with 2,4-dinitrofluorobenzene for 24 h (Infante & Davies, 1965).

Glycolysis in human muscle biopsies may also be followed by natural abundance ^{13}C NMR (see Figure 3). Based on the peak assignments by Canioni, Alger, and Shulman (1983) and Bárány et al. (1984), the following carbon resonances are identified: C−1, lactic acid (21.0 ppm), C−6, α, β-glucose, glycogen (61.5 ppm), C−2, lactic acid (69.3 ppm), C−4, α, β-glucose (70.3 ppm), C−2, C−5, α-glucose and C−5, glycogen (72.2 ppm), C−3, α-glucose (73.5 ppm), C−2, β-glucose (75.1 ppm), C−3, β-glucose, and C−5, β-glucose (76.6 ppm), C−1, α-glucose (92.9 ppm), C−1, β-glucose (96.6 ppm), and C−1, glycogen (100.6 ppm). Figure 3 compares the ^{13}C spectra of a normal muscle (bottom) with that of a muscle from a patient with osteosarcoma. More glycogen and glucose are present in the normal muscle than in the muscle from the patient. On the other hand, if one compares the peak heights of the C−2 lactic acid carbons (69.3 ppm) with that of the carbons of the external dioxane

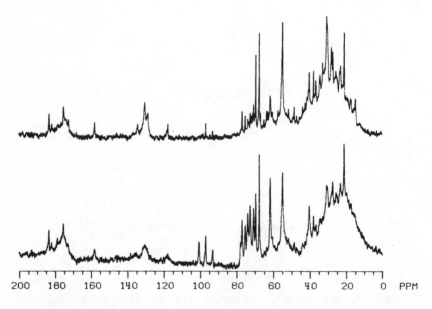

Figure 3. Natural abundance ^{13}C NMR spectra of human leg muscle biopsies from osteosarcoma (upper trace) and hip operation (lower trace). Both muscle samples were extracted with isopentane to remove neutral fats (Bárány et al., 1984), and 3600 transients were collected in both cases. The signal at 67.4 ppm in both spectra is from dioxane in a coaxial capillary.

standard (67.4 ppm), it is evident that the muscle from the diseased leg produced more lactic acid than the muscle from the normal leg.

In various diseases, we observed a decrease in the sugar content of human muscle and in its ability to generate lactic acid. Muscle from a myopathic patient contained uniformly less glycogen, glucose, and lactic acid (see upper part of Figure 4) than muscle from a normal subject (see bottom part of Figure 4). Glucose and lactic acid were barely detectable in the muscle of a cerebral palsy patient, as compared with normal muscle (see Figure 5). Finally, no glycogen or glucose was observed in the muscle of a Charcot-Marie-Tooth patient (see Figure 6), and the lactic acid content of this muscle remained low even after 8 hours of incubation at room temperature. (In the upper part of Figure 6, compare the height of the 69.3 ppm peak with that of the reference 67.4 ppm peak).

Table 1 compares our ^{13}C NMR determination of lactic acid produced by various muscles during 1 h incubation at 37°C. Several major differences are apparent. Frog, rat, or chicken skeletal muscles generate almost 3 times as much lactic acid as normal human muscles. Lactic acid production by human muscles roughly equals that of the rat soleus or heart. Diseases such as cerebral palsy or Duchenne dystrophy greatly reduce or abolish lactic acid production in muscle.

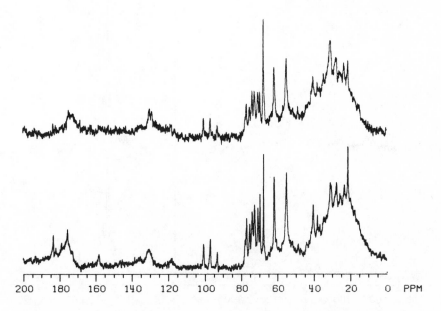

Figure 4. Natural abundance ^{13}C NMR spectra of human leg muscle biopsies from a patient whose disease was diagnosed as type II atrophy (upper trace) and from a hip operation (lower trace). Both muscle samples were extracted with isopentane, and 3600 transients were collected.

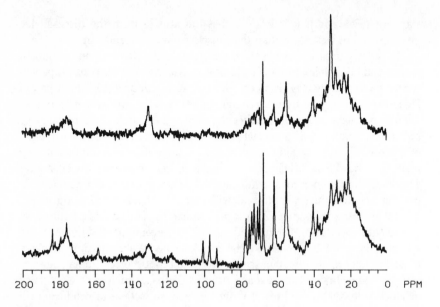

Figure 5. Natural abundance ^{13}C NMR spectra of human leg muscles from a cerebral palsy patient (upper trace) and hip operation (lower trace). Both muscle samples were extracted with isopentane, and 3600 transients were collected.

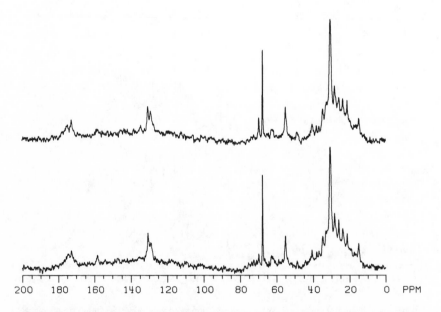

Figure 6. Natural abundance ^{13}C NMR spectra of a human leg muscle from a patient with Charcot-Marie-Tooth disease diagnosis. Spectra were recorded 3 h (bottom trace) and 8 h (upper trace) after the biopsy, and 1500 transients were collected in each case.

Table 1. Lactic Acid Production by Various Muscles, Determined by ^{13}C NMR

Muscle	μmol/h/g fresh weight/37°C	n
Human, normal	31 ± 7	8
Human, scoliosis	30 ± 10	8
Human, myopathic and neuropathic	21 ± 16	7
Human, cerebral palsy	7 ± 6	4
Human, Duchenne dystrophy	< 0.1	2
Frog, gastrocnemius	77 ± 10	8
Rat, gastrocnemius	96	2
Rat, soleus	34	2
Rat, heart	35	2
Chicken, pectoralis	84 ± 15	4
Chicken, heart	34	2

Supported by the Muscular Dystrophy Association, Shriners Hospital for Crippled Children, the National Institute of Health (RR01077) and the National Science Foundation (CHE-79-16109).

The rate of lactic acid production by normal human muscles or muscle from scoliotic patients is about 30 μmol/h/g. According to the data of Saltin and Gollnick (1983), 1 g human muscle contains 78-85 μmol glucose units in glycogen, corresponding to 156-170 μmol lactic acid in glycogen. Thus, normal human muscles hydrolyze about 20% of their glycogen at 37°C in one hour.

The rate of lactic acid production in muscles from myopathic or neuropathic patients decreases to 20 μmol/h/g on the average. However, the range is as wide as 8-55 μmol, clearly indicating the heterogeneity of this group. This rate decreases greatly in cerebral palsy to 7 μmol/h/g, whereas no lactic acid is detectable in muscles of Duchenne dystrophic children. The large differences in the lactic acid content between normal and diseased human muscles are related to differences in their glycogen and glucose content. For instance, cerebral palsy muscle contains significantly less sugar than a normal muscle (see Figure 5). This suggests that the disease affects the enzymes that are involved in the synthesis of glycogen. In addition, diseased human muscles may be deficient in the glycolytic enzymes that hydrolyze glycogen to lactic acid.

Fast skeletal muscles of frog, rat, and chicken generate as much as 77-96 μmol lactic acid h/g 37°C. From the glycogen content of rat muscle, 41-43 μmol glucose units/g (Saltin & Gollnick, 1983), it appears that all the glycogen was hydrolyzed by the rat gastrocnemius muscles during the 1 h incubation at 37°C.

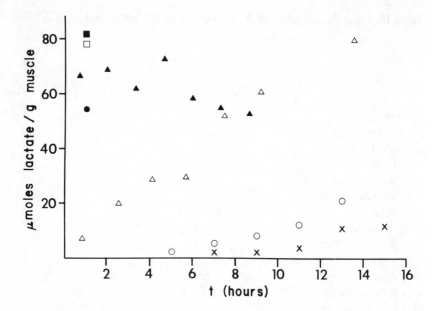

Figure 7. Lactate production in resting and caffeine-treated frog gastrocnemius muscle as a function of temperature and time: resting muscle at 22°C (x), 24°C (o), 28°C (Δ) and 43°C (□); caffeine-treated muscle at 24°C (●), 31°C (▲) and 32.5°C (■). The temperature of the muscle was controlled as described by Doyle, Chalovich, and Bárány (1981) and was measured by a hand thermometer after the scanning was completed. (Reproduced with permission for Doyle & Bárány, 1982.)

Indeed, our ^{13}C NMR spectra showed the absence of glycogen and glucose in these muscles. In contrast, our ^{13}C spectra revealed significant amounts of glycogen and glucose in incubated rat soleus and heart. These muscles liberated 34-35 μmol lactic acid/h/g 37°C, which is about 60% of their maximal capacity to generate lactic acid (28-30 μmol glucose units in glycogen) (Saltin & Gollnick, 1983).

We have used frog muscle to follow the temperature dependence of lactate production (see Figure 7). The rate of lactate production was 2.0 μmol/h/g muscle at 24°C and 6.5 μmol/h/g muscle at 28° C, giving a Q_{10} of about 8. This suggests that one reaction in the glycolytic sequences has an abnormally high activation energy. The lactate content is maximal, 82 μmol/g at 43°C in resting muscle at the earliest time of determination (20 min).

The lactate content of caffeine-treated muscle is significantly greater than that of the corresponding resting muscle at room temperature and appears to be maximal at the first time interval measured, decreasing after 5 h. This is due to the oxidation of lactate with the aid of the O_2 present in the muscle.

Studies with ¹H NMR

¹H is the most sensitive nucleus for application of NMR to intact tissue. Figure 8 shows the ¹H NMR spectrum of intact chicken pectoralis muscle recorded with one single transient, or in 0.7 sec. The muscle was stored frozen and was allowed to thaw before taking the spectrum. Freezing and thawing of muscle is known to hydrolyze glycogen, and this is evidenced in Figure 8 by a huge 1.30 ppm resonance from the methyl protons of lactic acid.

Figure 9 illustrates the accumulation of lactic acid in frog muscles under anaerobic conditions, as indicated by the increase in the resonance areas of the 1.30 ppm and 4.10 ppm peaks: The latter corresponds to the $-C\underline{H}OH$ proton of lactic acid.

From the spectra shown in Figures 8 and 9, one can estimate the lactic acid concentration to be 76 mmol/kg wet weight in the chicken muscle (see Figure 8), and 4 and 27 mmol/kg wet weight in the fresh and aged frog muscle (see bottom and top parts of Figure 9, respectively). With ¹H NMR, Seo, Yoshizaki, and Morimoto (1983) found less than 1 mmol lactate/kg in the resting

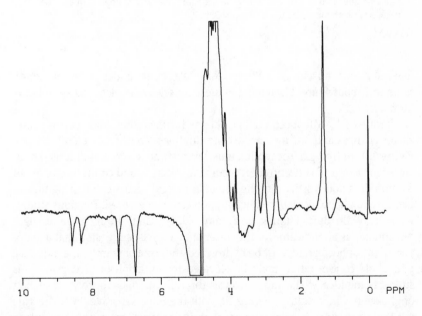

Figure 8.   ¹H NMR spectrum (470 MHz) of intact chicken pectoralis muscle recorded with only one transient.

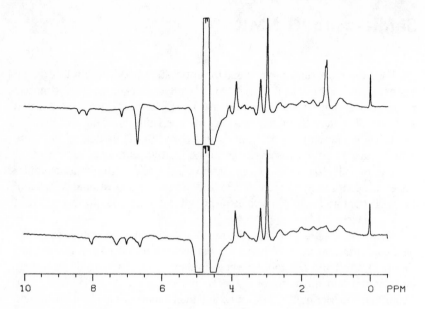

Figure 9. ¹H NMR spectrum of two fresh frog gastrocnemius muscles (bottom) and of the same two muscles after 12 h of anaerobic storage in the NMR tube at 25°C (top). Sixty-four transients were collected both for the bottom and top spectra.

femoral biceps muscles of bullfrogs, *Rana catesbeiana,* under anaerobic conditions and about 4 mmol lactate/kg in these muscles after electrical stimulation for 5 sec.

Because ¹H NMR spectra can be obtained with accumulation of a few transients, changes in tissue metabolite concentrations can be followed rapidly (see Figure 10). In frog gastrocnemius muscle under anaerobic conditions, an increase in lactic acid concentration occurs immediately and continues for about 8 hours. It is noteworthy that the rise in lactic acid occurs before a significant decrease in phosphocreatine concentration can be measured. Previous studies with ³¹P NMR (Burt, Glonek, & Bárány, 1976), using the increase of sugar phosphates as an indicator for the onset of glycolysis, suggested that a major part of phosphocreatine must be hydrolyzed and, concomitantly, the inorganic phosphate concentration must be elevated for initiation of glycolysis. This supports the idea of starting glycolysis through the phosphorolysis reaction of glycogen. The results of Figure 10, with the more sensitive ¹H NMR, rule out this possibility. It would appear that under anaerobic conditions in frog muscle, glycolysis is initiated by the reduction and NAD⁺, and the resultant NADH reacts with pyruvic acid to form lactic acid.

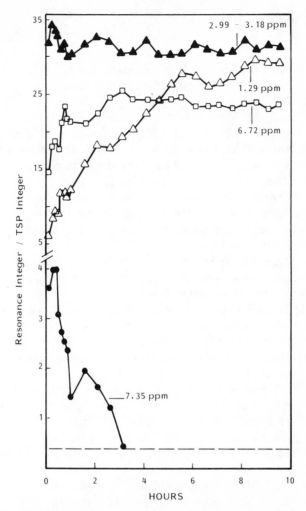

Figure 10. ^{1}H NMR determination of changes in the relative levels of lactic acid (Δ, 1.29 ppm), creatine (□, 6.72 ppm), phosphocreatine (●, 7.35 ppm), and the sum of total creatine, carnitine, and α-glycerophosphorylcholine (▲, 2.99-3.18 ppm) as a function of time of storage of frog gastrocnemius muscle under anaerobic conditions at 20°C. Each data point is derived from a spectrum accumulated with 256 transients (7 min). The dotted line at the bottom of the figure indicates the limit of detection. (Reproduced with permission for Arús, Bárány, Westler, & Markley, 1984a.)

Acknowledgment

We thank Timothy G. Blechl for his expert assistance and Donna M. Lattyak for typing the manuscript.

References

Arús, C., Bárány, M., Westler, W.M., & Markley, J.L. (1984a). ¹H NMR of intact muscle at 11 T. *Federation of the European Biochemistry Society Letters,* **165,** 231-237.

Arús, C., Bárány, M., Westler, W.M., & Markley, J.L. (1984b). ¹H NMR of Intact Tissues at 11.1 T *Journal of Magnetic Resonance,* **57,** 519-525.

Bárány, M., Doyle, D.D., Graff, G., Westler, W.M., & Markley, J.L. (1984). Natural abundance of ¹³C NMR spectra of human muscle, normal and diseased. *Magnetic Resonance in Medicine,* **1,** 30-43.

Burt, C.T., Glonek, T., & Bárány, M. (1976). Analysis of phosphate metabolites, the intracellular pH, and the state of adenosine triphosphate in intact muscle by phosphorus nuclear magnetic resonance. *Journal of Biological Chemistry,* **251,** 2584-2591.

Canioni, P., Alger, J.R., & Shulman, R.G. (1983). Natural abundance carbon-13 nuclear magnetic resonance spectroscopy of liver and adipose tissue of the living rat. *Biochemistry,* **22,** 4974-4980.

Dawson, M.J., Gadian, D.G., & Wilkie, D.R. (1978). Muscular fatigue investigated by phosphorus nuclear magnetic resonance. *Nature,* **274,** 861-866.

Doyle, D.D., Chalovich, J.M., & Bárány, M. (1981). Natural abundance ¹³C NMR spectra of intact muscle. *Federation of the European Biochemistry Society Letters,* **131,** 147-150.

Doyle, D.D., & Bárány, M. (1982). Quantitation of lactic acid in caffeine-contracted and resting from muscle by high resolution natural abundance ¹³C NMR. *Federation of the European Biochemistry Society Letters,* **140,** 237-240.

Infante, A.A., & Davies, R.E. (1965). The effect of 2,4-dinitrofluorobenzene on the activity of striated muscle. *Journal of Biological Chemistry,* **240,** 3996-4001.

Kushmerick, M.J. (1983). Energetics of muscle contraction. In L.D. Peachey, R.H. Adrian, & S.R. Geiger (Eds.), *Handbook of physiology: Sec. 10. Skeletal muscle* (pp. 189-236). Bethesda, MD: American Physiological Society.

Nassar-Gentina, V., Passonneau, J.V., Vergara, J.L., & Rapoport, S.I. (1978). Metabolic correlates of fatigue and of recovery from fatigue in single frog muscle fibers. *Journal of General Physiology,* **72,** 593-606.

Needham, D.M. (1971). *The biochemistry of muscular contraction in its historical development.* Cambridge, MA: University Press.

Saltin, B., & Gollnick, P.D. (1983). Skeletal muscle adaptability: Significance for metabolism and performance. In L.D. Peachey, R.H. Adrian, & S.R. Geiger (Eds.), *Handbook of physiology: Sec. 10. Skeletal muscle* (pp. 555-631). Bethesda, MD: American Physiological Society.

Seo, Y., Yoshizaki, K., & Morimoto, T. (1983). A ¹H-nuclear magnetic resonance study on lactate and intracellular pH in frog muscle. *Japanese Journal of Physiology,* **33,** 721-731.

Discussion

Dr. Stein was interested in the quality of the data obtained by even single sweeps with the proton NMR in measuring lactate; part of the improvement must be due to replacing one carbon atom with three hydrogen atoms, thus increasing the concentration, but he did not feel that this was the sole reason for the sharper and more intense resonance. Dr. Bárány replied that proton NMR is much the most sensitive form of presently available NMR techniques because the proton gyromagnetic ratio is the highest of all biologically important nuclei and the natural abundance of protons is 99.98%. Thus proton NMR is 5,676 times more sensitive than natural abundance carbon NMR and fifteen-fold as sensitive as phosphorus NMR. The improvement is due not to the replacement of one carbon atom with three protons but to the high sensitivity of the proton NMR over carbon NMR. The General Electric (previously Nicolet) narrow bore NMR obtains very high resolution for protons by running at 360 or 470 MHz. Carbon NMR, which is based on the natural abundance of 13 C, suffers from the fact that 12 C has no magnetic moment, and thus the measurements are based on 13 C, which represents only 1.1% of carbon. In order to work with this extremely small concentration, decoupling of the protons bound to the carbons is required. If the proton attached to the carbon is irradiated, the proton spin is decoupled from the carbon spin and the sensitivity of the carbon resonance is increased (maximally threefold). New developments in NMR for proton-carbon decoupling are leading to great reductions in the irradiation power required and thereby avoiding any damage of biological tissues.

Dr. Newsholme wondered whether it was fair to assume that the lactate measured with NMR necessarily yielded an index of glycolysis; as described in Dr. Bárány's talk, it is more an in vitro technique in which samples of muscle are placed in the magnetic field than an in vivo technique. The muscle being studied is necessarily at rest, and results obtained in this state have a limited application to what happens during muscle contraction. For example, if an insect flight muscle was found not to produce lactate, one would infer that there is no glycolysis, and yet many insects depend almost totally on glycolysis. Dr. Bárány made several points in reply. First, perhaps he should have emphasized that the measurements he presented were all carried out on muscle biopsies. Second, as the muscle is placed in the NMR tube, no metabolite leaves the system; therefore, no lactic acid was lost in these experiments. Third, he did not feel that there was any conversion of lactic acid into other metabolites. For example, there is no alanine formation, which would be readily detected by proton NMR; pyruvic acid formation would also be detected by 13 C NMR. Finally, although *in vitro* NMR is not able to solve all the problems which control muscle metabolism *in vivo*, it quantitates the level of muscle metabolites accurately and helps to obtain a better understanding of what is going on, particularly in ischemic situations in which not only is the extent of glycolysis measured but damage of the muscle membrane may also be detected.

Dr. Gollnick followed up Dr. Newsholme's question to comment that he doubted if the measurements gave a good indication of the potential of the tissue for anaerobic production of lactate. The value obtained, approximately 0.5 μ moles per gram per minute would compare to peak values obtained during heavy exercise as high as 30. Dr. Bárány reemphasized that the lactate formation rate is so low because the muscles are not stimulated and resting metabolism is all that is being measured. However, if metabolism is stimulated with caffeine, lactic acid is produced rapidly and all the glycogen and glucose are broken down. In such experiments the total glycogen and glucose in the muscles appears to be within the range of measurements made by other techniques. Also, the method is capable of identifying differences in the glycolytic capacity of slow and fast muscles; previously, slow and fast muscles were characterized only through differences in myosin ATPase activity. In general, based on lactic acid production, human muscle appears to behave as a rather slow muscle, consistent with myosin ATPase measurements. Dr. Gollnick countered by pointing out that many human muscle fibers would be classified as typical fast twitch fibers with metabolic characteristics that correspond to fast muscles. If the maximal glycolytic potential is to be measured, then a closed anoxic system was required. Dr. Bárány pointed out that he was not using a single criterion to conclude that the main bulk of human muscle is a slow muscle; his own measurements of myosin ATPase activity were important in this regard. In the NMR preparation the system is a closed one and there is no oxygen present; rat muscle is able to degrade all the glycogen and produce lactic acid much faster than human muscle. Dr. Wilkie felt that the argument was pointless in that Dr. Bárány had emphasized that he was working with postmortem material and with caffeine stimulated muscle that bypasses the action potential and calcium release mechanisms. His own group, studying intact human muscles, had obtained values of lactate production of 30 mmols/kg/min similar to that found with other methods. Recently he has been using 31 P NMR to study brain metabolism in intact infants; he would like to use 13 C and proton NMR to get better quality spectra, but too much energy is involved in decoupling the protons in the case of 13 C NMR, and the water suppression techniques that Dr. Bárány used also involve decoupling energy that will be turned into heat, theoretically leading to problems in performing studies on infant brains. Dr. Bárány replied that the newer NMR machines were capable of producing high quality records with less and less energy.

Dr. Jones found it interesting that a peak for fatty acids was shown on one of the slides (this is not described in the paper), and he wondered whether this enabled muscle fat utilization to be measured in such situations as Mc-Ardle's syndrome, where glycogen is unavailable for energy metabolism. Dr. Bárány answered that his group had carried out studies on hibernating frogs, in which glycogen and ATP fall during the winter. When muscle is placed in the NMR tube, peaks are seen that are not seen in other situations and are related to fatty acids, most likely produced by the degradation of phospholipids. This is indicated by results with 13 C NMR, which allows differentiation between phospholipid and neutral fat for the origin of fatty acid. The peak height ratio of the 130 to 128 ppm resonances is about 1 for the fatty acid of phospholipid but 4 for that of neutral fat. The peak height ratio, close to 1, in the 13 C spectrum of the starving frog shows that the fatty acid is derived from phospholipid.

References

Bárány, M. (1967). ATPase activity of myosin correlated with speed of muscle shortening. *Journal of General Physiology,* **50** (Suppl., Pt. 2), 197-218.

11

Application of Principles of Metabolic Control to the Problem of Metabolic Limitations in Sprinting, Middle Distance, and Marathon Running

E.A. Newsholme
University of Oxford

Knowledge of the factors involved in the provision of energy for muscle and those that might limit performance has been accrued largely through the work of physiologists and biochemists who are primarily interested in chemical and biophysical apsects of energy provision. Another field of biochemistry, which has only recently been applied to exercise, is that of regulation and integration of metabolism and metabolic pathways. Application of knowledge from this field to the question of the control of fuel supply for exercising muscle leads to some new insights into metabolic limitations in sprinting, middle distance running, and the marathon. For further details on these points, readers are recommended to consult Newsholme and Leech (1983a, 1983b).

Simple observations concerning athletic performance raise very important questions about the limitations in these running events. In a short sprint (60-100 m) the maximum speed of the runner is around 23 mph, which is achieved within a few seconds. However, the sprinter can maintain this high power output only for very short periods and is exhausted well within 60 s. The marathon runner runs at a speed of only about half of that of the sprinter (11-12 mph) but maintains it for about 9,000 s, or about 150 times longer than the sprinter. Can knowledge of metabolic regulation explain this difference? A further important point is that the training regime recommended by most coaches for middle and long distance runners is quite different. Is it possible to explain this difference?

Integration of Metabolism and Limitations in Sprinting

To understand the metabolic limitations in sprinting, it is important to appreciate that sprinting probably evolved as an escape reaction and consequently involves a violent burst of effort, which is needed only for a short time. The obvious requirement for such an activity is the immediate availability of energy to power maximum muscular activity. This is achieved more effectively from anaerobic metabolism. If the energy was obtained from aerobic metabolism, a large flow of blood would have to pass through the muscles continuously, placing a heavy work load on the heart. (Aerobic muscles do not suffer from this problem because their blood supply is much reduced at rest and takes several minutes to increase fully when the muscles are exercised—delay not acceptable in an escape mechanism.) A further advantage in shifting to anaerobic metabolism is that mitochondria are no longer required, and this makes even more space available in the fibre for myofibrils, which means more power and therefore more speed and a greater chance to escape from the predator. Similarly, only a few arteries and veins are required so that more space is available for muscle fibres and hence a greater power output by the muscle.

Fuels for Sprinting

Our knowledge of metabolic biochemistry tells us what fuels can be used under anaerobic conditions: These are phosphocreatine and glycogen in the muscle (see Table 1). Phosphocreatine may be considered as the "fast fuel." It is present in muscle at a high concentration, providing an immediate reserve for the resynthesis of ATP. In a single reaction, catalysed by the enzyme creatine kinase, phosphocreatine phosphorylates ADP to form ATP and thus replenishes the ATP used in contraction. (After the exercise, phosphocreatine is resynthesised by reversal of the same reaction.) It can be calculated that the amount of phosphocreatine in muscle of man provides energy for about 5 s of full-speed sprinting (i.e., about 50-60 m). Its particular importance is that it can be used instantaneously to regenerate ATP, thus allowing time for the more complex glycolytic process to come into operation.

The conversion of glycogen to lactic acid can occur in the absence of oxygen and can generate ATP. Because a large amount of glycogen is stored in the muscle, considerably more ATP can be produced from degradation of glyco-

Table 1. Fuels of the sprinter

Sprint distance (m)	Major fuel used
100	Phosphocreatine plus glycogen
200	Glycogen
400	Glycogen plus glucose

gen than from the utilization of phosphocreatine. However, there are two drawbacks. First, in the absence of oxygen, each molecule of glucose l-phosphate produced from glycogen is converted not to pyruvate for entry into the Krebs cycle but to two molecules of lactate plus almost two protons. Unless removed, these protons will alter the internal environment of the muscle fibre and result in fatigue and exhaustion. Secondly, for every glucose unit in glycogen that is converted to lactic acid, only three molecules of ATP are produced compared with the 39 that would have been produced if it had been fully oxidized to carbon dioxide and water (see Table 2). The solution to this problem is simply for muscle to possess a high capacity for glycolysis and to use this capacity to compensate for the reduced efficiency. Indeed, the muscle fibres of sprinters possess a high capacity for glycolysis. Unfortunately, this exacerbates the problem of proton accumulation because, to produce sufficient ATP to power contraction, the rate of glycolysis must approach maximal so that large quantities of protons rapidly accumulate.

Table 2: Yield of ATP From Various Fuels Under Aerobic and Anaerobic Conditions

Fuel	Conditions	ATP Yield (mol) per mol of Fuel Utilized
Glucose	Aerobic, complete oxidation	38
Glucose	Anaerobic, conversion to lactate	2
Glycogen	Aerobic, complete oxidation	39
Glycogen	Anaerobic, conversion to lactate	3
Palmitate	Aerobic, complete oxidation	129

It seems very likely that for 100-m sprinters all the ATP is generated from phosphocreatine degradation plus anaerobic glycolysis, but for the 200- and especially the 400-m sprint, the importance of the oxidative processes increases. It seems likely that for the total energy required by the 400-m run, about 50% will be obtained from the oxidation of pyruvate, which has been derived from glucose or more likely glycogen. Despite this the rate of formation of lactate will be about tenfold greater than that of the oxidation process so that the accumulation of protons is still large. There are two advantages in having some of the energy produced aerobically. First, the generation of ATP is much more efficient so that less glycogen is degraded to provide the ATP. Secondly, and probably more importantly, to provide sufficient oxygen, the blood supply to the muscle must increase, allowing protons in the form of lactic acid to diffuse out of the muscle into the bloodstream where it can be removed. The importance of this phenomenon in delaying the onset of fatigue is described below.

Protons and Athletic Performance

Knowledge of the cause of fatigue in sprinters is of interest not only to the handful of competitive sprinters but to almost all athletes: It is the cause of fatigue in almost all popular sports and other physical activities. In relation to the number of people involved, it is vastly more important than fatigue in marathon runners—despite the extensive coverage of this latter subject in running journals. The person returning home from a job involving physical activity, the woman who has taken the dog for a walk, the man who has chopped logs for the fire, the father who has played a few vigorous games with his children— all suffer from the same cause of fatigue as does the Olympic 400-meter champion: the accumulation of protons.

Protons readily combine with negatively charged ions, including those present in proteins, as follows:

$$\text{protein}^- + H^+ \rightarrow \text{protein} - H$$

Many proteins have special functions in the cell (such as catalysis), which depend on their being in a particular state of ionisation. An increase in the concentration of protons can alter this state so that their function is impaired, in some cases irreversibly. The importance of the increase in proton concentration is emphasized by the simple fact that we have enough muscle glycogen and a sufficient capacity of anaerobic glycolysis to produce a massive quantity of protons—sufficient to kill ourselves in less than 1-2 min. A calculation shows that during an exhaustive 400-m race, enough protons might be produced from the conversion glycogen to lactate to lower the pH of the blood and muscle to below pH 2.0. But measurements show that the muscle pH actually falls from pH 7.0 to about pH 6.0, and that of the blood from pH 7.4 to about pH

6.9. The difference is explained by the existence of buffers that remove protons and so reduce the extent of a pH change. Buffers are present in muscle fibres themselves; they include proteins, phosphate, bicarbonate, and some amino acids and peptides. However, the largest buffer in the body is found in the blood and extracellular fluid; this is the bicarbonate/carbon dioxide system. The bicarbonate ion combines with a proton from a molecule of carbonic acid:

$$HCO_3^- + H^+ \rightarrow H_2CO_3$$

This buffer system, fortunately, is much more efficient than would appear from this reaction. The product of the reaction between bicarbonate and protons, carbonic acid, is broken down in the bloodstream and in the lungs to produce carbon dioxide and water in a reaction catalysed by the enzyme carbonic anhydrase.

$$H_2CO_3 \rightarrow H_2O + CO_2$$

The complete buffer reaction can therefore be described as follows:

$$HCO_3^- + H^+ \rightarrow H_2CO_3 \rightarrow CO_2 + H_2O$$

The system is further improved because the carbon dioxide is removed from the body via the lungs, whereas the bicarbonate ion is added to the blood by the kidneys. Hence, the buffering system is a dynamic one, converting the dangerous protons into water and carbon dioxide.

The efficiency of this buffer system together with the efficiency of aerobic metabolism explains why, except perhaps for the 100-m sprint, it is enormously advantageous from a metabolic point of view to increase the flow of blood to the muscle. It is likely that in races under 5,000 m, and indeed even in this race, some of the energy is obtained from conversion of glycogen to lactate plus protons so that the buffering system described above is vitally important.

How does an increase in proton concentration in muscle result in fatigue? The answer in biochemical terms is still not known, although there are many hypotheses. Protons may interfere in the link between the nervous stimulation of muscle and contraction (the excitation-contraction coupling process). Calcium ions are known to be intimately involved in this link within the muscle so that it would not be too surprising if a high concentration of protons (H^+) interfered with the biochemical actions of calcium ions within the muscle.

Limitations in Sensitivity of Control Mechanisms in Sprinting

One major problem in sprinting is that the enormous demand for energy, which is supplied by the inefficient process of glycolysis, requires that the rate of the process of glycolysis must increase by more than 1,000-fold during sprinting. This causes a major problem for the control of enzymes that catalyse non-equilibrium reactions, namely phosphorylase, 6-phosphofructokinase, and pyruvate kinase. It is likely that one important factor in improving sensitivity is the operation of substrate cycles between glycogen and glucose l-phosphate, phosphoenolpyruvate and pyruvate, and fructose 6-phosphate and fructose bisphosphate (Newsholme & Leech, 1983b). The latter cycle is used to illustrate the principle.

The presence of fructose diphosphatases in a wide variety of muscles from many different species in the animal kingdom has led to the suggestion that this enzyme plays a role in the regulation of glycolysis via the operation of a substrate cycle between fructose 6-phosphate and fructose diphosphate. The role of this cycle in muscle of human subjects is considered to be to increase the sensitivity of metabolic control at the level of fructose 6-phosphate phosphorylation to changes in the concentrations of the regulators of 6-phosphofructokinase. Because of the problem of hyperthermia, which results from high rates of cycling, it is suggested that when the subject is in the basal metabolic state, the rate of cycling will be very low. However, when exercise is anticipated, the rate of cycling will be raised so that the sensitivity of the metabolic control system is increased. Thus, it is predicted that for the sprinter in his blocks, the blood levels of the stress hormones, epinephrine and norepinephrine, will be raised to increase markedly the rate of cycling. Evidence has now been obtained that the rate of this cycle can be increased by catecholamines—at least in rat muscle incubated *in vitro* (Challiss, Arch, & Newsholme, 1984). A high cycling rate/flux ratio for the phosphorylation of fructose 6-phosphate while the sprint runner is in his blocks waiting for the gun is important because the reaction will now be very sensitive to changes in the concentrations of the regulators of phosphofructokinase. Once the sprint is under way, the rate of ATP hydrolysis will increase markedly; this will lead to decreases in the concentrations of creatine phosphate, ATP, and citrate, and to increases in the concentrations of AMP, phosphate, and NH_4^+. This, in turn, will increase the activity of phosphofructokinase toward its maximum. Such a procedure will ensure that the rate of energy production via anaerobic glycolysis will increase precisely to the high rate required to satisfy the demand for ATP utilization by the contractile process. It is suggested that one reason for the remarkable performances of elite sprint runners is that metabolic control mechanisms are so well developed they provide maximum sensitivity when required in the control of the energy-producing pathways in muscle. Some aspects of the training of sprinters, particularly "start-training," may in fact be increasing the capacity of such cycles and perhaps their sensitivity to hormones such as the catecholamines.

Integration of Metabolism and Metabolic Limitations in the Marathon

The provision of fuels for the marathon probably differs from that of every other race. The energy required by the marathon runner is obtained by oxidation of the two major fuels, carbohydrate and fat. Knowledge of the biochemical mechanism for mobilization of fatty acids and the relationship between carbohydrate and fat metabolism should be of importance to every athlete and every coach.

Carbohydrate

Carbohydrate is stored in the body in both the liver and muscle as a polymer of glucose that is known as glycogen. In muscle, glycogen can be degraded to a compound that enters directly into the energy-producing system. In the liver, glycogen is broken down to glucose, which is released into the blood-stream where it is available as a fuel for all organs of the body, including muscle. It is important to appreciate that some organs have an absolute requirement for glucose so that the level of this fuel in the blood be maintained. If blood glucose was used at a high rate for any sustained period by muscle, it could lower the blood glucose concentration sufficiently to cause hypoglycemia, in which the function of the brain is jeopardized. This means that as the glucose is used by muscle, it must be replaced by glucose released from the liver.

The liver contains about 100 g and muscle about 350 g of glycogen. The demand for energy by an elite marathon runner is such that if it could be provided only from glycogen, it would last for *less than* 90 minutes. The available evidence suggests that liver glycogen runs out before muscle glycogen and that physical exhaustion coincides with muscle glycogen stores reaching low levels. Further, it is known that the time taken to exhaustion is directly proportional to the amount of glycogen in the muscles at the beginning of the run. Nonetheless, since the total marathon distance cannot be run on glycogen, an additional fuel must be used at the same time as the carbohydrate. This fuel is fatty acid.

Fat

Fat is composed of triglyceride molecules, which are stored in fat cells in adipose tissue. Unlike most other tissues, adipose tissue does not occur as a discrete organ but is widely distributed throughout the body (e.g., beneath the skin; around the major organs; in men, at the front of the abdominal cavity; and in women, in the breasts, upper thighs, and buttocks). In complete contrast to the stores of carbohydrates, there are sufficient triglyceride reserves in the average man to last for three days and three nights of marathon running. So why does exhaustion occur so early in the marathon? To answer this question, we must understand how the fat store is made available to the muscle and what limits its rate of utilization.

The triglyceride molecules in the fat cell must be broken down to fatty acids before they leave the cell to enter the blood. Unfortunately, they are insoluble in the blood and can only be transported in combination with albumin, one of the blood proteins. This is identical in principle to the transport of oxygen in combination with hemoglobin in the blood. It is this combination of protein and fatty acids that restricts the rate of utilization of this fuel. The albumin combines tightly with the fatty acid molecules when they are released by the fat cell, and in this form they are transported to the muscle via the bloodstream. Although the binding is tight, the complex breaks up in the blood during passage through working muscles. This is because of the continual oxidation and thus very low concentration of fatty acids within the muscle cells. This transport mechanism is very effective because a large quantity of fatty acid can be transported rapidly from the adipose tissue stores to the muscle. However, a price must be paid. The price is a limitation in the rate of fatty acid oxidation by muscle. This is caused by the low rate of diffusion of fatty acids from the albumin complex into the muscle cell and hence the low concentration of fatty acids in the muscle. Evidence suggests that this low rate of diffusion restricts fatty acid oxidation by muscle to such an extent that it can provide only a proportion, about 50%, of the maximum demand for energy by muscle. The evidence in support of this view is as follows:

- If the body's store of carbohydrate is depleted prior to a run (e.g., a low carbohydrate diet), endurance is decreased; that is, despite the large stores of fat, exhaustion occurs very early in an endurance event after the runner has been on a low-carbohydrate diet.
- If the body's store of carbohydrate is increased prior to a run (e.g. by a high carbohydrate diet), endurance is increased. Most marathon runners attempt various dietary tricks to increase the glycogen level in the muscle prior to a run.
- In ultradistance running (that is, distances greater than the marathon), the power output gradually declines to about 50% of the maximum as fat becomes the dominant fuel in the later stages of the run.
- The maximum ability to take up oxygen during running is about half of what is expected in patients suffering from an inability to oxidise glucose and who are, therefore, dependent solely on fatty acid oxidation.

The general conclusion is, therefore, that fatty acids *are* used during sustained running but that the maximum rate at which they can be used is limited to about 50% of the maximum rate of energy utilization required to support maximum running speed. The difference is made up by oxidation of carbohydrate, either in the form of muscle glycogen or glucose from the bloodstream.

Controlling the Correct Mixture of Fuels

The facts presented so far lead us to the view that the marathon runner should be using a mixture of fuels, fat, and carbohydrate for the whole of the race. At first sight, however, this presents difficulties. Prior to the race the concentration of fatty acids in the bloodstream will be low because the athlete will be rested and will have eaten, at least some hours before the start of the race, and will have been on a high carbohydrate diet prior to the race so that most tissues will be using glucose. Even during the race the concentration of fatty acids in the blood, although it will rise, will not exceed that of glucose, so one might very reasonably think that glucose would be used in preference to fatty acids. But it isn't. When glucose and fatty acids are both available to the muscle, the fatty acids are oxidized in preference. Even more important to the runner is the fact that a control system ensures as much fatty acid oxidation as possible takes place, up to about 50% of the maximum oxygen uptake, but that the remainder of the energy is generated by the oxidation of blood glucose or muscle glycogen. It is a mechanism that always allows a mixture of fuels, carbohydrate, and fat to be burnt provided both are available. The advantage of this is that it "spares" carbohydrate so that the limited stores will last longer.

The importance of the mechanism is further emphasized by the fact that an elite runner, using only glucose as a source of energy, requires more than 5 g of glucose each minute to maintain the speed of 11-12 mph. This rate of glucose utilization would remove all the glucose from the bloodstream (about 3 g) in less than one minute.

Exhaustion occurs in the marathon runner when the glycogen store in the muscle is totally depleted. This means that ATP can no longer be synthesized from oxidation of carbohydrate; it can be obtained only from the oxidation of fatty acid. But the latter can provide only about half the energy required. The pace must be decreased by 50%. This means that for an elite runner, with a normal pace of 11-12 mph, the pace will fall to 5-6 mph or just above fast walking. This, for the elite runner, is exhaustion.

The long training runs (20-plus miles) are so necessary for the marathon runner because this trains the metabolic mechanism for the precise mobilization of fatty acids from adipose tissue and for the regulation of the rate of glucose utilization in relation to the rate of fatty acid oxidation. Failure of either of these mechanisms could result in higher rates of utilization of glycogen and hence an earlier onset of fatigue.* The integration between carbohydrate and fat metabolism also explains one further fact that is well known to marathon runners and coaches. A period of starvation for at least 4 h (some runners prefer to starve for 12 h) is advantageous; only water should be taken. Even fluid containing sugar or carbohydrate should be avoided. The reason for this is that ingestion of any carbohydrate increases the rate of secretion of insulin, which raises the plasma level of this hormone, and this prevents the mobilization of fatty acid from adipose tissue. This means that more glycogen has to be used in the early part of the marathon, and thus increases the risk that glycogen stores will be depleted well before the end of the marathon.

Metabolic Integration and Limitations in Middle Distance Running

Runners of distances below about 3,000 m probably make use of both aerobic and anaerobic processes; that is, glucose will be completely oxidized via Krebs cycle but, in addition, some glycogen will be degraded to lactate. Some lactate and proton production can occur without the risk of fatigue because the better blood supply in middle distance runners will allow continuous removal of lactic acid into the blood where it can be effectively buffered and eventually removed by oxidation in other muscles such as the heart or reconverted to glucose via gluconeogenesis in the liver. This will allow the sprint type of fibres to contribute to the power output of the middle distance runner and, because they have a greater power output than the endurance fibres, it may be advantageous for middle distance runners to possess muscles with both types of fibers.

Physiological studies suggest that the rate of oxygen consumption of the muscles in 5,000- and 10,000-m runners probably limits performance. Consequently, much of the training is directed towards improving the blood supply to the muscles. One biochemical factor is, in addition, of considerable importance: For the same amount of ATP generation, the oxidation of fat requires about 10% more oxygen than does the oxidation of carbohydrate so that oxidation of fat would be detrimental to performance. Consequently, unlike the marathon runner, the middle distance runner should *not* mobilize the fat stores. If the blood fatty acid level is elevated, this will ensure that some fatty acid is oxidized and, because of the control mechanisms described above, fewer

---

*It is likely that, in normal sedentary man who eats three good meals a day, there is not normally any reason to mobilize fatty acid from the fat stores, except in stress. Long runs or periods of starvation that deplete liver glycogen stores are essential to "train" the fatty acid mobilization mechanism.

carbohydrates will be used. To maintain the same power output, a greater rate of oxygen consumption will need to occur or, if this is not possible, some energy will need to be obtained by the less efficient anaerobic system. Either will be detrimental to performance. One factor that causes mobilization of fatty acids is stress and nervous tension. Before an important race, nervous stress should be controlled as far as possible by the middle distance runner.

This may explain the benefits that are claimed for relaxation exercises and yoga performed by some athletes prior to such races. Another factor that causes mobilization of fatty acids is a period of starvation, whereas carbohydrate intake decreases the rate of fatty acid mobilization. It is therefore suggested that, in contrast to the practice of marathon runners, a small quantity of carbohydrate should be ingested perhaps 30-60 min before the race.

References

Challiss, R.A.J., Arch, J.R.S., & Newsholme, E.A. (1984). The rate of substrate cycling between fructose 6-phosphate and fructose 1, 6-bisphosphate in skeletal muscle. *Biochemical Journal, 221*, 153-161.

Newsholme, E.A., & Leech, A.R. (1983a). *The runner: Energy and endurance.* Roosevelt, NJ: Fitness Books.

Newsholme, E.A., & Leech, A.R. (1983b). *Biochemistry for the medical sciences.* Chichester, England: John Wiley & Sons.

Discussion

Dr. Green opened the discussion by questioning the widely held belief that the higher the exercise intensity the greater the proportion of carbohydrate utilization. The studies of Essén, Hagenfeldt, and Kaijser (1977) showed that if the duration and intensity of the work bout are carefully chosen, a substantial utilization of free fatty acids may be shown to occur. Some years ago his own group published a study in which subjects exercised at 90% to 95% of VO_2max for 6 min with 54 min of rest. The exercise was carried out once every hour for 12 h with no carbohydrate replacement allowed to force muscles into a low glycogen state; plasma free fatty acids increased, and although oxygen uptake did not change, carbon dioxide output fell, indicating a high proportion of free fatty acid utilization. Thus, there is no doubt that fats can be used in heavy exercise, but there may be a limit to the extent that they may provide fuel for exercise, and the duration of exercise also appears to play a part. Dr. Hultman added that some of the studies have indicated that about 50% of the body's maximal fuel utilization may come from free fatty acids, but he also wondered where the limitation was. Although the circulation and diffusion might be limiting factors in supplying free fatty acids from adipose tissue, muscles have a lot of intracellular fat that is available for energy. Dr. Newsholme agreed and argued that if the limitation was the entry of fatty acids into muscle, then the capacity to use them, the beta oxidation capacity, would not in fact significantly exceed this delivery when adipose tissue lipolysis and blood flow were maximal. So even though intramuscular triglycerides are available, they are not in this situation additive to free fatty acids supplied from the blood stream and cannot be used at a higher rate than that of exogenous fatty acid. Because of the huge store of triglycerides in adipose tissue, it seems likely that this would be the usual source and the intramuscular pathway would be used only when the supply was inadequate for the needs. Intramuscular triglycerides would not be used in addition to exogenous fatty acids due to the site of the biochemical rate-limiting process.

Dr. MacDougall made the point that training increased muscle fat, and Dr. Howald had shown that muscle triglycerides may be almost completely depleted after long distance races. He asked if there were estimates of the total fat available in muscle. Dr. Howald indicated that his group measured intracellular lipid using morphometric methods and found a content in untrained muscle of only 0.5%. There is about 1.0% in well-trained long distance runners, about 2.0% in ultra-marathon runners, and 3.0% in top-class professional cyclists. In one study of runners taking part in a 100 km run, they showed a 75% decrease in intracellular fat after the race. In addition to these differences in fat storage, the enzymes involved in beta oxidation of free fatty acids are also increased with endurance training. Dr. Newsholme asked how much of the total energy needs might be provided by intracellular fat in a marathon runner; Dr. Howald estimated it to be about 25% of the total fat oxidized, with the rest coming from adipose tissue. Dr. Hultman mentioned that muscle biopsies taken before and after marathon runs were examined for fat content by chemical means, but the variability was so high that it was impossible to show utilization reliably.

Dr. Bárány had measured free fatty acids in human muscle by gas chromatography and found values of 1 micromole per g of muscle, compared to about 100 micromoles of glucose. With 14 C-labelled fatty acids, they found that little goes into the muscle under resting conditions compared to the liver. He doubted that fatty acids would be readily mobilized from neutral fats and then enter muscle in significant amounts in a running leg. Dr. Newsholme did not agree and quoted the studies of Wahren and his collaborators in Stockholm who have shown marked uptake of free fatty acids by the muscles (Felig & Wahren, 1975; Hagenfeldt & Wahren, 1972). These measurements suggested that about 65% of the total oxygen requirements were being provided by fatty acids, but of course these studies were done at only moderate workloads. Dr. Bárány expressed surprise at this conclusion in that there appeared to be enough glycogen in order to provide all the energy needs for running. Dr.

Newsholme replied that if one does these calculations, it is clear that in addition to muscle glycogen, fat is required in order to run a marathon (Newsholme & Leech, 1983). The extent to which the glycogen stores may be expanded by various dietary manoeuvres is still a controversial area; there is not doubt that glycogen loading may be extremely effective in terms of improving endurance, probably increasing liver glycogen as well as muscle glycogen. Dr. Hultman has shown that liver glycogen is extensively mobilized in running.

Dr. Green brought up the question of the role played by beta receptors in glycogenolysis and the substrate cycling that Dr. Newsholme described. He also asked if cycling occurred mainly in fast twitch fibers. Dr. Newsholme did not know of any direct evidence that muscles increase their oxygen consumption under the influence of catecholamines. There is no doubt that total oxygen uptake may be increased by injecting beta agonists, and several pharmaceutical firms would like to make their fortune through the marketing of agents that would increase oxygen consumption and act as antiobesity agents.

Dr. Green wondered whether there was any possibility that the forward reaction in a cycle could be in excess of a backward reaction at rest, thus leading to an excess of lactic acid before exercise occurred; several subjects studied by his group had high resting muscle lactate concentrations. Dr. Newsholme felt that this was quite likely.

Dr. Hultman pointed out that various agents that stimulate fatty acid mobilization, such as caffeine, heparin, and fat ingestion, decrease glycogen utilization. Beta blockade and nicotinic acid have the opposite effect. He wondered to what extent acetate formation could be a limiting reaction. Dr. Newsholme pointed out that there was normally a delay in the mobilization of fatty acids; for example, in Dr. Wahren's work it took 2 to 3 hr to increase plasma free fatty acid levels to a maximum of around 1.8 m mol/litre. If fat mobilization can be increased, carbohydrates will be spared.

Dr. Stauber asked if the limitation of free fatty acid use was in relation to diffusion distance from the capillary into the cell and if there might be specific sites of fat utilization. Dr. Newsholme pointed out that in a cross-section of muscle many mitochondria are seen close to the capillaries, and it seems likely that free fatty acids would be used just below the surface. Of course, there is possibly a transport protein system inside the muscle that encourages movement of free fatty acid within the muscle fiber, but that is really unknown. Capillary density of muscle would also be important in relation to muscle fiber size.

Dr. Stauber wondered why Dr. Newsholme had not commented on protein utilization, as Dr. J. Norbury has shown through constant infusion studies in humans that during a marathon run we may burn up to one third of the liver proteins. Dr. Newsholme found that an interesting question but wondered which tissues would be using the proteins. Is amino acid oxidation by muscle occurring or does gluconeogenesis by the liver occur to produce glucose under these conditions? He felt that gluconeogenesis from amino acids might add an extra dimension to the system that had not been addressed quantitatively yet. If amino acid oxidation does occur in muscle, the major amino acids oxidized are the branched chain amino acids. The maximum capacity of branched chain amino acid dehydrogenases has been measured in skeletal muscle and shows that these reactions could contribute no more than a few percent of the total energy requirements (Newsholme & Leech, 1983).

Dr. Thoden felt there was no question that there is a great potential for muscle to take up fatty acids; turnover studies have shown that about 20% of the total fuel for a marathon run may come from blood-borne fatty acids with little effect of a glycogen super compensation diet. Dr. Newsholme pointed out again that this could indicate that a significant amount of triglycerides in muscle was being used, which might possibly cause a dilution of the radioactive label. Recent studies in his laboratory have shown that there is a significant amount of cycling going on between triglycerides and fatty acids within the muscle itself. Consequently labelled free fatty acids find their way into triglycerides and therefore do not take part in metabolism and are not seen as labelled carbon dioxide. The rate of the process was thought to be rather slow. Dr. Thoden pointed out that he had calculated that 15% to 16% of energy needs came from free fatty acids in blood, and that allowing for recycling this might go up to 20% to 25%, still a low proportion of the total. Dr. Newsholme suggested that this was very low compared to the findings of Felig and Wahren (1975).

References

Essén, B., Hagenfeldt, L., & Kaijser, L. (1977). Utilization of blood-borne and intramuscular substrates during continuous and intermittent exercise in man. *Journal of Physiology* (London), **265**, 489-506.

Felig, P., & Wahren, J. (1975). Fuel homeostasis in exercise. *New England Journal of Medicine*, **293**, 1078-1084.

Hagenfeldt, L., & Wahren, J. (1972). Human forearm muscle metabolism during exercise. *Scandinavian Journal of Clinical and Laboratory Investigation*, **30**, 429-436.

Newsholme, E.A., & Leech, A.R. (1983). *Biochemistry for the medical sciences*. Chichester, England: John Wiley and Sons.

Newsholme, E.A., & Leech, A.R. (1983). *The runner*. Roosevelt, NJ: Fitness Books.

12

Power Output of Man; The Contributions Made by Lars Hermansen

Bengt Saltin, Philip D. Gollnick, Loring B. Rowell, and Ole M. Sejersted
University of Copenhagen

Exercise physiology can be many things. For some, it describes the stress and demands of performing various forms of physical activity or sports. For others, it defines and measures man's ability to perform mechanical work. It is also the study of the adaptive response of an organ as it is repetitively used in a particular physical activity or when it becomes inactive. Exercise physiology also uses work to stress bodily functions, thereby giving us a unique tool to study both regulatory mechanisms and the limits of regulation.

Looking back in time to the beginnings of exercise physiology, one can see that its founders covered many of the different aspects in the field and, in fact, made very significant contributions in all of these. Today, specialization and methodological developments have made it difficult for most researchers to try to cover more than one facet of the broad area of exercise research. Lars Hermansen, in keeping with the Scandinavian tradition in human physiology, was one of the last, perhaps the last, who contributed significantly to all the more important fields of exercise physiology. Starting with intact man and assessing the maximal oxygen uptake of various ethnic groups, he then carefully investigated methods of determining maximal aerobic power, as well as studying the limiting factors in the oxygen transport chain and the regulation of the circulation. Man's ability to perform work is not only a function of oxygen uptake and an aerobic energy yield: anaerobic energy metabolism can also play a very important role in work performance. No one has studied the magnitude of the anaerobic capacity of man and the broad range of consequences and physiological implications of lactate accumulation as thoroughly as Lars. In this review, we will try to give some insight into Lars' broad contributions to the study of human physiology, bearing in mind the themes of the symposium of human muscle power and the factors underlying maximal performance.

Man and His Environment

In the sixties, many biologists took an interest in how various ethnic groups had adapted to their environment. At this time, Lars had just finished his M.Sc. degree in animal physiology at Oslo University and was recruited by Kristian Lange Andersen to join him and Robert Elsner in the search for mechanisms and range of human adaptations. They studied man living in remote areas, exposed to low temperatures, and dependent on hunting and fishing for survival. The studies included measurements of physical working capacity as well as energetic and circulatory responses to cold exposure. The very first study in a long series was to investigate arctic indians living in Northern Canada (Elsner, Lange Andersen, & Hermansen, 1960). They were studied in the fall and then restudied in the early spring after a long, cold winter. The metabolic response to sleeping one night at a room temperature of 2-4°C as well as various skin temperatures were determined. In this study, little to no seasonal variation was observed in the cold stress responses. Indeed, not only were the metabolic rates during the cold stress the same in the fall and spring, but skin temperatures of fingers, toes, and torso were similarly low in both studies. In fact, the overall results reported in this study, as well as those from many other similar investigations, led to the conclusion that man living in the arctic or similar climates was not particularly cold acclimatized (i.e., neither metabolism nor blood flow to the limbs was elevated in the cold, and skin temperatures were as low as those of urban man exposed to cold). The lack of demonstrable cold adaptation in arctic man can probably be explained, at least in part, by the fact that clothing has been and is the decisive factor for survival in the arctic. The determination of physical working capacity of man has been an integrated part of this worldwide biological programme. Studies have included not only people living in remote areas for generations, but also sedentary man living in industrialized countries (Lange Andersen, Elsner, Saltin, & Hermansen, 1962; Hermansen & Lange Andersen, 1965; Lange Andersen & Hermansen, 1965; Hermansen & Ekblom, 1966). It demonstrated that maximal oxygen uptake of a person was clearly linked to physical demands in daily life (Lange Andersen et al., 1962), and it was found that discreet differences in job tasks in a village or family were reflected in the observed level of physical working capacity. The largest effects were observed following voluntary physical activity in the daily life of urban man. Just as clear was that any change in the activity level of a person was soon manifested in a changed maximal oxygen uptake. Thus, man's fitness level was shown to be largely acquired, not simply inherited.

In this area of interest, Lars also made very elaborate studies on Norwegian school children living in rural and urban areas (Hermansen, 1973). Children of 10 or 13 years of age were selected and followed twice a year for three years, resulting in a detailed mapping of growth and physical working capacity in the years of adolescence through adulthood. It was demonstrated that Norwegian school children of both sexes were extremely fit; mean values of maximal oxygen uptake for both sexes average above 50 ml/kg $\times$ min^{-1} and approached and surpassed 60 ml/kg $\times$ min^{-1} in the older boys in the rural communities. Based on weight-adjusted maximal oxygen uptake values, it was found that Norwegian males peaked at an age of 16-19 years, whereas females reached their peak as early as 11-13 years. The maximal oxygen uptake (in 1 $\times$ min^{-1}) in females increased until the age of 16-18, but not enough to compensate for a weight gain. When school children from rural and urban areas were compared, a tendency for larger body weights and oxygen uptakes was observed in the rural areas, suggesting that more daily activity associated with living in the country made the children slightly fitter. Thus, the conclusion was that a physically active life was important during adolescence for fitness, although in a country like Norway, very few if any school children were in the risk zone of being underdeveloped physically due to lack of exercise.

How to Determine "True" Maximal Oxygen Uptake

During the studies of possible adaptations in primitive and urban man, Lars became interested in some basic methodological questions that had implications to our understanding of what limits maximal oxygen uptake $\dot{V}O_2$max. A series of experiments were conducted to evaluate differences between various forms of exercise and maximal oxygen uptake (Hermansen & Saltin, 1969; Hermansen, Ekblom, & Saltin, 1970). Exhaustive cycle exercise gave an average of 8% lower values for maximal oxygen uptake than running on a treadmill. In particular, running uphill was shown to be a safe and efficient way of eliciting the highest $\dot{V}O_2$max. An explanation of why running gave higher $\dot{V}O_2$max values than cycling was difficult to find; a difference in the muscle mass involved extensively in each mode of exercise was unlikely. One important observation was that the oxygen pulse was significantly higher during submaximal and maximal exercise when running. This could have been due to a larger stroke volume or a larger oxygen extraction. Steps were, therefore, taken to study central hemodynamics during running and cycling, and at all exercise levels stroke volume was found to be slightly larger ($\approx 5\%$) in running than in cycling. At submaximal exercise intensities, cardiac output was essentially the same in both forms of exercise, resulting in a slightly lower heart rate during running at a given oxygen uptake than during cycling. During maximal exercise, the larger stroke volume in running gave rise to a slightly larger cardiac output, as heart rate was similar in cycling and running. Any answer to the crucial question of why stroke volume was larger in running than cycling could hardly be given. Filling pressures were not measured, but there was no obvious reason why they should differ. Another possibility could have been a lower arterial blood pressure; in fact, a tendency for it to be lower in running was observed. Thus, the afterload would seem to be less in running than in cycling. Furthermore, the work of the heart, as judged by the double product (HR $\times$ BP), was quite similar in the two exercise forms during maximal exercise. The overall conclusion then was that a critical minimal amount of muscle is involved in the exercise (leg-exercise), and any additional mass of muscle is not crucial for achieving a true $\dot{V}O_2$max. This was nicely confirmed in experiments in which subjects during exhaustive uphill walks on the treadmill added work by vigorously using ski poles; even though significantly higher $\dot{V}O_2$max values were obtained, the magnitude of this difference was only 2% and was therefore of little practical or biological significance (Hermansen, 1973)

What Limits Maximal Oxygen Uptake?

Detailed studies of several links in the oxygen transport from the sea of oxygen surrounding us to muscle mitochondria where it has its crucial role as a hydrogen acceptor are included in Lars' thesis work. In subjects with extremely high $\dot{V}O_2$max values, pulmonary ventilation was in the range of 200 l/min or above (Hermansen, 1973; Ekblom & Hermansen, 1968). This level of ventilation has been regarded as inefficient from two standpoints: One is that a large percentage of the oxygen uptake may be consumed by the respiratory muscles, and the other is the risk of desaturation of arterial blood, due to the very short transit time of the erythrocytes in the lungs. Both these objections can be argued against based on Lars' findings. First, power output was closely related to maximal oxygen uptake, even at the very highest pulmonary ventilation; this would not be the case if a large fraction of the oxygen was consumed by the respiratory muscles. Second, to the most critical question about complete saturation a clearcut answer can be given: That is, in all subjects arterial oxygen saturation was above 94% at peak exercise. The conclusion was drawn that ventilation could be excluded as a limiting factor.

What became so apparent from these studies, in which maximal cardiac output was determined in subjects representing a large range of $\dot{V}O_2$max values, was that a very close relationship existed between arterially-delivered oxygen and maximal oxygen uptake. Furthermore, as the values for heart rate and arterial oxygen content were quite similar in all subjects, the main determinant for the maximal oxygen uptake was the stroke volume. Bearing this in mind the heart became a likely candidate for limiting maximal oxygen uptake in man. Further support for this idea also came from longitudinal studies of the effect of physical conditioning on maximal oxygen uptake and central hemodynamics.

The role of the periphery was also evaluated, and some of the very first data on capillarization of muscles in man were produced by Lars. He could demonstrate that trained individuals had more capillaries per fibre than un-trained ones (Hermansen & Wachtlova, 1971) and that the best-trained subjects had the lowest peripheral resistance. The question then was whether the degree of vasodilation in the body during exhaustive short-term exercise was deter-mined by the capacity of the heart or whether the heart was able to supply an output sufficient to maintain arterial blood flow, regardless of the degree of vasodilation. Partly because of his findings on the importance of muscle mass for achieving a maximal oxygen uptake, Lars believed that the degree to which peripheral vascular beds could dilate was much larger than the capacity of the heart to fill them with a flow. Thus, according to Lars the heart was the limiting factor for maximal oxygen uptake, and the key to regulation was to maintain arterial blood pressure.

Reflex Control of the Circulation

For one year (1975-76) Lars Hermansen was a visiting scientist in the Depart-ment of Physiology and Biophysics at the University of Washington School of Medicine in Seattle. Lars was the recipient of a grant from the Fogarty Foundation and from the Perkins Fund of the American Physiological Society. For those of us who worked together with Lars in Seattle, his stay was an un-forgettable one.

Lars' arrival in Seattle coincided with the first experiments on a muscle reflex affecting the circulatory response to exercise (Rowell, Hermansen, & Blackmon, 1976). This reflex was presumed to be of a metabolic nature and thought to originate from chemosensitive nerves in skeletal muscle. The ques-tion was asked whether such reflexes could be graded in proportion to the degree of muscle ischemia or to the magnitude of metabolite accumulation in the working muscle. The first approach was to grade the intensity of leg exer-cise and measure the degree to which blood pressure rose during recovery when the circulation to the legs was occluded at the moment the exercise ceased. Lars argued for a protocol in which the intensity of exercise was kept constant, but the degree of ischemia was increased by occluding blood flow to the legs 10, 20, or 30 sec *before* the exercise stopped. As the occlusions con-tinued into post-exercise recovery, a graded pressor response to ischemia in working muscles was observed. Arrest of the circulation to resting muscle had no effect on blood pressure. It was further observed that the ischemic muscle pressor response was modulated during and after exercise by a vigorous arterial baroreflex that appeared to oppose the elevation in pressure in some cases and to support it in others, depending on the heart rate responses. This suggested that the operating point of the baroreflex must be changed, and subsequent studies supported this view.

Another area of study during Lars's stay in Seattle was related to the question of how arterial pressure was maintained when competing demands for skin and muscle blood flow exceeded the heart's ability to supply these tissues with a flow (Brengelmann, Johnson, Hermansen, & Rowell, 1977). We observed that skin blood flow, measured in the forearm, consistently approached an upper limit at values about one half of those measured at the same core temperature in the same subjects during supine rest. Our conclusion was that the break in the relationship of skin blood flow to internal temperature coincided with the point at which vasoconstrictive stimuli for blood pressure regulation began to overwhelm the progressive vasodilator influence of a rising core temperature. Although this study raised some important and still unanswered questions, it revealed that exercising, heat-stressed humans quickly reach a point when cutaneous blood flow and temperature regulation are sacrificed in order to maintain blood pressure.

Maximal Anaerobic Power

The assessment and significance of an anaerobic power in man was of great interest to Lars. Consequently, he devoted considerable effort to its measurement and its relevance to work capacity (Hermansen, 1969, 1971, 1977; Gollnick & Hermansen, 1973). His basic concept was that during high intensity exercise, a sizeable portion of the ATP consumed comes from metabolic processes that do not require an immediate consumption of oxygen. For an exercise that requires an energy consumption that is less than maximal, there exists in the early stages of the metabolic adjustment to exercise a delay in the rate of rise in $\dot{V}O_2$ such that a portion of the energy is derived from "anaerobic" mechanisms, which are usually named the "oxygen deficit." When exercise intensity exceeds the $\dot{V}O_2$max, a major portion of the energy must come from the anaerobic mechanism. Thus, the capacity of muscle to consume ATP during exercise exceeds that of the aerobic process; this is due in part to a limitation in the oxygen delivery system, which cannot keep pace. Quantitating the oxygen deficit is difficult, especially during exhaustive exercise. Lars and his group "solved" the problem by letting the subjects perform at various submaximal and maximal speeds on the treadmill (Hermansen & Medbo, 1984). By measuring the oxygen uptake throughout the exercise period, the oxygen consumed at any speed as well as the oxygen deficit could be estimated. This method demonstrated that the oxygen deficit could amount to a value as high as or higher than the $\dot{V}O_2$max of the subject. It was further shown that two minutes of exercise were needed to fully utilize a person's maximal anaerobic capacity. With both vigor and clear thinking, Lars attacked the problem of assessing anaerobic capacity and the mechanisms responsible for it, a problem replete with technical difficulties.

The phosphagens (ATP and CP) and the production lactate (La) are the most obvious sources of anaerobic energy. Because the phosphagen pool in muscle can account for only a small portion of maximal anaerobic energy production, Lars turned his attention to La production as the major source of anaerobic ATP production. This effort encompassed the areas of maximal La production, La removal after exercise, La as a substrate for glycogen synthesis by muscle, La production and pH, and pH and tension developing capacity of muscle.

Maximal Lactate Production

Instrumental in the continuation of this line of investigation was the development of the protocol of repeated exercise bouts, separated with short rest intervals, which results in the accumulation of very high concentrations of La in blood and muscle (Hermansen & Stensvold, 1972; Hermansen & Osnes, 1972; Osnes & Hermansen, 1972). Well aware that the concentration of La in blood or muscle does not account for all the La produced during a given period of exercise, and that with short-term exercise the distribution of La throughout the body is non-uniform, Lars demonstrated that the La concentration in blood could be driven up to levels between 22 and 32 mM with little difference observed between males and females. In spite of the many technical difficulties, he persisted in his efforts to find the role of La in muscle metabolism. He demonstrated that during exercise at altitude the onset of La production was shifted to the left of the $\dot{V}O_2$-La concentration relationship (Hermansen & Saltin, 1966). This was shown to be due to the reduction in the $\dot{V}O_2$max that occurs with exercise as a result of the lowered oxygen-carrying capacity of the blood; the latter is, in turn, produced by the depression in the PO_2 of atmospheric air because of the drop in barometric pressure at altitude. It was also demonstrated that the La production was linked to the percent of the $\dot{V}O_2$max (Hermansen & Stensvold, 1972). An important contribution to the study of the control of metabolism was made with the finding that, with training, the point of onset of La accumulation in blood was shifted to the right of the relative intensity—La curve, and that this shift was independent of the percent of the $\dot{V}O_2$max at which the exercise was being performed.

Lactate Removal

It is an old observation that the La in blood declines exponentially towards its rest value after exercise. Lars directed his attention to the mechanism responsible for this decline, asking the fundamental question: What is the fate of La after the termination of exercise? One of his earliest efforts in this field demonstrated that exercise during recovery enhanced the rate of La removal from blood (Hermansen & Stensvold, 1972; Hermansen et al., 1975). These findings had important practical implications for those wishing to speed up a return to the resting state after exercise. An analysis of the data concerning La removal from blood following exercise convinced Lars that it was not possible to account for all the La being cleared on the basis of its oxidation in other tissues or through glycogen synthesis via the Cori cycle in the liver. Indeed, the postexercise oxygen uptake could not account for the total amount of oxygen that would be required for this process. He was further impressed by the old reports of a synthesis of glycogen and a disappearance of La in the isolated muscles of frogs, and so forth, during recovery periods when oxygen was available to the tissue. From these older data, and his observations of a lack of concordance between the rate of La disappearance and its maximal rate of oxidation, he postulated that human skeletal muscle was capable of synthesizing glycogen directly from La. The first step in these studies was an examination of the venous-arterial difference for La across the leg following exercise that produced a large increase in blood La (Hermansen & Vaage, 1977). These data indicated that the rate of La release from the muscle was slow and that a significant amount of the La may have been removed from within the muscle by processes other than a release via diffusion. To continue these studies, muscle biopsies were taken from the leg muscles of subjects before and at intervals after completion of a series of heavy exercise bouts that produced major increases in blood La. Analysis of these samples revealed that the La concentration dropped rapidly in parallel with a rise in glycogen concentration. These data have opened the intriguing prospect that skeletal muscles possess the capacity to directly salvage the energy remaining in La by its resynthesis to glycogen (Hermansen & Vaage, 1979). These initial observations will undoubtedly spawn activity in this field.

Lactate Production and pH

Based on the magnitude of La production with repeated bouts of heavy exercise, it could be expected that a major shift in blood and muscle pH would occur. Lars launched some of the pioneering studies in this field (Hermansen & Osnes, 1972; Osnes & Hermansen, 1972). He demonstrated that muscle pH declined from a resting value of just below 7.0 to as low as 6.3. At the same time blood pH (including capillary blood) declined only to 7.1. These data illustrate the separation between intramuscular pH and that recorded in blood.

pH and Tension Developing Capacity of Muscle

The logical question that Lars asked after observing the large decrease in muscle pH as a consequence of heavy exercise was, "Does this have any effect on the contractile activity of muscle?" This work was performed while Lars was in Seattle, where he collaborated with Sue Donaldson. They designed and conducted experiments to determine the effects of low pH on the contractile characteristics of different types of skeletal muscle fibers (Donaldson & Hermansen, 1978; Hermansen, 1979). The ideal model for these studies was the isolated skinned fibres where diffusion barriers are eliminated. Using muscle fibres isolated from different types of muscle, they demonstrated that a reduction in pH from 7.0 to 6.5 produced a reduction in maximal tension from 12% to 30% with type II fibres being more sensitive to the reduced pH than the type I or cardiac muscle fibres. Of further interest was that the low oxidative type II fibres were more sensitive to a lowering of pH than the high oxidative type II fibres.

The studies to explain muscle fatigue and exhaustion were expanded by including studies on the interaction during intense exercise between lactate and pH changes on the one hand, and electrolyte shifts on the other (Sejersted, Medbo, & Hermansen, 1981; Sejersted et al., 1984; Sejersted, Medbo, Orheim, & Hermansen, 1984). Already in the very first studies it could be demonstrated that the efflux of K^+ from the exercising muscles was so large that an altered K^+ homeostasis in the muscle and the body were factors of major significance in the explanation of reduced muscle function. In the middle of these studies came Lars' untimely death, and the continuation of this project and others that Lars had begun will now have to depend on his young and very active collaborators.

Lars Hermansen: The Person, His Goals and Principles

Several in this meeting have met Lars Hermansen, and many have had the opportunity to work with him. We all know what an open and very friendly person Lars was, and many of us were privileged to be his close friends. Lars was a person who could inspire and stimulate, and he was always ready with help. Lars will be remembered for all this as well as his scientific contributions. But there is something more, not easy to define or describe. Maybe it is best exemplified by his struggle during his last years. Lars worked at the National Institute of Occupational Health in Oslo. The improvement of the work environment of people has, surprisingly enough, only recently been the focus of attention and today it has top priority in many industrialized countries. Although improvements have been achieved, many serious problems still remain unsolved and new ones are created due to modern technology. Despite the very dramatic reduction in the use of man for mechanical power output in industry during the last 150 years, discreet muscle disorders of the neck, shoulder, and back are major causes for complaints, sick leave, and early retirement (Hermansen, 1981). The problems are easy to register, but the fact that solutions may be far away is not so easy for workers or their representatives to understand or accept. Lars was concerned and deeply involved in tackling these problems. He realized that without knowing the cause for sore and aching muscles it was difficult to find any long lasting cure. His research strategy—for which he fought—was to learn more about the basic mechanisms of muscle function, and it thus became a struggle for basic science to gain acceptance in an applied field. This problem is not new. T.H. Huxley described it beautifully when in 1880 he gave the opening address at Birmingham's Institute of Technology:

> I often wish that this phrase, "applied science," had never been invented. For it suggests that there is a sort of scientific knowledge of direct practical use, which can be studied apart from another sort of scientific knowledge, which is of no practical utility, and which is termed "pure science." But there is no more complete fallacy than this. What people called applied science is nothing but the application of pure science to particular classes of problems. It consists of deductions from those general principles, established by reasoning and observation, which constitute pure science. No one can safely make these deductions until he has a firm grasp of the principles; and he can obtain that grasp only by personal experience of the operations of observation and of reasoning on which they are founded.

Our thanks go to Lars for the person he was, for his science, and for defending the very basic principles on which science has to rely, and on which all of us depend.

References

Brengelmann, G.L., Johnson, J.M., Hermansen, L., & Rowell, L.B. (1977). Altered control of skin blood flow during exercise at high internal temperatures. *Journal of Applied Physiology, 43*, 790-794.

Donaldson, S.K.B., & Hermansen, L. (1978). Differential, direct effects of H^+ on Ca^{2+}—activated force of skinned fibres from the soleus, cardiac and adductor magnus muscle of rabbits. *Pflügers Archives, 376*, 55-65.

Ekblom, B., & Hermansen, L. (1968). Cardiac output in athletes. *Journal of Applied Physiology, 25*, 619-625.

Elsner, R.W., Lange Andersen, K., & Hermansen, L. (1960). Thermal and metabolic responses of Arctic Indians to moderate cold exposure at the end of winter. *Journal of Applied Physiology, 15,* 659-661.

Gollnick, P.D., & Hermansen, L. (1973). Biochemical adaptations to exercise: anaerobic metabolism. In J.H. Wilmore (Ed.), *Exercise and Sports Sciences. Reviews.* Vol. 1. New York: Academic Press.

Hermansen, L. (1969). Anaerobic energy release. *Medicine and Science in Sports,* 1, 32-38.

Hermansen, L. (1971). Lactate production during exercise. In B. Saltin (Ed.), *Muscle metabolism during exercise.* New York: Plenum.
ation.

Hermansen, L. (1973). Oxygen transport during exercise in human subjects. *Acta Physiologica Scandinavica* (Suppl. 399).

Hermansen, L. (1977). Anaerobic energy metabolism during exercise. Norsk Idrettsmedisinsk Kongress, Beitostolen. *Snytex Terapi-serie nr. 2.*

Hermansen, L. (1979). Effect of acidosis on skeletal muscle performance during maximal exercise in man. *Bulletin de Physio-Pathologie Respiratoire,* 15, 229-238.

Hermansen, L. (1981). Muskel-skjelettsykdommer-Et stort sosialt og okonomisk problem. *Jernindustri nr.* 3, 91-95.

Hermansen, L., & Ekblom, B. (1966). Physical fitness of an arctic and a tropical population. In K. Evang & K. Lange Andersen (Eds.), *Physical activity in health and disease.* Oslo, Norway: Universitetsforlaget.

Hermansen, L., Ekblom, B., & Saltin, B. (1970). Cardiac output during submaximal and maximal treadmill and bicycle exercise. *Journal of Applied Physiology,* 29, 82-86.

Hermansen, L., & Lange Andersen, K. (1965). Aerobic work capacity in young Norwegian men and women. *Journal of Applied Physiology,* 20, 425-431.

Hermansen, L., Maehlum, S., Pruett, E.D.R., Vaage, O., Waldum, H., & Wessle-Aas, T. (1975). Lactate removal at rest and during exercise. In H. Poortmans (Eds.), *Prolonged Physical Exercise* 7, 101-105. Basel: Birkhauser Verlag.

Hermansen, L., & Medbo, J.I. (1984). The relative significance of aerobic and anaerobic processes during maximal exercise in man. In P. Marconnet & J. Poortmans (Eds.), *Medicine and sports science: Vol. 17. Physiological chemistry of training and detraining.* Basel: Karger.

Hermansen, L., & Osnes, J.-B. (1972). Blood and muscle pH after maximal exercise in man. *Journal of Applied Physiology,* 32, 304-308.

Hermansen, L., & Saltin, B. (1966). Blood lactate concentration during exercise at acute exposure to altitude. In R. Margaria (Ed.), *In exercise at altitude.* Amsterdam: Excerpta Medica Monograph.

Hermansen, L., & Saltin, B. (1969). Oxygen uptake during maximal treadmill and bicycle exercise. *Journal of Applied Physiology,* 26, 31-37.

Hermansen, L., & Stensvold, I. (1972). Production and removal of lactate during exercise in man. *Acta Physiologica Scandinavica,* 86, 191-201.

Hermansen, L., & Vaage, O. (1977). Lactate disappearance and glycogen synthesis in human muscle after maximal exercise. *American Journal of Physiology, 233*, E422-E429.

Hermansen, L., & Vaage, O. (1979). Glyconeogenesis from lactate in skeletal muscle. *Acta Physiologica Scandinavica,* Suppl. **18**, 63-79.

Hermansen, L., & Wachtlova, M. (1971). Capillary density of skeletal muscle in well-trained and untrained men. *Journal of Applied Physiology,* **10**, 860-863.

Lange Andersen, K., Elsner, R.W., Saltin, B., & Hermansen, L. (1962). *Physical fitness in terms of maximal oxygen intake of nomadic Lapps* (Tech. Documentary Rep. AAL TDR-61-53). Fort Wainwright, AK: Arctic Aeromedical Laboratory.

Lange Andersen, K., & Hermansen, L. (1965). Aerobic work capacity in middle-aged Norwegian men. *Journal of Applied Physiology,* **20**, 432-436.

Osnes, J.-B., & Hermansen, L. (1972). Acid-base balance after maximal exercise of short duration. *Journal of Applied Physiology,* **32**, 59-63.

Rowell, L.B., Hermansen, L., & Blackmon, J.R. (1976). Human cardiovascular and respiratory responses to graded muscle ischemia. *Journal of Applied Physiology,* **41**, 693-701.

Sejersted, O., Medbo, J.I., & Hermansen, L. (1981). Metabolic acidosis and changes in water and electrolyte balance after maximal exercise. In *Metabolic acidosis.* London: Pitman.

Sejersted, O., Medbo, J.I., Orheim, A., & Hermansen, L. (1984). Relationship between acid-base status and electrolyte balance after shortlasting maximal exercise. In P. Marconnet & J. Poortmans (Eds.), *Medicine and sports sciences: Vol. 17. Physiological chemistry of training and detraining.* Basel: S. Karger.

Sejersted, O., Hargens, A.R., Kardel, K., Blom, P., Jensen, O., & Hermansen, L. (1984). Intramuscular fluid pressure during isometric contractions in humans. *Journal of Applied Physiology,* **56**, 287-295.

Section $\overline{5}$

Fatigue

13

Excitation Frequencies and Sites of Fatigue

B. Bigland-Ritchie, F. Bellemare, and J. J. Woods
John B. Pierce Foundation Laboratory

P ower output is determined by the strength of muscles and their speed of movement; sustained power output is therefore limited by the rate at which muscle strength diminishes. For running, optimum performance depends on selecting a speed appropriate for the distance to be run so that the final speed is not reduced by fatigue (Hill, 1922).

Most forms of exercise are carried out at submaximal levels. Initially there is little undue sense of effort. Only later is performance reduced. This has led to the concept, often shared by physiologists, that fatigue is delayed in onset and is to be regarded as a semipathological state separate from so-called "normal" activity. But as soon as exercise commences, physiological changes that may contribute to fatigue occur at many sites within the muscle and nervous system. These changes should therefore be considered as a normal part of most forms of neuromuscular activity.

Fatigue is often defined as "an inability to generate the required or expected force" (Edwards, 1981). However, for maximum contractions the required force is the most that an individual can do, and this declines from the onset of activity. Even if a subject who works at some constant submaximal level periodically makes a brief maximal effort, the force he can produce declines progressively until, at the limit of endurance, the initially submaximal work load is now the best he can do. We therefore prefer to define neuromuscular fatigue as any reduction in the maximum force generating *capacity*, regardless of what type of work is being done.

Fatigue is commonly regarded as a failure of normal physiological function. Perhaps it should rather be thought of as a protective mechanism for survival.

Whenever the energy cost of exercise exceeds the rate of energy supply, muscle ATP stores are depleted. Functionally, it is imperative that some process limit the extent to which this can occur, thus preventing the onset of irreversible muscle rigor and protecting the subsequent recovery process (Edwards, 1981). Similarly, it is equally essential that, when exercising to the point where limb muscles are exhausted, fatigue of respiratory muscles does not prevent continued breathing against a load that remains elevated until the accumulated oxygen debt has been repaid.

Sites of Fatigue

Voluntary contractions depend on a chain of events within the central nervous system and muscle, any of which may become impaired. These include the excitatory drive to the higher motor centers (i.e., motivation or effort); the balance between the excitatory and inhibitory pathways converging on the lower motor neuron pool; changes in spinal motor neuron excitability; the integrity of electrical transmission from the nerve to muscle, and over the muscle sarcolemma and t-tubular system; effective excitation/contraction coupling; availability of muscle energy supplies; and the accumulation of metabolites that may interfere with both the metabolic and electrical events. During fatigue changes occur at all these sites. The rate limiting factors determining force production may depend on the type of exercise performed and the physiological characteristics of the particular muscles employed.

We have studied fatigue induced in different muscles by various forms of isometric exercise to determine to what extent loss of force generating capacity is due to an inability of the central nervous system to fully activate fatigued muscle than to a reduction of contractile power within the muscle fibers themselves. We have also measured changes in the pattern of motor drive and considered the functional consequences of these in relation to the complementary changes in the muscle contractile properties.

Measurement of Muscle Activation by the CNS

Human muscle strength is normally measured as the force generated by maximal voluntary efforts. Traditionally, however, many have believed that even in the absence of fatigue, the central nervous system is not capable of recruiting and maximally activating all motor units, and that with continued activity, the degree to which the muscle can be excited decreases progressively—that is, central fatigue (Asmussen, 1979). In some muscles this can be tested by comparing the force of the voluntary contraction with that from supramaximal tetanic nerve stimulation. Where this has been possible, equal forces have been generated under both conditions (Merton, 1954; Bigland-Ritchie, Jones, Hosking, & Edwards, 1978). However, few human muscles have readily available motor nerves, and tetanic stimulation is too painful to be tolerated by patients or the average naive subject. A simpler objective method is required.

In 1954 Merton used both tetanic nerve stimulation and the twitch occlusion method for assessing the degree of muscle activation. When the adductor pollicis muscle was stimulated with single shocks during voluntary contractions of graded intensity, the amplitude of the superimposed twitch declined in proportion to the voluntary force. During maximal contractions, where the force matched that from tetanic nerve stimulation, no twitch increment could be detected. Thus, all motor units must already have been fully activated by voluntary effort.

This method has many advantages. Single shocks are relatively painless and can be applied percutaneously directly over the muscle surface. It also provides an objective evaluation of muscle strength which is independent of the degree of voluntary effort (Bellemare & Bigland-Ritchie, 1984). We have found that, after suitable practice, no superimposed twitches could be detected during maximal contractions of the human quadriceps, soleus, biceps brachii (Bellemare, Woods, Johansson, & Bigland-Ritchie, 1983), or diaphragm muscles (Bellemare & Bigland-Ritchie, 1984). Belanger and McComas (1981) report similar findings for the ankle dorsiflexors, although small superimposed twitches could generally still be detected during maximal contractions of the plantarflexors. These critieria therefore show that for most human muscles, in the absence of fatigue, voluntary effort can recruit all motor units to respond with maximum force. However, if loss of force during fatigue is due to failure of motor drive, then superimposed twitches should reappear.

We have used this method to evaluate changes in the degree of muscle activation during fatigue of intermittent submaximal contractions executed over various periods of time. If, at the limit of endurance when a maximal effort is required to reach the target force, no superimposed twitch can be detected, then the central nervous system is still capable of generating full muscle activation.

Central and Peripheral Fatigue

For many years climbing Everest or running a 4-min mile seemed physiologically impossible. Yet once one person achieved such a goal, others quickly followed. Psychological factors are obviously important. In normal life, including competitive athletics, continued maximum power output is probably always partially limited by a reduction in the central neural drive. But can this be overcome?

Sustained Maximal Isometric Contractions

Merton (1954) found that the force of maximal voluntary contractions of the adductor pollicis muscle declined by more than 50% when sustained for 1-3 min. This force could not be restored by supramaximal nerve stimulation, and superimposed twitches remained occluded. No reduction was seen in the muscle mass action potential (M wave) evoked by single maximal shocks to the motor nerve. He therefore concluded that the loss of force was not due to failure of neuromuscular transmission or to a reduction in the central motor drive, but could be attributed entirely to failure of the muscle contractile system. We have subsequently confirmed this observation (Bigland-Ritchie, Kukulka, Lippold, & Woods, 1982; Bigland-Ritchie, Johansson, Lippold, & Woods, 1983). However, we found that maximum force could be sustained only by highly motivated and trained subjects using visual force feedback and given loud vocal encouragement. Indeed, in similar experiments on the quadriceps (Bigland-Ritchie et al., 1978), we found that most subjects could maintain maximum force throughout and those who could not were always able to restore it during brief "super efforts."

Perhaps the most convincing evidence for the maintenance of full muscle activation and the integrity of neuromuscular transmission comes from the report by Merton, Hill, and Morton (1981) that the loss of force during a sustained maximum voluntary contraction cannot be restored by massive direct stimulation of the adductor pollicis muscle fibers themselves. The stimulus currents used were so great that even conduction over the muscle surface membrane may have been bypassed. Moreover, Merton et al. (1981) found no decline in the muscle mass action potential evoked by periodic stimulation of the human motor cortex during fatiguing maximal voluntary contractions. These two important observations seem to demonstrate the absence of any physiological mechanisms limiting electrical propagation during fatigue at any site in the motor pathway, either within the central nervous system or on the periphery.

Thus, for sustained maximal contractions the available evidence suggests that the CNS is capable of maintaining full muscle activation and that loss of force can then be attributed solely to failure of the muscle contractile system. However, one must be cautious before assuming that this conclusion applies equally to fatigue of other muscles, or when induced by different forms of exercise.

Intermittent Submaximal Contractions at 50% MVC

Recently we have investigated the central and peripheral causes of fatigue induced over longer periods of time by intermittent submaximal contractions of the adductor pollicis, quadriceps, and diaphragm muscles. Although these contractions were still largely isometric, this form of exercise is closer to the type of rhythmic activity normally employed in daily life.

Contractions were held for 6 s at a target force of 50% MVC and repeated 6 times per min (duty cycle 0.6). Once per min the subject made a brief (3 s) MVC to measure maximum force generating capacity. Periodically, the muscle was stimulated between contractions with either single shocks or 8 pulses at 50 Hz to measure muscle contractile failure, and with single shocks during contractions to measure changes in the degree of CNS muscle activation from the amplitude of the superimposed twitch.

Figure 1 shows results from the adductor pollicis muscle. Before fatigue the MVC force matched that from 2-3 s of supramaximal tetanic nerve stimulation. The force from 8 pulses at 50 Hz did not generate full tetanic force. No superimposed twitch could be detected during a maximal voluntary effort. During the fatiguing exercise the target force superimposed twitches declined rapidly in amplitude, disappearing completely by the time a maximum effort was required. No twitches could be detected at any time when superimposed on the periodic maximal contractions. The MVC force declined in parallel with that from brief trains of 50 Hz tetanic nerve stimulation, and at the end of the experiment it still matched that from longer periods of stimulation. The target force integrated surface EMG increased progressively to match that of the MVC at the time when a maximal effort was first required to reach the target force, and the time when the target force superimposed twitch disappeared (approximately 10 min).

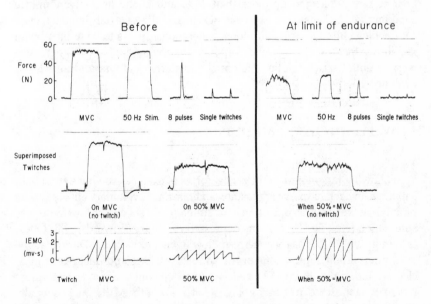

Figure 1. Mechanical and electrical responses of the adductor pollicis before and at the limit of endurance following fatigue from 50% initial MVC intermittent contractions (see text).

Similar results were also obtained for intermittent contractions of the quadriceps muscle executed at either 50% or 30% MVC. In these experiments the muscle was stimulated from electrodes over the muscle surface. The force during maximal voluntary efforts declined linearly and in parallel with that from 50 Hz stimulation. This, together with the absence of MVC superimposed twitches, the disappearance of the target force superimposed twitches, and the increase in the surface EMG to MVC values suggest that maximum muscle activation could be achieved throughout (Bigland-Ritchie, Bellemare, & Woods, 1983).

For fatigue of the diaphragm, the results were rather different (Bellemare, Furbush, & Bigland-Ritchie, 1984). Subjects learned to breathe so that the force generated and the pattern of contractions were similar to those of the limb muscle experiments. The strength of contractions was assessed from changes in the transdiaphragmatic pressure (Pdi) using the conventional esophageal and gastric balloon technique (Milic-Emili, Head, Turner, & Glauser, 1964). The muscle was stimulated percutaneously by maximal single shocks delivered bilaterally to both phrenic nerves between and during voluntary contractions of the required intensity. Electrical activity was monitored from thoracic surface electrodes over the area of apposition and also directly from esophageal electrodes. Fatigue was induced either by breathing against a variable airway resistance or by repeated expulsive maneuvers to increase abdominal pressure.

Once more the amplitude of the evoked M waves remained unchanged, indicating no failure of electrical transmission. But the twitches elicited between breaths rarely declined by more than 25%, and at the limit of endurance superimposed twitches were still evident. Thus, in this case only limited muscle contractile failure was seen and force generation appears to be limited by an inability to increase the neural drive. This was accompanied by a progressive recruitment of activity in the intercostal and sternocleidomastoid muscles as evidenced by their EMG.

Low Frequency Fatigue

Following fatigue induced by most forms of exercise, the force from both supramaximal tetanic nerve stimulation and maximum voluntary effort recovers rapidly. However, that in response to either single shocks or low frequency stimulation (e.g., 20 Hz) remains depressed for hours (Edwards, Hill, Jones, & Merton, 1977). This has been termed "low frequency fatigue." During fatigue from intermittent contractions of the adductor pollicis and quadriceps muscles, we found that the twitches elicited between contractions declined more rapidly than the force from trains of pulses at 50 Hz or the MVC, but less rapidly than the target force superimposed twitches. The twitch amplitude fell rapidly at first and then tended to stabilize late in the exercise, whereas the target force superimposed twitches continued to fall to zero. Typically a 50% reduction in MVC was accompanied by a 75% reduction in twitch amplitude. A similar disproportionate decline in twitch amplitude was also seen in fatigue of the diaphragm.

Low frequency fatigue has been attributed to impaired excitation/contraction coupling. It is suggested that each action potential fails to release the normal amount of calcium so that fewer cross bridges are available for force generation. However, if a train of impulses arrives in quick succession, then the calcium accumulates in the sarcoplasm and full force (all that is still available) can develop.

Excitation Rates During Fatigue

Stimulation Experiments

Most fatigue studies are made on isolated muscles. But it is difficult to relate these findings to what may occur during natural activity because the response of different motor unit types is highly dependent on the excitation rates employed. In voluntary contractions these probably vary widely between different motor units, but all can apparently respond with full tetanic force.

The stimulus rate required for maximum force generation by any motor unit depends on its contractile speed. In the cat, twitches from slow units start to fuse when excited at about 5 Hz and reach tetanic fusion at 25-30 Hz, whereas fast units may require 80-100 Hz (Wuerker, McPhedran, & Henneman, 1965). Even within the slow fatigue resistant group, a threefold range of contractile speeds has been reported for both the cat (Burke, 1981) and man (Buchthal & Schmalbruch, 1970). Thus, stimulation rates that are sufficient for tetanic fusion in fast twitch units are markedly supratetanic for the slower ones. Electrical propagation failure develops rapidly if the excitation rates are high (i.e., "high frequency fatigue," Edwards, 1981). This can easily be demonstrated when stimulating whole human muscle (Naess & Storm-Mathisen, 1955; Bigland-Ritchie, Jones, & Woods, 1979). We suggested that this may result, at least in part, from depletion of $Na+$ and/or accumulation of $K+$ in the t-tubules and extracellular spaces because similar effects can be demonstrated by changing the extracellular electrolytes in isolated muscles stimulated directly. But propagation failure can be avoided if the stimulus rate is progressively reduced. Indeed, fatigued muscle generates more force when stimulated at lower excitation rates (Jones, Bigland-Ritchie, & Edwards, 1979; Jones, 1981). However, Merton et al. (1981) have shown that the rate of force loss for adductor pollicis muscle is proportional to the number of impulses and independent of their frequency of delivery.

Voluntary Contractions

When first recruited, motor units generally commence firing at about 8 Hz (Monster & Chan, 1977). In small hand muscles, most are recruited at relatively low force levels (Milner-Brown, Stein, & Yemm, 1973; Kukulka & Clamann, 1981), but in others new units are progressively activated throughout the entire force range (Kukulka & Clamann, 1981). Thus, during submaximal contractions some may be firing at minimum rates while others will have already reached near tetanic frequencies. Few studies report motor neuron firing rates exceeding 25-30 Hz in voluntary contractions. However, with conventional recording techniques, clear identification of spike trains from single units during high force contractions is difficult.

Using tungsten microelectrodes in the absence of fatigue, we were able to record single fiber potentials from a large population of motor units during maximal voluntary contractions of different human muscles (see Figure 2A). These were compared with their respective contractile speeds (Bellemare et al., 1983). Contraction maximality was tested by the absence of superimposed

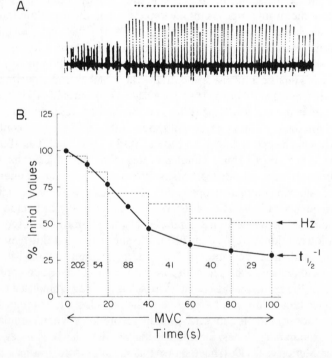

Figure 2. A) A train of spikes recorded from a single motor unit during a maximal voluntary contraction. Intervals were counted during the 1-5 s shown. B) Changes in motor neuron firing rates (Hz) and relaxation rates (t 1/2) during a series of maximal voluntary contractions sustained for 100 s. The number of units recorded is shown for each time period.

twitches. For the faster muscles, biceps brachii and adductor pollicis, firing rates ranged from 12-50 Hz with mean values close to 30 Hz. Preliminary data suggest similar values also apply to quadriceps (unpublished observation). Presumably, the units that require the higher excitation rates (up to 50 Hz) are those with the faster contractile speeds. Similarly, the slowest units are probably tetanically activated at only 15-20 Hz. This suggestion is supported by the finding that during maximal contractions of the slow soleus muscle, the mean firing rates were only 10.7 ± 2 Hz. Thus the central nervous system seems to have the "wisdom" to provide each motor unit type with a range of firing rates compatible with its contractile properties. By not exceeding the minimum rates required by each for maximum force production, the sensitivity of motor control is protected and the risk of electrical propagation failure reduced.

Changes in Neural Firing Rates and Contractile Speed During Fatigue

Sustained maximal contractions are usually accompanied by a progressive decline in the integrated surface EMG, and a reduction in the frequency of motor unit potentials has been reported (Marsden, Meadows, & Merton, 1971; Grimby, Hannerz, & Hedman, 1981). This has supported the concept that loss of force results from either failure of neuromuscular transmission (Stephens & Taylor, 1972) or a decline in motor drive (Asmussen, 1979). Yet the M waves remain intact and the force cannot be restored by tetanic nerve stimulation. Thus all units must remain active. However, fatigue is commonly associated with slowing of muscle contractile speed. We therefore suggested that this may reduce the frequency required for tetanic fusion such that the muscle may still be fully activated despite a reduction in motor neuron firing rates.

In a series of brief (10 sec) maximal contractions of the adductor pollicis muscle executed 1/min, the average firing rate of more than 200 units recorded from 5 subjects was 29.8 ± 6.4 Hz. During prolonged maximal effort both force and firing rates declined. Between 30-60 sec and 60-90 sec after the onset of the contractions, the rates were 18.8 ± 4.6 Hz (n = 65) and 14.3 ± 4.4 Hz (n = 38), respectively. As in previous experiments, periodic monitoring of the evoked M wave showed no sign of neuromuscular block (Bigland-Ritchie, Johansson, Lippold, Smith, & Woods, 1983). Similar results were also obtained when the number of spikes per unit time were recorded from small groups of fibers during sustained maximal efforts. In both sets of experiments the decline in mean motor neuron firing rate paralleled, and appeared to account for, that of the surface EMG.

In twitches recorded before and immediately after a 60 s MVC, we found no significant change in twitch contraction time, but relaxation time was prolonged by about 50% (Bigland-Ritchie, Johansson, Lippold, & Woods, 1983). When stimulated at a given subtetanic rate (e.g., 7 or 10 Hz), the force generated after fatigue increased as did the degree of tetanic fusion despite a substantial fall in the maximum tetanic force. Thus, changes in fusion frequency during fatigue are clearly related to changes in muscle relaxation rate.

Accurate measurements of relaxation rates are difficult. These were therefore measured throughout each 60 s MVC both as the maximum relaxation rate (MRR) and as the half-relaxation time (t 1/2) during the exponential phase of force decay (Wiles, Young, Jones, & Edwards, 1979). Both measurements showed that fatigue was accompanied by a twofold to threefold slowing in relaxation rate; that is, the percent change in contractile speed equalled or exceeded the simultaneous changes in motor unit firing rates (see Figure 2B). Thus, during this type of fatigue, the reduction in motor neuron firing rates need not necessarily reduce the degree of tetanic fusion. However, it remains to be seen whether similar parallel changes in contractile speed and motor neuron firing rates occur in other muscles when fatigue is induced by different forms of exercise.

Functional Speculations

Although psychological factors probably play an important part in determining power output in normal types of exercise, for fatigue of limb muscles in those situations so far examined, it seems that the natural tendency to "let off" centrally can be overcome. The central nervous system remains capable of generating maximum muscle activation so that the reduced strength results only from changes within the muscle contractile system. However, our current evidence suggests that this may not be the case for fatigue of the respiratory muscles. We found that in the absence of fatigue the diaphragm, like most other muscles, can be fully activated by voluntary effort. This no longer seems possible after fatigue. An inability to drive respiratory muscles into substantial contractile failure may make functional sense. At the time when limb muscles may be exhausted, respiratory muscles must continue to work against a substantially elevated load.

"High frequency fatigue" results from failure of peripheral electrical transmission in response to high frequency stimulation. Muscles fatigued by voluntary contractions become markedly more susceptible to this, but we have never seen evidence that propagation failure occurs spontaneously during any type of voluntary activity, probably because the motor neuron firing rates decline.

The term "low frequency fatigue" refers to the disproportionate reduction in the amplitude of the response to low frequency stimulation (e.g., 1-20 Hz). It is evident during and following most forms of exercise, probably secondary to impaired excitation/contraction coupling. While this phenomenon may throw light on the physiological changes that accompany prolonged activity, it is unclear what role low frequency fatigue plays in force generation during voluntary contractions. It can hardly be a limiting factor in the MVC returns to its prefatigue level at the time when the twitch amplitude or response to 20 Hz stimulation has shown little recovery. This is even more puzzling because 20 Hz is not far below the excitation rates observed during high force voluntary contractions.

Our results define the upper limit of motor neuron firing rates that can be sustained by voluntary effort. They also suggest that in any muscle these firing rates, either before or after fatigue, do not exceed the minimum required for maximum force production. In either condition once maximum force is generated, no useful purpose is served by further increases in excitation frequency.

Figures 3A and B show the range of motor neuron firing rates recorded from the human adductor pollicis muscle during maximum efforts before and after a 60 s MVC, together with the corresponding relaxation rates. The force

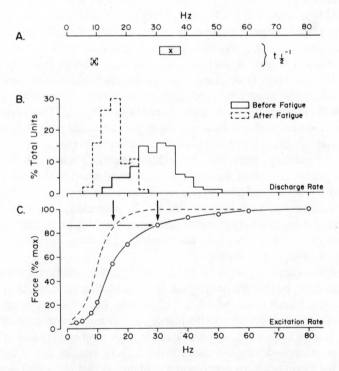

Figure 3. Adductor pollicis measurements at onset and termination of 60 s MVC. A) Relaxation rates, t 1/2 −1 (mean ± SD). B) Motor neuron firing rates. Arrows show mean rates recorded. C) % maximum force generated by nerve stimulation before fatigue (solid line) and predicted after contractile slowing (dotted line).

generated by the unfatigued adductor pollicis when the motor nerve is stimulated at comparable rates is shown below in Figure 3C (Edwards, Young, Hosking, & Jones, 1977). To generate maximum tetanic force in the unfatigued muscle, supramaximal shocks at 50-80 Hz must be delivered. Yet the same force can be produced in an MVC where the mean motoneuron discharge rate is only 30 Hz. Motor nerve stimulation at 30 Hz results in 85% of this force.

Thus, the remaining 15% of the force is probably generated by those units that fire at rates from 30-50 Hz, presumably those of highest recruitment threshold and fastest contractile speed. It also seems likely that those with the lower discharge rates (15-25 Hz) are the slowest low threshold units with tetanic fusion rates similar to those observed in the slow soleus muscle. After fatigue and contractile slowing, the mean motor neuron discharge rate declines to about 15 Hz. The now reduced maximum force still matches that from supramaximal tetanic nerve stimulation. Thus, if the same argument is applied, the relationship after fatigue between excitation frequency and relative force generation for the muscles as a whole has shifted toward the lower frequency range (see dotted line, Figure 3C). All motor units can remain fully activated despite a substantial reduction in motor neuron discharge rates. If the initial frequency required to generate full force in the unfatigued muscle was maintained, the frequency would become markedly supratetanic after contractile slowing. The decline in rate not only provides a safeguard against failure of neuromuscular transmission, but more importantly also serves to optimize force regulation by limiting the range of discharge rates so that they continue to correspond closely with those where force production can be modulated; that is, the steeper parts of the force-frequency response curve (see Figure 3C). These rates vary between different motor units according to the contractile properties of their individual constituent muscle fibers. Because these properties change with fatigue, a regulatory mechanism must exist within the CNS to match the motor neuron discharge rates to the changing contractile speed of the motor units they supply. Such regulation would require some sensory feedback from the individual muscles. Such a mechanism may be particularly important for the small hand muscles where all motor units are thought to be recruited in contractions of less than 50% MVC, above which rate coding becomes the sole means for further force regulation.

Fatigue is commonly regarded as a failure of physiological function. Perhaps it should rather be thought of as a protective mechanism for survival. A reflex mechanism, if such exists, which in limb muscles limits motor neuron firing rates to those which optimize performance (despite muscle contractile failure) may also serve to prevent comparable amounts of contractile failure in respiratory muscles. Reducing the motor drive to these muscles below those required for maximum force generation would ensure that at the end of a race, when limb muscles are exhausted, the respiratory system can continue to function against a heavy load. Moreover, for both systems, contractile failure prevents ATP depletion to levels at which recovery could no longer occur.

Acknowledgments

Much of this work was supported by USPHS grants NS 14576 and HL 30026, and by the Muscular Dystrophy Foundation.

References

Asmussen, E. (1979). Muscle fatigue. *Medical Science and Sports Reviews*, **11**, 313-321.

Belanger, A.Y., & McComas, A.J. (1981). Extent of motor unit activation during effort. *Journal of Applied Physiology: Respiratory, Environmental and Exercise Physiology*, **51**, 1131-1135.

Bellemare, F., & Bigland-Ritchie, B. (1984). Assessment of human diaphragm strength and activation using phrenic nerve stimulation. *Respiration Physiology*, **58**, 263-277.

Bellemare, F., Furbush, F., & Bigland-Ritchie, B. (1984). Localization of human diaphragm fatigue. *Federation Proceedings*, **43**, 530.

Bellemare, F., Woods, J.J., Johansson, R., Bigland-Ritchie, B. (1983). Motor unit discharge rates in maximal voluntary contractions of three human muscles. *Journal of Neurophysiology*, **50**, 1380-1392.

Bigland-Ritchie, B., Bellemare, F., & Woods, J.J. (1983). Central and peripheral fatigue of intermittent submaximal contractions. *Neuroscience Abstracts*, **9**, 631.

Bigland-Ritchie, B., Johansson, R., Lippold, O.C.J., Smith, S., & Woods, J.J. (1983). Changes in motoneurone firing rate during sustained maximal voluntary contractions. *Journal of Physiology* (London), **340**, 335-346.

Bigland-Ritchie, B., Johansson, R., Lippold, O.C.J., & Woods, J.J. (1983). Contractile speed and EMG changes during fatigue of sustained maximal voluntary contractions. *Journal of Neurophysiology*, **50**, 313-324.

Bigland-Ritchie, B., Jones, D.A., Hosking, G.P., & Edwards, R.H.T. (1978). Central and peripheral fatigue in sustained maximum voluntary contractions of human quadriceps muscle. *Clinical Science and Molecular Medicine*, **54**, 609-614.

Bigland-Ritchie, B., Jones, D.A., & Woods, J.J. (1979). Excitation frequency and muscle fatigue: Electrical responses during human voluntary and stimulated contractions. *Experimental Neurology*, **64**, 414-427.

Bigland-Ritchie, B., Kukulka, C.G., Lippold, O.C.J., & Woods, J.J. (1982). The absence of neuromuscular transmission failure in sustained maximal voluntary contractions. *Journal of Physiology* (London), **330**, 265-278.

Buchthal, F., & Schmalbruch, H. (1970). Contraction time and fiber types in intact human muscles. *Acta Physiologica Scandinavica*, **79**, 435-452.

Burke, R.E. (1981). Motor units: Anatomy, physiology, and functional organization. In *Handbook of physiology: The nervous system* (Sec. 1, Vol. 11, Part 1, Chap. 10, pp. 345-422). Bethesda, MD: American Physiological Society.

Edwards, R.H.T. (1981). Human muscle function and fatigue. In R. Porter & J. Whelan (Eds.), *Human muscle fatigue: Physiological mechanisms* (pp. 1-18). London: Pitman Medical.

Edwards, R.H.T., Hill, D.K., Jones, D.A., & Merton, P.A. (1977). Fatigue of long duration in human skeletal muscle after exercise. *Journal of Physiology* (London), **272**, 769-778.

Edwards, R.H.T., Young, A., Hosking, G.P., & Jones, D.A. (1977). Human skeletal muscle function: Description of tests and normal values. *Clinical Science and Molecular Medicine*, **52**, 283-290.

Grimby, L., Hannerz, J., & Hedman, B. (1981). The fatigue and voluntary discharge properties of single motor units in man. *Journal of Physiology* (London), **316**, 545-554.

Hill, A.V. (1922). The maximum work and mechanical efficiency of human muscles and their most economical speed. *Journal of Physiology* (London), **56**, 19-41.

Jones, D.A. (1981). Muscle fatigue due to changes beyond the neuromuscular junction. In R. Porter & J.Whelan (Eds.), *Human muscle fatigue: Physiological mechanisms* (pp. 178-198). London: Pitman Medical.

Jones, D.A., Bigland-Ritchie, B., & Edwards, R.H.T. (1979). Excitation frequency and muscle fatigue: Mechanical response during voluntary and stimulated contractions. *Experimental Neurology*, **64**, 401-413.

Kukulka, C.G., & Clamann, H.P. (1981). Comparison of the recruitment and discharge properties of motor units in human brachial biceps and adductor pollicis during isometric contractions. *Brain Research*, **219**, 45-55.

Marsden, C.D., Meadows, J.C., & Merton, P.A. (1971). Isolated single motor units in human muscle and their rate of discharge during maximal voluntary effort. *Journal of Physiology* (London), **217**, 12P-13P.

Merton, P.A. (1954). Voluntary strength and fatigue. *Journal of Physiology* (London), **128**, 553-564.

Merton, P.A., Hill, D.K., & Morton, H.B. (1981). Indirect and direct stimulation of fatigued human muscle. In R. Porter & J. Whelan (Eds.), *Human muscle fatigue: Physiological mechanisms* (pp. 12-126). London: Pitman Medical.

Milic-Emili, J., Head, J.J., Turner, J.M., & Glauser, F.M. (1964). Improved technique for estimating pleural pressure from esophageal balloon. *Journal of Applied Physiology*, **19**, 207-211.

Milner-Brown, H.S., Stein, R.B., & Yemm, R. (1973). The orderly recruitment of human motor units during voluntary isometric contractions. *Journal of Physiology* (London), **230**, 359-370.

Monster, A.W., & Chan, H. (1977). Isometric force production by motor units of extensor digitorum communis muscle in man. *Journal of Neurophysiology*, **40**, 1432-1443.

Naess, K., & Storm-Mathisen, A. (1955). Fatigue of sustained tetanic contractions. *Acta Physiologica Scandinavica*, **34**, 351-366.

Stephens, J.A., & Taylor, A. (1972). Fatigue of maintained voluntary muscle contraction in man. *Journal of Physiology* (London), **220**, 1-18.

Wiles, C.M., Young, A., Jones, D.A., & Edwards, R.H.T. (1979). Relaxation rate of constituent muscle fibre types in human quadriceps. *Clinical Science*, **56**, 47-52.

Wuerker, R.B., McPhedran, A.M., & Henneman, E. (1965). Properties of motor units in a heterogeneous fast muscle (m. gastrocnemius) of the cat. *Journal of Neurophysiology*, **28**, 85-99.

Discussion

Dr. Faulkner commented that he had measured the force-frequency relationship for small bundles of human soleus fibers and it matched Dr. Bigland-Ritchie's prediction. He then asked whether a possible reason for a difficulty in exerting maximal transdiaphragmatic pressure (Pdi) might be that none of us are accustomed to generating maximum tensions. He also wondered whether training would improve this. Dr. Bigland-Ritchie replied that some of their subjects needed training but most learned to achieve maximum contraction; her subjects were very dedicated and interested students, but she felt that when one is unable to do something, it does not prove anything. Because of this question, she abandoned resistive breathing because of the possibility of intercostal muscle action, instead using expulsive movements during which the diaphragm is acting against the abdomen and measurements of gastric pressure. This experimental procedure produced, however, the same results.

Dr. Grimby thought that possibly there might be some contradiction between his findings that ordinarily trained subjects do not maintain tonic firing for more than a limited number of seconds and Dr. Bigland-Ritchie's statement that motor units drop out. He felt that it was mainly a matter of definition, in that it is possible by extraordinary motivation to maintain tonic firing in high threshold units for a minute or perhaps more; this requires such motivation that he doubted if it happened in everyday life. Dr. Bigland-Ritchie agreed and also felt that visual feedback helped to avoid central fatigue in such studies.

Dr. Chance wondered what the signal for the loss of transmission effectiveness was and asked whether the muscle pH profile of this phenomenon had been established. He felt this to be particularly important in those patients who have peripheral vascular problems and must live with the metabolic consequences of ischemia, leading to a sensitivity to fatigue in relation to biochemical depletion of energy reserves. Dr. Bigland-Ritchie had not studied this, but Dr. Faulkner pointed out that Edman (1970), in studies of single fibers, has shown that a reduction in pH may produce the same effects as those shown by Dr. Bigland-Ritchie; however, this was a correlation and did not establish any cause and effect mechanisms. Dr. Bigland-Ritchie pointed out that changes in extracellular sodium and potassium mimic the effects of increasing frequency of stimulation.

Dr. Edgerton felt that the results obtained by his group were different, perhaps due to the different forms of muscle contraction that were being studied; he wanted details of how the quadriceps was stimulated in order to obtain maximum force. Dr. Bigland-Ritchie pointed out that the quadriceps was not stimulated maximally, but that she used the technique already established by several researchers, including Dennie-Brown, Merton, and McComas, which does not require maximum stimulation of the motor nerve. Percutaneous stimulation over the surface of the muscle is used to stimulate a constant fraction of muscle. All that is required is a big enough twitch to establish that there is a decline in the output; the technique is used to predict the maximum force output characteristics. Dr. Edgerton wondered where the tension was coming from. Dr. Bigland-Ritchie replied that it was only those motor units not fully activated by the central nervous system; if they are maximally activated, then no response is obtained. Dr. Edgerton wondered how valid this approach was, and Dr. Bigland-Ritchie referred him to the studies of Merton (1954) and of Dr. McComas, (Belanger & McComas, 1981); she felt it was valid in fatiguing muscle because the twitch tension was small and the antidromic impulse led to a silent period. Dr. Edgerton felt that it was unreasonable to expect that full activation in the twitch was obtained, when it is difficult to get maximum activation even in animal muscle, such as the rat soleus. Dr. McComas stated that he found the interpolated twitch technique very useful, but problems may occur when the voluntary contraction is almost maximal and one is searching for the presence or absence of a superimposed twitch; the signal to noise ratio then may be small. For this reason his group uses a voltage clamp on the amplifier, which is released just before the stimulus, and the twitch is observed using a fast sweep on the oscilloscope. Dr. McComas then pointed out that the force-frequency curve for the human soleus indicates that maximum tension is obtained at a stimulus rate of about 50 Hz, whereas the dorsiflexors, which are faster muscles, are activated only at 90 Hz. The higher frequency may be less important in exercise; Rack and Westbury (1969) in animal muscle isolated fascicles of nerve and used a sychronous stimulation to obtain a smoother tetanus at lower frequencies. Dr. Bigland-Ritchie suggested that the technique was most effective at the lower end of the force-frequency relationship and, thus, in the ranges employed in everyday life.

Dr. Winter admitted to some confusion and wondered what was happening at different levels: the twitch, the firing frequency, and the maximal voluntary contraction. Maximal voluntary force falls, pointed out Dr. Winter, in a sustained contraction, but the twitch amplitude increases at a faster rate. He also thought that the half-relaxation time was also slowed. Dr. Bigland-Ritchie pointed out that the half-relaxation time was actually greater. Although she did not know what happened to the area under a twitch, the high frequency units changed at the same rate as voluntary force. Single twitches demonstrated the development of what has come to be known as low frequency fatigue, but it is not clear what accounts for this, particularly as it may last for 24 hr after exercise, at a time when normal voluntary activity has been regained.

References

Belanger, A.Y., & McComas, A.J. (1981). Extent of motor unit activation during effort. *Journal of Applied Physiology: Respiratory, Environmental and Exercise Physiology*, **51**, 1131-1135.

Edman, K.A.P. (1970). The rising phase of the active state in single skeletal muscle fibres of the frog. *Acta Physiologica Scandinavica*, **79**, 167-173.

Merton, P.A. (1954). Voluntary strength and fatigue. *Journal of Physiology* (London), **123**, 553-564.

Rack, P.M.H., & Westbury, D.R. (1969). The effects of length and stimulus rate on tension in the isometric cat soleus muscle. *Journal of Physiology* (London), **204**, 443-460.

14

Biochemical Causes of Fatigue

Eric Hultman and Hans Sjöholm
Huddinge University Hospital, Huddinge Sweden

After more than 100 years of extensive research, the etiology of fatigue is still essentially unknown. Ernst Simonson, in the introduction of his book *Physiology of Work Capacity and Fatigue* (1971), states, "Fatigue, generally defined as transient loss of work capacity resulting from preceding work, is one of the most fundamental problems both for research and for practical application. Fatigue limits performance in normal conditions and even more so in disease. It produces a general feeling of discomfort and frustration and interferes with well-being."

This statement refers to two aspects of "fatigue": firstly, "objective fatigue," which is frequently defined as a reversible decrement in performance such as occurs and can be measured in a nerve-muscle preparation during stimulation or during work with a finger ergograph; and secondly, the subjective sensation of fatigue, which can limit exercise performance by an individual.

The definition of fatigue proposed by the organizers of the Fifth International Symposium on Biochemistry of Exercise (1982) was "the inability of a physiology process to continue functioning at a particular level and/or the inability of the total organism to maintain a predetermined exercise intensity." Two other definitions are the following: "failure to maintain a required or expected force" (Edwards, 1981) and "failure to maintain the required or expected power output" (Ciba Symposium, 1981).

Although many experimental studies of isolated muscles use decline in force as the definition of fatigue, the generally accepted layman's definition of fatigue in human exercise is the failure to maintain an expected power output.

Fatigue as a Decrease in Expected Power Output

Maximum Rates of Energy Production and Substrate Utilization in the Field

Estimates of the maximum theoretical rates of energy production from different substrates are presented in Table 1. The maximum rate of high energy phosphate ($\sim$ P) generation from phosphagen utilization is clearly the highest, but the amount available is very small. This is in contrast to fat, whose rate of $\sim$ P generation is ten times lower but whose total body store is almost unlimited.

Table 2 gives the rates of utilization and the amounts needed during various types of track events (adapted from Fox, 1984). It can be seen that a 100 m sprint will necessitate the utilization of the phosphagen store. Theoretically phosphagen utilization could meet the total energy requirements, both in terms

Table 1. Muscle Metabolite Concentrations Before and After Intermittent Work

| Metabolite | Sampling Time | | | | |
	Rest	Post 1	Post 2	Post 3	Post 4
ATP	5.2	3.14	2.93	2.98	3.24
+ SEM	0.37	0.34	0.50	0.30	0.39
CP	14.26	4.23	1.22	1.69	0.60
$\pm$ SEM	0.65	0.92	0.26	0.54	0.22
Lactate	1.43	28.9	34.7	27.0	35.1
$\pm$ SEM	0.25	2.7	1.6	2.4	1.8
Glycogen	85.8	67.6	52.8	54.8	51.8
$\pm$ SEM	9.4	2.8	2.1	3.1	6.0
G-6-P	0.52	6.86	4.73	1.84	1.92
$\pm$ SEM	0.11	0.28	0.57	0.22	0.29
F-6-P	0.12	1.23	0.80	0.24	0.29
$\pm$ SEM	0.03	0.11	0.14	0.03	0.06
F-16-BP	0.27	1.22	0.62	0.45	1.10
$\pm$ SEM	0.06	0.46	0.34	0.09	0.26

Concentrations are in mmol/ks wet weight muscle.
The four bouts of maximal cycling exercise were of 30 s duration, with 4 min recovery between each. The total work accomplished in 30 s decreased from 20.8 $\pm$ 3.13 kj in the first bout to 15.2 $\pm$ 2.94, 11.8 $\pm$ 2.33, and 11.8 $\pm$ 1.87 in bouts 2, 3, and 4, respectively. Muscle biopsies were taken by the Bergström technique immediately after each bout.

Table 2. Energy Turnover rate, ~ P mol•min⁻¹ and available amount, ~ P mol (in 70 kg man).

Activity: Running	Energy need[1] Rate	 Amount	Available from substrates[2] Max rate	 Amount
100 m	2.6	0.43	4.4	0.67 ATP + PCr[3]
400 m	2.3	1.72		
800 m	2.0	3.43	2.35	1.50 Glycolysis[4]
1500 m	1.7	6.0	0.85-1.14	84 Gluc. ox.[5]
Marathon	0.9-1.0	150.0	0.4-0.6	4000 Fat ox.[6]

[1]Calculated from Fox (1984)
[2]Calculated for a muscle mass of 28 Kg.
[3]Values taken from Bergström, Harris, Hultman, & Nordesjö (1971) and Hultman, & Sjöholm (1983b).
[4]Values taken from Hultman (1967) and Bergström et al. (1971). Maximum amount of lactate accumulation tolerated by the body is 1 mol of lactate (Margaria, Cerretelli, & Mangili, 1964).
[5]Rate calculated assuming a maximum rate of oxygen utilization available for glycogen (glucose) oxidation of 3 - 4 l O_2•min⁻¹.
[6]Calculated from McGilvery (1973) and Pernow & Saltin (1971).

of rate and amount of ~ P required. However, in practice some anaerobic glycolysis will occur even within the first few seconds of running. Again because of the high rate of energy demand, the phosphagens will be utilized during a 400 m sprint, but here the total amount required will necessitate a contribution from anaerobic glycolysis as well (i.e., there is no possibility of phosphagen alone meeting the total energy requirements). At the other end of the energy spectrum, a marathon runner is able to meet the rate of energy demand from the oxidation of glucose, but the total store of carbohydrate is not sufficient and has to be supplemented by the use of fat as an additional energy source. If the runner is not particularly well trained and has a low capacity to oxidize fat, then he will not be able to sustain the required energy output after depletion of the body's carbohydrate reserves, leading to a loss of power and an experience of fatigue.

Fatigue at Maximum Work Rates

Fatigue—defined as the inability to sustain a required power output—will occur at maximum work rates if the local supply of phosphagen is exhausted, despite the availability and utilization of other energy sources. It was, however, recently shown that glycolysis begins within the first second of maximum exercise (Hultman & Sjöholm, 1983b). Muscle contraction in this case was achieved by electrical stimulation. From measurement of metabolite levels in biopsy samples, it was calculated that during the first 1.26 s the rate of ATP utilization was 11 mmol•kg^{-1} dry muscle^{-1}.s^{-1} (2.6 mmol•kg^{-1} wet muscle), 80% of which was derived from PCr degradation and 20% from lactate production. From 1.26–2.52 s of stimulation, the contribution of ATP from lactate production averaged 50%. Similar results have been reported by Boobis, Williams, and Wootton (1983) for supramaximal ergometer exercise. During the first 6 s of exercise, lactate formation accounted for a minimum of 50% of the ATP resynthesized. At this point the power output decreased in spite of a PCr content corresponding to 65% of the basal level.

Continuation of the exercise resulted in a further decrease of the PCr store and increasing acidosis. At the end of exercise there was also a decline in the level of ATP itself. This may be secondary to pH decrease, which will be discussed later. Decline in power output during sustained "maximal" exercise is thus due to a number of factors rather than to the total depletion of a single energy source.

Fatigue at Submaximal Work Rates

Glycogen. During prolonged exercise at submaximal work loads, the initial utilization of anaerobic ATP production via PCr degradation and glycolysis will decrease along with time due to the increase in blood flow and delivery of oxygen to the muscles. This will increase the capacity of the muscles to oxidize pyruvate, resulting in increased ATP production and a lower rate of lactate formation. In turn this leads to a decreased rate of glycogen degradation (Hultman & Bergström, 1973).

During prolonged work there is also an increase in FFA release from adipose tissue, and the increase in blood FFA stimulates its uptake and utilization by the muscle. Thus, the use of fat as energy substrate will increase with time at these work loads. If the work load is between 65% and 85% of the subject's VO$_2$max, eventually the whole glycogen store will be utilized, and at this point power output will decrease to a level where the energy demand rate can be met by oxidation of fat (i.e., < 65% of VO$_2$max).

It has been repeatedly shown that the performance time at these high work loads is dependent upon the size of the muscle glycogen stores before exercise, and also that these stores can be varied by a combination of exercise and diet. For instance, exercise time during standardized cycle work to exhaustion varied from one to three hours in subjects fed either a carbohydrate-free or carbohydrate-rich diet during the three days before the test (Bergström, Hermansen, Hultman, & Saltin, 1967).

Glucose. Blood glucose decrease can also be a cause of fatigue due to effects on the CNS during prolonged exercise, that is, after a preceding diet low in carbohydrate (Bergström et al., 1967; Hultman & Nilsson, 1971; Hultman,

1978) or during very prolonged exercise periods without food intake. The normal glycogen store in the liver ($\approx$ 500 mmol glucose units) is sufficient to provide glucose to the body for several hours of heavy exercise.

Fat. The available stores of lipid in normal men are very large, and fat as a substrate is not limiting for prolonged exercise. Increased availability of fat to the working muscle can be achieved by stimulation of lipolysis in adipose tissue by heparin injection, caffeine intake, or a decreased blood level of insulin. This will decrease the utilization of glycogen and increase performance capacity relative to the size of the available glycogen store. Inhibition of lipolysis—for example, following insulin increase or administration of nicotinic acid or a β-blocking agent—will increase the use of glycogen, thereby producing earlier fatigue in exercise situations that are dependent upon the availability of glycogen (Pernow & Saltin, 1971).

Fatigue as a Decrease in Force

Fatigue, or decrease in force, is a reduction of the number of simultaneously attached cross-bridges in the force generating state. Obviously, decreased release of Ca^{2+} to the sarcoplasm or reduced affinity for Ca^{2+} by troponin C will result in a decrease in the force by decreasing the number of cross-bridges formed. A decrease in the supply of substrate for myosin ATPase, or a reduction of the activity of myosin ATPase, will also promote fatigue by decreasing the rate of cross-bridge turnover.

In 1929, Hill and Kupalov suggested that decreased intracellular pH due to lactate accumulation could be a major factor causing fatigue. Spande and Schottelius (1970), on the other hand, proposed that decrease in phosphocreatine (PCr) should be considered as the main fatigue factor. Studies with the nondestructive NMR technique by Dawson, Gadian, and Wilkie (1978) have suggested, however, that decrease in tension is proportional to increases in the concentrations of hydrogen ions and of free ADP rather than to a decrease in the PCr content.

In the following, a series of experiments on animal and human skeletal muscle will be reported. The aim was to correlate metabolic changes with the development of fatigue during a variety of experimental procedures.

Electrical Stimulation of Rat Muscle, Single Twitches

The isolated fast-twitch extensor digitorum longus muscle (EDL) of the rat was stimulated electrically for several minutes at 2 Hz. All the experiments were carried out under anaerobic conditions. The muscles were maintained in a moist chamber during stimulation and not in Ringer solution in order that all products of metabolism should remain within the muscle (Sahlin, Edström, Sjöholm, & Hultman, 1981).

One series of muscles was poisoned with iodoacetic acid (IAA) in order to block glycolysis and prevent formation of lactic acid. The only source of ATP resynthesis was PCr. Force decreased to 50% in 1 minute with a parallel decrease in PCr. When PCr was depleted, irreversible rigor developed concomitantly with a progressive decrease in ATP. Clearly there was no inhibition of Ca^{2+} activation in the IAA poisoned muscle. The results demonstrate that an insufficient rate of ATP supply can lead to a progressive decline in force.

Unpoisoned EDL-muscles with intact glycolysis behaved differently. They fatigued at a much slower rate, and when the PCr store was depleted, more than 80% of the force was still preserved. There was only a marginal decrease in ATP, and there was no development of rigor in the unpoisoned muscle. The availability of glycolysis as energy source made the muscles more fatigue resistant and the decline in force was proportional to the accumulation of lactic acid, not to the decrease in PCr content (see Figure 1). As force development had virtually ceased long before complete utilization of glycogen, the likely explanation would seem to be inhibition of the contractile process by decrease in muscle pH. This inhibition of the contractile process also seems to protect the muscle from rigor development, which likely would have ensued when either the glycogen store had been depleted or the glycolysis had been inhibited by decreased pH. Rigor development seems to occur when ATP supply or

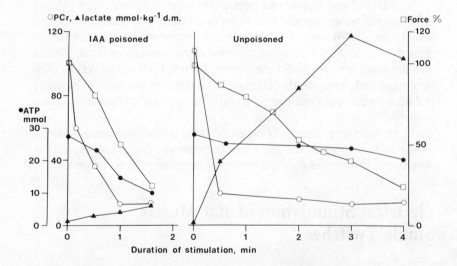

Figure 1. Force (□) as % of initial and contents of phosphagens and lactate in IAA-poisoned and unpoisoned EDL muscles of rat during electrical stimulation at 2 Hz.

myosin ATPase activity are compromised but Ca^{2+} activation remains unchanged (as in the iodoacetate poisoned muscle or in patients with phosphorylase deficiency). In normal muscle, decreasing pH seems to protect against the development of rigor. In order to examine the pH hypothesis for fatigue, EDL-muscles were exposed to 30% CO_2 (Sahlin, Edström, & Sjöholm, 1983). This resulted in a decrease in intracellular pH to around 6.65, which is equivalent to that seen after exhausting exercise. Force declined to 55% of control. However, the increase in H^+ ions also displaced the creatine kinase equilibrium with decreased PCr and increased inorganic phosphate (P_i). Thus, the fall in tension could have been a direct pH effect, but the decrease in PCr and increase in P_i could alternatively or additionally have been the cause. Edman and Mattiazzi (1981) observed a similar decrease in tension of single frog fibers that were exposed to high CO_2 atmospheres. They noted that tension and cross-bridge turnover rate decreased in parallel, implying a causal relationship. This could be due to product inhibition of the myosin ATPase by increase in P_i and H^+, or a direct effect on the enzyme activity of decreased pH (Schädler, 1967), or blockade of Ca^{2+} binding sites by H^+ ions (Fabiato & Fabiato, 1978).

Electrical Stimulation of the Human Quadriceps Femoris Muscle

Electrical stimulation with surface electrodes or intramuscular threads in combination with the muscle biopsy technique makes it possible to relate contractile and metabolic changes to each other independent of the subject's voluntary effort (Hultman, Sjöholm, Jäderholm-Ek, & Krynicki, 1983; Hultman, & Sjöholm, 1983a).

Tetanic contraction of the quadriceps femoris muscle can be performed continually or intermittently. 70% of the maximum force is produced at a stimulation frequency of 20 Hz (Sjöholm, Sahlin, Edström, & Hultman, 1983).

Intermittent Tetanic Contraction

In the following studies the muscles were repeatedly stimulated at 20 Hz for 1.6 s, pauses of 1.6 s being allowed between stimulations. The circulation to the leg was occluded by the application of a tourniquet around the upper part of the quadriceps muscle 30 s before start of the electrical stimulation. Force was measured continuously by a strain gauge connected to a strap round the ankle, and biopsy samples were taken after 13, 26, 39, and 52 trains of stimulations. The corresponding contraction times ranged from 20.6 to 83 s.

The force produced by the knee extensors decreased continuously during stimulation, measuring only 19% of the initial after 83 s. The main metabolic

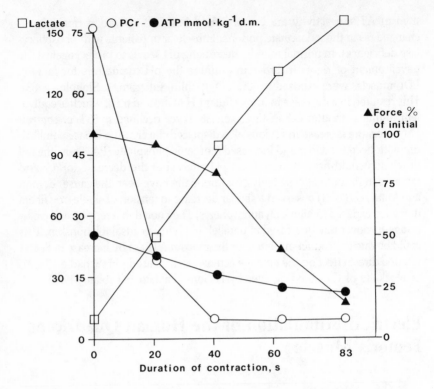

Figure 2. Force (▲) in % of initial and contents of phosphagens and lactate of the quadriceps femoris muscle during intermittent stimulation with occluded circulation. Muscle biopsies were performed before and after 13, 26, 39, and 52 tetanic contractions with a duration of 1.6 s each. Rest interval between contractions was 1.6 s. Total contraction time is given in the figure.

changes are shown in Figure 2. The PCr store was practically emptied within 40 s of contraction, whereas lactate production continued, reaching values up to 170 mmol·kg^{-1} d.m. The ATP content decreased to a mean value of 37% of the resting level, ranging from 8.9 to 13.8 mmol·kg^{-1} d.m. after 83 s of contraction. IMP increased in parallel to the fall in ATP. The total adenine nucleotide + IMP content remained essentially unchanged. Figure 3 shows the contribution of ATP from the different energy sources during the contraction period. Total ATP turnover rate was 6.30 mmol·kg^{-1} d.m.·s^{-1} initially and decreased to 1.8 mmol during the last 20 s period. The decrease in turnover rate during the period 20-40 s is due to exhaustion of The PCr store, whereas the rate of glycolysis remains relatively constant. The decrease in force seems to parallel the decay in available energy stores. There is also a continuous utilization of ATP itself, which is highest during the second and third period but decreases presumably due to lack of adenine nucleotide during the last seconds of contraction. The rate of glycolysis decreases in this period, also. As

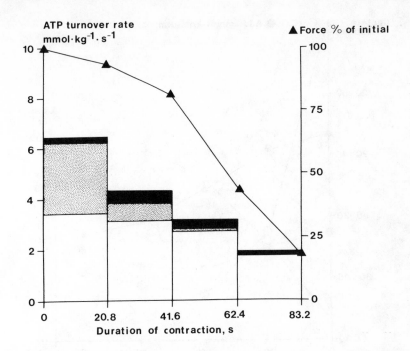

Figure 3. Force and ATP turnover rate during the intermittent stimulation shown in Figure 2. ATP turnover rates in mmol·kg⁻¹ dry muscle·s⁻¹ were calculated from changes in the ATP store (■) from degradation of PCr (▨) and from glycolysis (□).

a whole this figure gives the impression that the energy yielding processes are maximally used and that power decline is related to decreased energy production, possibly mediated through a decrease in the ATP/ADP ratio and/or accumulation of lactate and H⁺ ions, rather than to a primary inhibition of excitation as suggested by Merton, Hill, and Morton (1981).

In the control experiment using the contralateral leg of the same subjects, the same stimulation procedure was followed, but in this case there was no occlusion of the circulation (see Figure 4). The decrease in force and the utilization of the different energy sources were similar to those described previously during the first 40 s of contraction, but thereafter force decay was much less and the accumulation of lactate lower, which showed the effect of increasing blood flow. The decrease in PCr and ATP during the first 40 s changed to a small increase with continuation of the contraction. Seemingly with intact circulation, energy production from anaerobic and aerobic utilization of carbohydrate is sufficient to maintain force and also increase the content of energy rich phosphagens. Thus, the decrease in force in this case must be caused by factors other than a lack of available energy, possibly by the accumulation of H⁺ ions.

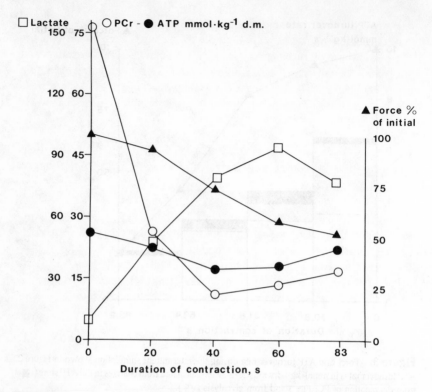

Figure 4. The same experiments and symbols as in Figure 2 but with open circulation.

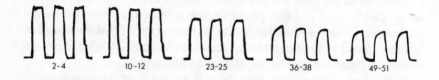

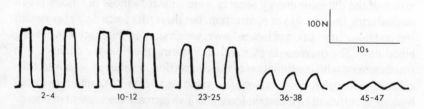

Figure 5. Force registration during the intermittent stimulation. The figures denote the consecutive numbers of the tetanic stimulations. Upper line denotes open circulation; lower line, occluded circulation.

Figure 5 shows a typical picture of force registration at different times during the intermittent stimulation without and with occluded circulation. Note the difference in shape of the twitches during the later part of the contraction period with occluded circulation. There is a pronounced delay in attaining maximum force of the tetanic twitches and also a prolongation of relaxation time. The delay in initial force production is probably a sign of inhibition of myosin AT-Pase activity.

Relations Between Force and Individual Energy Rich Phosphagens and Lactate

Figures 3 and 4 show that force was well maintained as long as PCr was available but decreased thereafter. This bears out the results described by Nassar-Gentina, Passonneau, Vergara, and Rapoport (1978) in single frog fibers. The relation is less obvious in muscle with intact circulation in which, as explained above, some resynthesis of PCr occurred with continued stimulation. No direct relation, however, was found between force and PCr; seemingly force can vary between 10% of 85% of initial with a PCr store of only 10 mmol·kg^{-1} d.m.

ATP decrease was related to force attainment, a sharp decrease in force occurring when 30% or more of the ATP had been lost. A 30%-40% loss of ATP corresponds to the maximum decrease we have earlier observed during heavy dynamic exercise (Hultman, Bergström, & McLennan Anderson, 1967).

It is interesting to note that the ATP content in the study with occluded circulation declined to very low values, the lowest observed being 8.9 mmol or 37% of the basal value. The IMP content in this sample was 14.8 mmol·kg^{-1} and the total nucleotide content was 27.3 mmol·kg^{-1} d.m. There was no tendency of rigor development in these studies (see Figure 6).

There was also a relation between force and ATP/ADP quotient (see Figure 7), which was most pronounced in the anoxic state. A similar relationship was also found between lactate content and force (see Figure 8). During anoxia the decay in force is closely related to lactate accumulation above 80 mmol·kg^{-1} d.m. Both are also related to time of contraction. A relation is also seen in aerobic muscle, but the accumulation of lactate and decrease in force are less pronounced. The relation between ATP and lactate is shown in Figure 9. The results suggest a linear relationship between ATP and lactate with lactate contents above 50 mmol·kg^{-1} d.m.

This last finding can probably be explained on the basis of increased activity of AMP deaminase when pH is falling, resulting in a decrease in the total adenine nucleotide pool. AMP deaminase has a pH optimum of 6.5 (Setlow & Lowenstein, 1967) that corresponds to the pH of exhausted muscle. During contraction decrease in ATP was mirrored by increase in IMP, and overall IMP was linearly related to increase in lactate (see Figure 10).

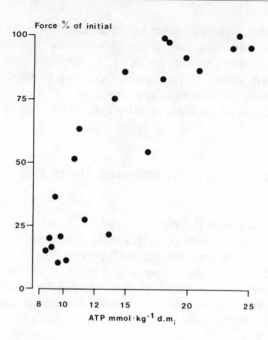

Figure 6.   Force in % of initial in relation to ATP content in muscle during the intermittent stimulation with occluded circulation.

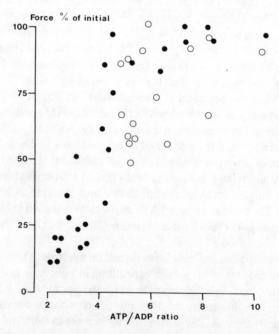

Figure 7.   Force in % of initial in relation to ATP/ADP ratio: occluded circulation (●), open circulation (o).

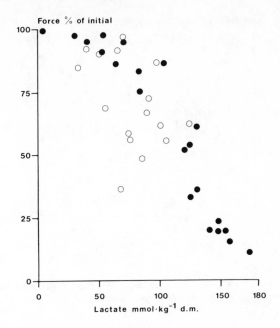

Figure 8. Force in % of initial in relation to lactate content during the intermittent stimulation: occluded circulation (●), open circulation (o).

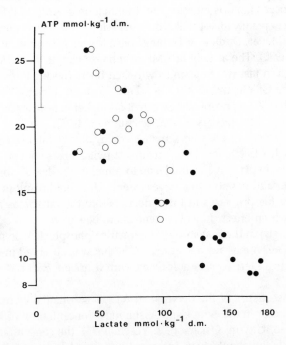

Figure 9. ATP in relation to lactate content in muscle tissue during the intermittent stimulation: occluded circulation (●), open circulation (o).

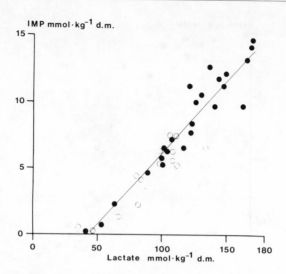

Figure 10. The relation between IMP and lactate content in the muscle tissue during the intermittent stimulation: occluded circulation (●), open circulation (o).

An intriguing possibility is that the large decrease in ATP, up to 60%, could be unevenly distributed between the two different muscle fiber types found in the quadriceps femoris muscle. The deamination of AMP to IMP has been shown to occur readily in fast-twitch but not in slow-twitch fibers during intense contraction (Meyer, Dudley, & Terjung, 1980; Meyer & Terjung, 1979; Meyer & Terjung, 1980). The activity of AMP deaminase in animal species is about twice as high in fast-twitch as in slow-twitch fibers (Bockman & McKenzie, 1983; Meyer, Gilloteaux, & Terjung, 1980; Winder, Terjung, Baldwin, & Holloszy, 1974). Also phosphorylase activity is higher in fast-twitch fibers than in slow-twitch fibers (Harris, Essén, & Hultman, 1976).

The differences in enzyme activities could, during intense contraction, produce a higher lactate formation rate in fast-twitch fibers with an earlier and larger decrease in pH, which would tend to stimulate the deamination of AMP to IMP earlier and possibly to a larger extent. This could result in inhibition of the contractile processes in these fibers before the muscle as a whole is fatigued. Such an effect, however, remains to be shown.

Interestingly, in the first study of energy rich phosphagens in man (Hultman et al., 1967) a massive decrease in ATP that was observed in one of the subjects during exercise was associated with a greatly reduced work performance.

As a consequence of the decrease in ATP, a substantial increase in free Mg^{+2} would occur in the cytoplasm. Assuming a concentration of 1 mmol•l^{-1} at rest (Veloso, Guynn, Oskarson, & Veech, 1973), the concentration at the end of stimulation should have increased to 5 mmol•l^{-1}. As Mg^{2+} competes with CA^{+2} for binding sites of troponin (Donaldson & Kerrick, 1975), an increase of Mg^{2+} to that extent could clearly decrease the number of active cross-bridges and thus contribute to loss of force.

Maintained Tetanic Contractions and Effect of pH Variation

In another study the quadriceps femoris was stimulated continuously for 75 s and 20 Hz. The force was well maintained as long as PCr was not utilized to completion (Hultman & Sjöholm, 1983a), but thereafter there was a relatively rapid force loss. A group of volunteers was given NH$_4$Cl orally to a total dose of 0.3 mmol·kg^{-1} body weight during 3 hr, the same dose used by Sutton, Jones, and Toews (1981) in a study of dynamic exercise. Before and after the NH$_4$Cl ingestion the subjects were tested with continuous electrical stimulation of the quadriceps femoris muscle for 75 s. The circulation to the leg was occluded. The administration of NH$_4$Cl decreased the blood pH to 7.25 but did not measurably decrease the muscle pH before stimulation. The pH after stimulation, however, was lower when the subjects had taken the NH$_4$Cl, mean values being 6.55 and 6.70, respectively, and the buffer capacity was apparently decreased; the mean control value was 68 slykes and after NH$_4$Cl, 54 slykes (Hultman, Del Canale, & Sjöholm, 1985). Concomitant with the lower pH, force was also lower (see Figure 11), supporting the view that isometric force is in-

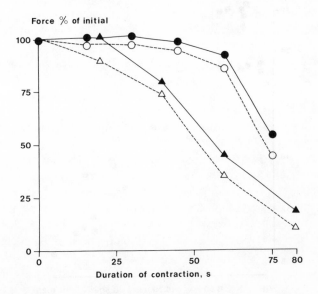

Figure 11. Force of the quadriceps femoris muscle in % of initial during continuous electrical stimulation (● o) and during intermittent stimulation (▲ △). Filled symbols denote control study; open symbols, after NH$_4$Cl ingestion. The blood circulation was occluded in both studies.

fluenced by intracellular pH. Additionally, two subjects performed intermittent isometric contractions during 84 s, as described above, before and after NH$_4$Cl administration. In one subject, muscle pH following NH$_4$Cl decreased to as low as 6.25 at the end of the contraction period. This is, as far as we know, the lowest pH value observed in human muscle. At the same time, the ATP content declined to 8.9 mmol·kg^{-1} d.m. and the lactate content increased to 170 mmol·kg^{-1}. At the end of the 84 s, force was just 11% of the initial. The relation between ATP content and muscle pH is shown in Figure 12. The highest lactate value recorded in this study was 175 mmol·kg^{-1} dry muscle and was obtained with a combination of NH$_4$Cl ingestion and stimulation. This finding seems to contradict the opinion that pH inhibition of phosphofructokinase (PFK) activity is a reason for fatigue.

Comparison Between Energy Metabolism During Continuous Isometric Contraction and Intermittent Contraction

The effects of continuous (Hultman & Sjöholm, 1983a) and intermittent contractions have been compared using the same frequency of stimulation (20

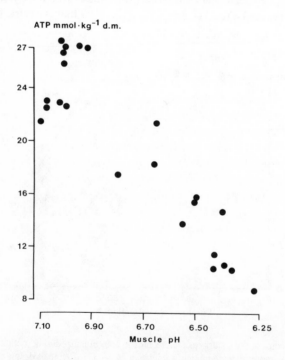

Figure 12.   ATP content and pH in the quadriceps femoris muscle before and after electrical stimulation with and without preceding NH$_4$Cl ingestion.

Hz) and with the same relative force (30% of MVC). Blood supply to the contracting muscles was occluded in both cases. During the first 40 s of contraction (for intermittent stimulation this included also 40 s of rest between the contraction periods), the rate of ATP turnover was 5.2 mmol•kg^{-1}•s^{-1} for continuous contraction and 6.3 for intermittent. Force decay was observed earlier during intermittent contraction, probably as an effect of the higher energy output.

It was found that the accumulation of hexosemonophosphates was continuous during continuous contraction and followed the increase in lactate, reaching values of 28 mmol glucose 6-phosphate per kg dry muscle at end of contraction, whereas in the intermittent model further accumulation of hexosemonophosphates had ceased after 20 s with mean values of 13 mmol•kg^{-1}. As lactate accumulation was the same in the two contraction models, it was reasoned that the difference in hexosemonophosphate accumulation was due to a lower activity of glycogen phosphorylase in the intermittent mode. We were subsequently able to show that phosphorylase a was increased to near 100% of the total phosphorylase within the first seconds of isometric contraction in both models and stayed high when the tetanic stimulation was continued for 50 s. However, when intermittent stimulation was applied, the initial increase in phosphorylase a activity was followed by a retransformation back to phosphorylase b within 20 s of contraction. At 50 s of the intermittent contraction only 3% of the phosphorylase remained in the a form. One possible explanation for this is that phosphorylase a is transformed to b during the 1.6 s interval between contractions and that the transformation back to a during contraction is slowed down when pH decreases. An inhibitory effect of pH decrease on the phosphorylase b kinase has been described earlier (Krebs, Graves, & Fischer, 1959; Chasiotis, Hultman, & Sahlin, 1983). Another possibility is that the Ca^{2+} content in the cytoplasm responsible for phosphorylase transformation is decreased during intermittent stimulation due to a pH effect upon Ca^{2+} transport, but that this effect is less pronounced during continuous stimulation when less Ca^{2+} is transported between the cytoplasm and sarcoplasmic reticulum. It is interesting to note that the rate of lactate formation seems to be insensitive to these differences in hexosephosphate concentration.

Summary

As discussed earlier there are two biochemical processes that could bring about fatigue in the force generating state, namely the formation and the turnover of myosin-actin cross-bridges. Formation is mediated by the release of Ca^{2+} ions from the sarcoplasmic reticulum and by their coupling to the troponin molecule. Both these processes are subject to interference by increased hydrogen ion concentration. In addition, Mg^{2+} ions will compete with Ca^{2+} in binding to the troponin molecule. Breakage of myosin-actin cross-bridges in an energy consuming process, the energy being generated from the splitting of ATP by myosin ATPase. The activity of this enzyme is decreased at low physiological pH and also by a low ATP/ADP ratio.

Both of these processes— formation and breakage— appear to be important, under different conditions of work, to the onset of fatigue. Thus, fatigue without decrease in pH, as seen in the iodoacetate poisoned muscle, is best explained by a decreased rate of cross-bridge turnover due to a lowered ATP/ADP ratio. A lowered ATP/ADP ratio can probably account also for the fatigue seen after complete emptying of the local muscle glycogen stores following prolonged exercise. Decrease in muscle pH under these work conditions will again be minimal and unlikely to affect either cross-bridge formation or breakage.

At the upper end of the energy spectrum, it is much more difficult to identify any one single factor as the primary cause of fatigue. Decreased ATP/ADP ratio is—as already noted for the iodoacetate study—one possibility, whereas decreased muscle pH is suggested by the NH_4Cl studies. We would like to emphasize that it is pH acting directly at the level of the contraction process itself rather than through the inhibition of energy production at the level of PFK. A further possibility is the actual depletion of ATP in the contracting muscle fibers. This occurs readily under conditions of maximal intermittent work output and at the extreme can result in a decrease in ATP by as much as 60%. At the moment it is not known if this occurs equally in all muscle fibers or is restricted to just one type. Neither do we have any information on the amount of ATP that must be present in a muscle cell for maintenance of force generation, but such a large decrease clearly cannot be overlooked when considering factors causing fatigue.

The mechanism behind the decrease in ATP is the deamination of AMP to IMP by AMP deaminase. Increased levels of AMP during contraction and fall in pH will increase the activity of AMP deaminase and thus the breakdown of adenine nucleotide. The precise role played by AMP deamination is uncertain, but clearly it is associated with maximum work rates performed under conditions of increasing acidosis. One effect of deamination will be to keep the cellular level of ADP low (ADP being linked to AMP via adenylate kinase) and thus help to maintain a high ATP/ADP ratio. This in turn will help in delaying the onset of fatigue (assuming the ATP/ADP ratio to be important here). Conceivably, therefore, adenine nucleotide deamination is a process for delaying fatigue development in the maximally working muscle. However, ultimately a price must be paid for this as a result of the fall in ATP.

Acknowledgments

This work was supported by grants from the Swedish Medical Research Council (02647) and the Swedish Work Environment Fund (81-0173).

The authors wish to thank the entire staff at the Department of Clinical Chemistry II for excellent collaboration in this investiagation.

References

Bergström, J., Harris, R.C., Hultman, E., & Nordesjö, L.-O. (1971). Energy rich phosphagens in dynamic and static work. In B. Pernow & B. Saltin (Eds.), *Advances in experimental medicine and biology* (pp. 341-355). New York: Plenum Press.

Bergström, J., Hermansen, L., Hultman, E., & Saltin, B. (1967). Diet, muscle glycogen and physical performance. *Acta Physiologica Scandinavica, 71*, 140-150.

Bockman, E.L., & McKenzie, J.E. (1983). Tissue adenosine content in active soleus and gracilis muscle of cats. *American Journal of Physiology, 244*, H552-H559.

Boobis, L.H., Williams, C., & Wootton, S.A. (1983). Influence of sprint training on muscle metabolism during brief maximal exercise in man. *Journal of Physiology* (London), *342*, 36-37P.

Chasiotis, D., Hultman, E., & Sahlin, K. (1983). Acidotic depression of cyclic AMP accumulation and phosphorylase *b* to *a* transformation in skeletal muscle of man. *Journal of Physiology* (London), *335*, 197-204.

Dawson, M.J., Gadian, D.G., & Wilkie, D.R. (1978). Muscular fatigue investigated by phosphorus nuclear magnetic resonance. *Nature, 274*, 861-866.

Donaldson, S., & Kerrick, W. (1975). Characterization of the effects of Mg^{2+} on Ca^{2+}—and Sr^{2+}—activated tension generation of skinned skeletal muscle fibers. *Journal of General Physiology, 66*, 427-444.

Edman, K.A.P., & Mattiazzi, A.R. (1981). Effects of fatigue and altered pH on isometric force and velocity of shortening at zero load in frog muscle fibres. *Journal of Muscle Research and Cell Motility, 2*, 321-334.

Edwards, R.H.T. (1981). Human muscle function and fatigue. In R. Porter & J. Whelan (Eds.), *Human muscle fatigue: Physiological mechanisms* (pp. 1-18). Ciba Foundation Symposium 82. London: Pitman Medical.

Fabiato, A., & Fabiato, F. (1978). Effects of pH on the myofilaments and the sarcoplasmic reticulum of skinned cells from cardiac and skeletal muscles. *Journal of Physiology* (London), *276*, 233-255.

Fox, E.L. (1984). *Sports physiology*. Saunders College Publishing.

Harris, R.C., Essén, B., & Hultman, E. (1976). Glycogen phosphorylase activity in biopsy samples and single muscle fibres of musculus quadriceps femoris of man at rest. *Scandinavian Journal of Clinical Laboratory Investigation, 200*, 99-105.

Hill, A.V., & Kupalov, P. (1929). Anaerobic and aerobic activity in isolated muscle. *Proceedings of the Royal Society of London: Series B, 105*, 313-328.

Hultman, E. (1967). Muscle glycogen in man determined in needle biopsy specimens: Method and normal values. *Scandinavian Journal of Clinical Laboratory Investigation, 19*, 209-217.

Hultman, E. (1978). Regulation of carbohydrate metabolism in the liver during rest and exercise with special reference to diet. In F. Landry & W.A.R. Orban (Eds.), *3rd International Symposium on Biochemistry of Exercise* (Vol. 3, pp. 99-126). Miami: Symposia Specialists.

Hultman, E., & Bergström, J. (1973). Local energy-supplying substrates as limiting factors in different types of leg muscle work in normal man. In J. Keul (Ed.), *Limiting factors of physical performance*. International Symposium at Gravenbruck, 1971, (pp. 113-125). Stuttgart G. Thieme Publishers.

Hultman, E., Bergström, J., & McLennan Anderson, N. (1967). Breakdown and resynthesis of phosphorylcreatine and adenosine triphosphate in connection with muscular work. *Scandinavian Journal of Clinical Laboratory Investigation, 19*, 56-66.

Hultman, E., Del Canale, S., & Sjöholm, H. (1985). Effect on induced metabolic acidosis on intracellular pH, buffer capacity and contraction force of human skeletal muscle. *Clinical Science, 69*(5), 505-510.

Hultman, E., & Nilsson, L.H. (1971). Liver glycogen in man, effect of different diets and muscular exercise. In B. Pernow & B. Saltin (Eds.), *Advances in Experimental Medicine and Biology* (pp. 143-151). New York: Plenum Press.

Hultman, E., & Sjöholm H. (1983a). Energy metabolism and contraction force of human skeletal muscle in situ during electrical stimulation. *Journal of Physiology* (London), *345*, 525-532.

Hultman, E., & Sjöholm, H. (1983b). Substrate availability. In H.G. Knuttgen, J.A. Vogel, & J. Poortmans (Eds.), *International Series on Sport Sciences. Biochemistry of Exercise* (Vol. 13, pp. 63-75).

Hultman, E., Sjöholm, H., Jäderholm-Ek, I., & Krynicki, J. (1983). Evaluation of methods for electrical stimulation of human skeletal muscle in situ. *Pflugers Archives, 398*, 139-141.

Krebs, E.G., Graves, D.J., & Fischer, E.H. (1959). Factors affecting the activity of muscle phosphorylase *b* kinase. *Journal of Biological Chemistry, 234*, 2867-2873.

Margaria, R., Cerretelli, P., & Mangili, F. (1964). Balance and kinetics of anaerobic energy release during strenuous exercise in man. *Journal of Applied Physiology, 19*, 623-628.

McGilvery, R.W. (1973). The use of fuels for muscular work, In H. Howald & J.R. Poortmans (Eds.), *Metabolic adaptation to prolonged physical exercise* (pp. 12-30). Basel: Birkhauser Verlag.

Merton, P.A., Hill, D.K., & Morton, H.B. (1981). Indirect and direct stimulation of fatigued human muscle. In R. Porter & J. Whelan (Eds.), *Human muscle fatigue: Physiological mechanism* (pp. 120-126). Ciba Foundation Symposium 82. London: Pitman Medical.

Meyer, R.A., & Terjung, R.L. (1979). Differences in ammonia and adenylate metabolism in contracting fast and slow muscle. *American Journal of Physiology, 237*, C111-C118.

Meyer, R.A., & Terjung, R.L. (1980). AMP deamination and IMP reamination in working skeletal muscle. *American Journal of Physiology, 239*, C32-C38.

Meyer, R.A., Dudley, G.A., & Terjung, R.L. (1980). Ammonia and IMP in different skeletal muscle fibers after exercise in rats. *Journal of Applied Physiology: Respiratory, Environmental and Exercise Physiology, 49*, 1037-1041.

Meyer, R.A., Gilloteaux, J., & Terjung, R.L. (1980). Histochemical demonstration of differences in AMP deaminase activity in rat skeletal muscle fibers. *Experientia, 36*, 676-677.

Nassar-Gentina, V., Passonneau, J.V., Vergara, J.L., & Rapoport, S.I. (1978). Metabolic correlates of fatigue and of recovery from fatigue in single frog muscle fibers. *Journal of General Physiology, 72*, 593-606.

Porter, R., & Whelan, J. (Eds.) (1981). *Human muscle fatigue: Physiological mechanisms.* Ciba Foundation Symposium 82. London: Pitman Medical.

Pernow, B., & Saltin, B. (1971). Availability of substrates and capacity for prolonged heavy exercise in man. *Journal of Applied Physiology, 31*, 416-422.

Sahlin, K., Edström, L., & Sjöholm, H. (1983). Fatigue and phosphocreatine depletion during carbon dioxide-induced acidosis in rat muscle. *American Journal of Physiology, 245*, C15-C20.

Sahlin, K., Edström, L., Sjöholm, H., & Hultman, E. (1981). Effects of lactic acid accumulation and ATP decrease on muscle tension and relaxation. *American Journal of Physiology, 240*, C121-C126.

Schädler, M. (1967). Proportionale Aktivierung von ATPase-aktivitat und Kontraktionsspannung durch Calciumionen in isolierten contraktilen Strukturen verschiedener Muskelarten. *Pflügers Archives, 296*, 70-90.

Setlow, B., & Lowenstein, J.M. (1967). Adenylate deaminase: II. Purification and some regulatory properties of the enzyme from calf brain. *Journal of Biological Chemistry, 242*, 607-615.

Simonson, E. (Ed.) (1971). *Physiology of work capacity and fatigue.* Springfield, IL: Charles T. Thomas.

Sjöholm, H., Sahlin, K., Edström, L., & Hultman, E. (1983). Quantitative estimation of anaerobic and oxidative energy metabolism and contraction characteristics in intact human skeletal muscle in response to electrical stimulation. *Clinical Physiology, 3*, 227-239.

Spande, J.I., & Schottelius, B.A. (1970). Chemical basis of fatigue in isolated mouse soleus muscle. *American Journal of Physiology, 219*, 1490-1495.

Sutton, J.R., Jones, N.L., & Toews, C.J. (1981). Effect of pH on muscle glycolysis during exercise. *Clinical Science, 61*, 331-338.

Veloso, D., Guynn, R.W., Oskarsson, M., & Veech, R.L. (1973). The concentrations of free and bound magnesium in rat tissue. *Journal of Biological Chemistry, 248*, 4811-4819.

Winder, W.W., Terjung, R.L., Baldwin, K.M., & Holloszy, J.O. (1974). Effect of exercise on AMP deaminase and adenylosuccinase in rat skeletal muscle. *American Journal of Physiology, 227*, 1411-1414.

Discussion

Dr. Jones opened the discussion period by presenting some data that he felt amplified Dr. Hultman's findings and also yielded some information with regard to the biochemical factors underlying fatigue. Studies carried out by McCartney, Heigenhauser, Sargeant, and Jones (1983) have employed the isokinetic cycle ergometer to examine maximal performance during 30 s of cycling. Muscle biopsies were taken at rest and following four successive maximal exercise bouts, with 4-min rest periods in between. The maximum work that subjects accomplished in the 30 sec fell between the first and the second and the second and the third bouts, but there was no change between the third and the fourth bouts, when severe fatigue was associated with a 50% to 60% reduction in the work accomplished in 30 sec. The muscle biopsy results (see Table 1) showed that glycogen utilization and lactate accumulation were negligible after the second bout; the changes in the concentration of G-6-P and F-6-P suggested that inhibition of phosphofructokinase, followed by phosphorylase, occurred in the later exercise bouts. This led to severe reductions in CP to virtually zero levels, even though almost full regeneration occurred during the 4 min of recovery between the bouts. Also, significant ATP reductions to about 60% of the basal values were found. The data were consistent with inhibition of rate limiting enzymes by a low muscle pH, leading to greater reliance on high energy phosphates.

Dr. Wilkie wondered what happened to inorganic phosphate in the heavy work that Dr. Hultman described, which involved ATP breakdown and regeneration. Dr. Hultman replied that although phosphate was not difficult to determine, the values in resting muscle, obtained by biochemical analysis, seem much higher, about 10 mmol/l i.c. water, than those obtained by NMR of about 2 mmol/l. He calculated the phosphate accumulation at the end of a maximum isometric contraction from the degradation of ATP and creatine phosphate and the uptake by hexosphosphates to 15-25 mmol/l. The calculated increases are then used to examine the activation of phosphorylase. Dr. Hultman felt no doubt that phosphate was an important controller of phosphorylase activity (Chasiotis, Sahlin, & Hultman, 1982; Chasiotis, Sahlin, & Hultman, 1983; Chasiotis & Hultman, 1983).

Dr. Chance pointed out that the accumulation of CO_2 and hydrogen ions would be expected to decrease the creatine phosphate/phosphate ratio due to the inhibitory effects of pH on the creatine kinase reaction. He wondered if the slope of the log CP/P ratio to pH, which should have a slope of 1.0, had been examined in this situation. There might be an additional effect revealed if the log of the phosphate potential was plotted against pH. Also, he felt that ATP/ADP ratios might be important in the interpretation; in iodoacetate treated muscle no pH change would occur. He hoped that such studies would reveal the thermodynamic relationship to cross-bridge activity. Dr. Hultman pointed out that although he had not shown the data, there was a good relationship of force and fatigue to changes in the ADP/ATP ratio. Dr. Wilkie pointed out that ADP in this study was the total ADP, which may be very different from the free ADP, which is important in acting as a regulator. There was a lot of ADP bound to actin and myosin.

Dr. Bárány wanted to emphasize that fatigue was related to shortage of ATP. The ultimate control of force was the ATP myosin binding site ratio, which was only 10; that is, only tenfold ratio of enzyme over substrate. To fully activate a tetanus, ATP is used at a rate of 4 mols/mol/sec, and replacing this with a binding factor of less than 10 is difficult. ATP has to diffuse to the active site, but this process is slow. Also, he felt that the breakdown of ATP would lead to the accumulation of phosphoric acid at the ATP site to produce a local fall in pH. As actin activated ATPase has an optimum pH of 7.4, as soon as muscle begins to contract the accumulation of phosphate may lead to pH falling below 7 and a considerable decrease in activity. Having said this, he felt that the most important topic that no one had addressed was the mechanisms by which fatigue was appreciated by the subject. Dr. Hultman felt that many factors, including accumulation of lactate and fall in pH, might be involved.

Dr. Hultman wondered what the effect of the accumulation of Mg^{2+} ions would be as they may increase from 1 to 5 m mol/kg. Dr. Bárány felt that this was likely to be a minor effect as only a very small fraction is free Mg^{2+}; more important might be the effect of a displacement of Ca^{2+} from troponin, as the small binding constant gives very little flexibility. Dr. Newsholme commented that as a fall in pH will influence the activity of phosphofructokinase, a stimulation of PFK activity by Ca^{2+} would reduce the effectiveness of the pH inhibition; although several of his colleagues were surprised that they had been unable to find stimulation of PFK by calcium, he felt it was a good job that this effect was not present. He also asked Dr. Hultman whether the fall in ATP, which had been shown in stimulated and ischemic muscle, occurred during voluntary contraction. Dr. Hultman replied that in their first paper that examined changes in CP and ATP (Hultman, Bergström, & McLennan Anderson, 1967) one of their subjects was unable to continue exercising for more than 5 min and was found to have extremely low PC concentration and also an ATP concentration that was about 40% of the basal value. Thus, he felt sure that ATP depletion did occur, particularly during very heavy short-term exercise. He mentioned that Roger Harris in Newmarket, England, found that even though race horses were allowed sufficient time for ATP resynthesis between runs, there was only 50% of the initial ATP left after the third run. These findings were similar to those presented by Dr. Jones.

References

Chasiotis, D., Sahlin, K., & Hultman, E. (1982). Regulation of glycogenolysis in human muscle at rest and during exercise. *Journal of Applied Physiology*, **53**, 708-715.

Chasiotis, D., Sahlin, K., & Hultman, E. (1983). Regulation of glycogenolysis in human muscle in response to epinephrine infusion. *Journal of Applied Physiology, 54*, 45-50.

Chasiotis, D., & Hultman, E. (1983). The effect of circulatory occlusion on the glycogen phosphorylase-synthetase system in human skeletal muscle. *Journal of Physiology, 345*, 167-173.

Hultman, E.M., Bergström, J., & McLennan Anderson, N. (1967). Breakdown and resynthesis of phosphorylcreatine and adenosine triphosphate in connection with muscular work. *Scandinavian Journal of Clinical Laboratory Investigation, 19*, 56-66.

McCartney, N., Heigenhauser, G.J.F., Sargeant, A.J., & Jones, N.L. (1983). A constant-velocity cycle ergometer for the study of dynamic muscle function. *Journal of Applied Physiology: Respiratory, Environmental and Exercise Physiology, 55*, 212-217.

15

Resting (State 4) to Active (State 3) Transitions as Observed by ^{31}PNMR in Steady State Skeletal Muscle Exercise in Normal and Peripheral Vascular Diseased Human Subjects

B. Chance, T. Graham, J. Maris, and J.S. Leigh, Jr.
University of Pennsylvania

It is a great pleasure to be present among those who study human muscle power with a variety of techniques and insights to which I shall attempt to add the possibility of continuous in vivo monitoring by phosphorus nuclear magnetic resonance (^{31}PNMR). Perhaps my only real qualification as a member of this meeting is that of a one-time Olympic contestant in a sport in which the "seat of the pants" response time to split second decision making was more of a prerequisite than human muscle power. However, my research carried me to the study of mitochondrial energetics, particularly the quantitation of the control properties of mitochondria in terms of the ADP concentration necessary for half maximal respiratory activity (Chance & Williams, 1955). At the same time, my colleagues and I titrated the mitochondrial response to single muscle twitches that, when compared to the mitochondrial response to ADP, gave results consistent with the values of Fleckinstein and Davies (1956) on the requirements of ATP breakdown for a single muscle twitch (Chance & Connelly, 1957; Chance & Jobsis, 1959; Chance, Mauriello, & Aubert, 1962; Chance and Weber, 1963).

New technology may often lead to new research approaches, and the capability of NMR to quantitate the free inorganic phosphate concentration of the cytosol has been a boon to those who are either puzzled with analytical biochemistry or, as I have done, attempted to calculate the ratio of the free phosphate to the total phosphate (80:1 in a particular case) from considerations of effectiveness of reversed electron transfer (Chance & Hollunger, 1961). The particular interest in inorganic phosphate determinations is that the ratio of phosphocreatine (PCr) to inorganic phosphate (P_i) gives direct information related to the potential of the system to do work and, particularly in muscle contractions, the amount of energy expenditure in muscle power output. Thus, I shall, in this short communication, attempt to indicate how we evaluate arm exercise efficiency in terms of work output measured with the Cybex isokinetic ergometer and biochemical cost measured by the decrease of the parameter PCr/P_i, conveniently expressed as its reciprocol, which increases as the power output increases.

Experimental Method

Since 1978 we have been measuring arm exercise of humans in a magnet specified for that purpose affording a 7-inch bore (Chance, Eleff, Leigh, Sokolow, Sapega, 1981), which readily accommodates the arm and the ten-

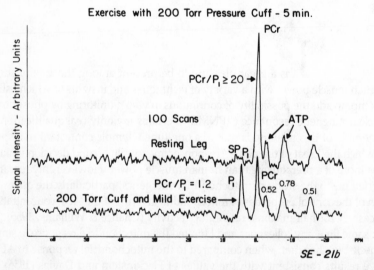

Figure 1. Example of phosphorus NMR spectra in rest and activity. Note the decrease of PCr and the rise of P_i in activity from very high and very low values, respectively. In this case, a tourniquet was employed to cause large drops of PCr/P_i ratio in mild exercise.   (SE-21)

sor/flexor muscle. The forearm can be laid directly on a probe that is electrostatically shielded so that the arm does not seriously detune the probe. The probe is then slid into the center of the magnet where the field is homogeneous. The PDP 11/23 computer controls the rf pulse to the coil, at the same time receiving the free induction decays of the nuclei involved (phosphorus), and Fourier transforms the figure, giving spectrum of the principal chemicals of the arm (see Figure 1). In addition to the computer console, data readout and printout modalities are provided as is a power supply for activating the room temperature shims, which are adjusted to afford a field homogeneous to one part in 10^7 over a diameter of a few inches. This equipment has been in reliable operation since the initial studies and has a performance such that a single measurement of phosphorus compounds requiring about 100 msec can be repeated at will every 5 sec (and thus can be gated to a synchronous muscle contraction with 100 msec time resolution) and the data readout under these conditions has a signal to noise ratio of approximately 10:1.

Experimental Data

The NMR spectrum of the human limb is shown in an example of Figure 1, where the resting spectrum shows characteristically the triplet of ATP peaks, the large PCr peak (usually 5 or 6 times the ATP peak) with a scarcely detectable P_i peak and a small sugar phosphate peak. The ratio of the peak values of PCr and P_i is over 10. In this particular case and in contrast to the studies below, ischemia has been induced by a pressure cuff together with mild exercise, which simulates violent exercise in the magnet with a nearly stationary leg. We see that PCr has fallen to a fraction of its initial value and that a complementary rise in P_i has occurred, maintaining the sum of PCr + P_i equal to a constant. Here the ratio of PCr/P_i is 1.15, and under these conditions the contributions to the error of this ratio from P_i and PCr are equal, while in the resting state, the error is mainly attributed to the low value of P_i. However, because PCr/P_i in the range of 1 to 3 is the normal range for a mild to strong exercise, the ratio determination is relatively accurate. It is relatively independent of the volume of muscle placed over the probe and of whether the muscle is pressed against the probe or slightly displaced from it as may occur in heavy exercise regimens. Our use of peak values is intended only for simplicity; curve fitting procedures will separate the areas of the two peaks, appropriately quantifying the ratios more accurately. However, in skeletal muscle, the change of the line shape of P_i and PCr with exercise seems small and the use of peak values has been of appropriate accuracy and, of course, of great convenience.

Theoretical Background

Although the chemical equations for muscle energy metabolism are well known, the expression that my colleagues and I (Chance & Williams, 1955; Bucher & Klingenberg, 1958) have developed from consideration of the reverse electron transfer properties of mitochondria, though not always used in considerations of muscle energy performance, is a simple expression of the equation of oxidative phosphorylation, expressed as an equilibrium constant.

PHOSPHATE POTENTIAL

$$K' = \frac{ATP}{ADP \times P_i}$$

$$K'' = \frac{PCr \times ADP}{Cr \times ATP}$$

$$\frac{ATP}{ADP} = \frac{1}{K''} = \frac{PCr}{Cr}$$

$$K'K'' = \frac{PCr}{P_i} \cdot \frac{1}{Cr}$$

$$K'K'' = \frac{PCr}{Pi} \cdot \frac{1}{Cr_o + P_i}$$

Because a second equilibrium constant is derived from the phosphocreatine equilibrium, it is possible to substitute for [ATP/ADP] = [PCr/Cr] and obtain a second equilibrium equation for thermodynamic performance involving PCr/P_i and the creatine concentration. Because creatine contains no phosphate, it gives no phosphorus NMR signal. It can be evaluated, however, from the sum of $[PCr + P_i]$ by proton NMR (if this is available) or from analytical chemical values for the muscle at rest. Because the components of the equilibrium of the creatine kinase equilibrium appear to be conserved within the muscle cytoplasm, it is legitimate to calculate increases of creatine appropriate to decreases of creatine phosphate by simply adding the increment of phosphate concentration to the initial creatine concentration as indicated in the bottom line of the equation.

Gyulai, Roth, Leigh, and Chance (1984; 1985) have explored whether or not this equation obtains in isolated mitochondria and if so what the maximum PCr/P_i might be obtainable at rest. One of their recent graphs is indicated in Figure 2, where the logarithm of PCr/P_i is plotted against the ATPase concentration as set by the amount of potato apyrase added to a suspension of mitochondria supplemented with phosphocreatine, inorganic phosphate, creatine, and creatine phosphokinase. It is seen that the straight line extrapolates to approximately 32 for PCr/P_i (agreeing reasonably well with the value of Figure 1) for a resting leg.

The progression of states for mitochondria represented from O ATPase to the maximum corresponds to a change in the character of metabolic control for ADP being rate limiting to electron transfer rate limiting, a state 4 to state 3 transition, the topic of this lecture. These states are represented and cor-

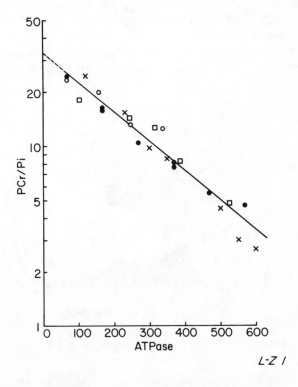

L-Z I

Figure 2. Experimental relationship between mitochondrial PCr/P_i and ATPase value plotted in semilogarithmic coordinates. (LZ −1)

METABOLIC STATES OF MITOCHONRIA
CELLS AND TISSUES

Fed	←Starved→	←	—Fed—		→	Substrate Level
Fatty Acid	←	—Citric Acid Cycle—			→	Substrate Type
←	—Normoxic—		→	←Anoxic→		Oxygen Supply
←	—Coupled—		→Uncoupled→	←Coupled→	Uncoupled→	Coupling
>10	<1	10	<0.1	>1.0	<0.1	PCr/Pi
medium	near 0	maximal	maximal	near 0	0	Respiration Rate
1	2	3	3u	4	5	Metabolic State

MT 446

Table 1. Table of metabolic states based upon studies of isolated mitochondria (Chance & Williams, 1955). (TG 19)

responding PCr/P$_i$ values are given in Table 1. These two states are of most interest here, other states of interest being those corresponding to starvation, for example, hypoglycemia (state 2), to hyperthermia (state 3), and finally to hypoxia (state 5). The latter state, of course, may be obtained under conditions of extreme exercise stress.

The mechanical coupling of the Cybex ergometer for arm exercise within the 7- or 10-in. magnet is represented in Figure 3 (Chance et al., 1983). The

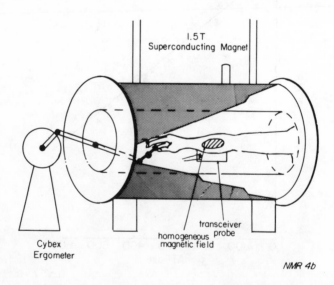

Figure 3. Coupling of NMR to Cybex ergometer with nonmagnetic materials. (NMR 4B)

mechanical advantage is 1:1 so that those familiar with exercise with the ergometer will recognize no change except that arm movements are restricted, and in the case of NMR the arm must be kept against the surface probe in order to avoid attenuation of the radio frequency signals. Furthermore, the coupling to the NMR is made of nonmagnetic material, and the Cybex ergometer is located far enough from the instrument that no interference with the magnetic field is observed.

Exercise Protocol

Portions of the protocol are clearly indicated by the bar graph (see Figure 4). The resting scan is followed by four intervals of increasing activity, in which visual feedback from the Cybex ergometer to the subject enables ramping of the exercise every 5 min according to the protocol in regular steps. Finally, when a high level of exercise has been reached, doubling of the number of events occurs every 5-min interval followed by an increase to 15 rpm at 1 Hz for the final level of activity. Following relaxation, continuous scanning occurs

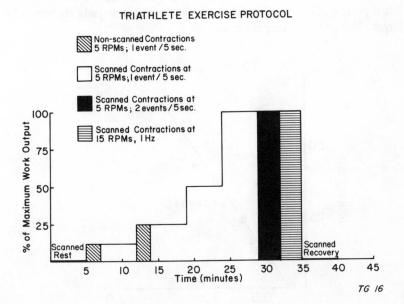

Figure 4. Exercise protocol.   (TG 16)

in order to follow the rate of recovery afforded by oxidative metabolism in the tissues.

Experimental Results

In order to identify an appropriate unit for the exercise performance in this range, we divide the power by the biochemical "cost," the latter in terms of 1 unit increase of P_i/PCr, and use this limit to compare the athletes' performances.

An example of the performance of an "elite" triathlete and rowing athlete is indicated in Figure 5. It is seen that the nature of the curve is similar to that obtained earlier (Chance et al., 1981) and to that for isolated mitochondria. The resting level corresponds to PCr/P_i of approximately 10. Increasing exercise regularly according to the protocol gives 4 points of increasing exercise that fits relatively well to a straight line, although in actuality this is an approximation of the initial portion of a rectangular hyperbola. The slope in this case corresponds to 47 Joules per min per 1 unit increase of P_i/PCr and approximately 0.8 Watts per unit increase of P_i/PCr.

Figure 6 represents a different kind of performance. The exercise has an initial portion similar to that of the previous one, the slope being somewhat larger (260) and a smaller slope thereafter.

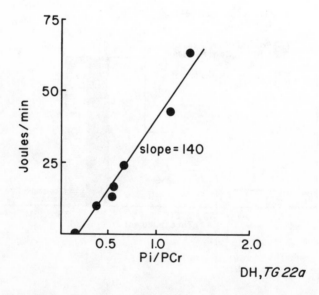

Figure 5. An example of the performance of an "elite" athlete who is capable of exercising with a linear relationship between power output and P_i/PCr.   (TG 22)

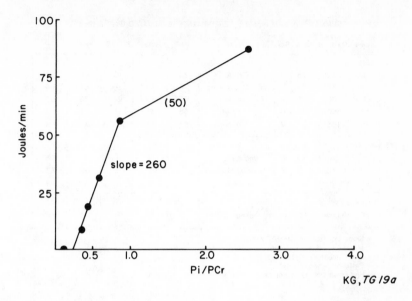

Figure 6. A top athlete who was able to continue with muscle performance in the region where oxidative metabolism reached its maximum and is supplemented by an aerobic glycolysis.

(TG 19)

Discussion

The results are generally two kinds: A nearly linear function including the resting intercept as published previously (Chance et al., 1981), the slope of the line being closely related to the metabolic recovery of the individual, a high slope indicates a high state of training, and vice versa. The dynamic range of the test seems rather large: Untrained individuals give values of 80, whereas trained individuals can give values over 200, a 3:1 ratio. Furthermore, trained individuals can exercise beyond the point at which lactic acidosis is highly significant. The initial slope is related to Figure 2 to be indicative of state 4 to state 3 transition for the mitochondria of the skeletal tissues. The second slope exhibited in Figure 6 is attributed to a combination of the intrinsic slope of the power versus P_i/PCr profile at values > 1, and the smaller increment of power output when respiration nears its V_{max} and glycolysis can supplement this by only a small quantity.[*] The limits of power versus P_i/PCr can vary between the maximum observed here (the 260 is the largest value we have observed) and a lower limit twentyfold less is established by a cytochrome b

---

[*]The uppermost asymptote or this second portion approaches a value that may be considered the work output permitted by mitochondrial oxidative capacity.

SUMMARY OF ARM MUSCLE PERFORMANCE EVALUATED BY ^{31}P NMR

Name	-Ath Relative	Age	Sex	Sport	$(V)O_2)_{max}$	Slope I$^+$	Slope 2$^+$	Max^o	$\frac{Pi+PCr}{ATP}$$^=$
Elite									
KG	(100)	25	M	Tri-Ath	84	88	18	87	5.7
DH	(70)	32	M	Tri-Ath/Rowing	74	48	–	67	8.4
ED	(65)	25	M	Tri-Ath	65	56	21	73	6.0
JD	(60)	37	M	Tri-Ath	55	36	11	73	5.8
BS	(55)	55	M	Tri-Ath	55	43	–	73	8.6
Moderate									
JK^x	Moderate	29	F	Olympic Yachting		14	4	30	5.3
JK*	Moderate	29	F	Olympic Yachting		27	3	20	7.3
TG	Moderate	22	M	Running		28	10	48	4.9
Untrained									
JT	Untrained	50	M	Sedentary		7	–	13	8.9

+ Slope Expression (J/min)/(Pi/PCr)
o Maximum Values in J/min
x Pre-Competing (3 Mon)
* Post-Competing (3 Day)
= Higher values are appropiate to more "white" fiber.

TG 24 b

Table 2. Summary of data comparing event performance and other parameters with NMR evaluated muscle exercise performance.   (MT 24)

deficient person in whom only glycolysis was available as an energy source to muscle contraction.

Table 2 summarizes these data and compares them to the slope of the naive individual.

Conclusions

It can be concluded that the exercise protocol described here has a large dynamic range, appears to be correlated to field performance, and may be used more incisively in further studies of exercise performance. This protocol may also be a useful correlate in the evaluation of fatigue.

References

Bücher, T., & Klingenberg, M. (1958). *Angew. Chem., 70,* 552.

Chance, B., & Connelly, C.M. (1957). A method for the estimation of the increase in concentration of adenosinediphosphate in muscle sarcosomes following a contraction. *Nature, 179,* 1235-1237.

Chance, B., Eleff, S., Leigh, J.S. Jr., Sokolow, D., & Sapega, A. (1981). Mitochondrial regulation of phosphocreatine/inorganic phosphate ratios in exercising human muscle: A gated ^{31}P NMR study. *Proceedings of the National Academy of Science* (USA), **78**, 6714-6718.

Chance, B., & Hollunger, G. (1961). The interaction of energy and electron transfer reactions in mitochondria: VI. The efficiency of the reaction. *Journal of Biological Chemistry*, **236**, 1577-1584.

Chance, B., & Jobsis, F. (1959). Change in fluorescence in a frog sartorius muscle following a twitch. *Nature*, **184**, 195-196.

Chance, B., Mauriello, G., & Aubert, X.M. (1962). In K. Rodahl & S.M. Horvath (Eds.), *Muscle in tissue* (pp. 128-145). New York: McGraw-Hill.

Chance, B., Sapega, A., Sokolow, D., Eleff, S., Leigh, J.S. Jr., Graham, T., Armstrong, J., & Warnell, R. (1983). Fatigue in retrospect and prospect: ^{31}P NMR studies of exercise performance. In H.G. Knuttgen, J.A., & J. Poortmans (Eds.), *Biochemistry of exercise* (Vol. 13, pp. 895-908). International Series in Sports Sciences. Champaign, IL: Human Kinetics.

Chance, B., & Weber, A.M. (1963). The steady-state of cytochrome b during rest and after contraction in frog sartorius. *Journal of Physiology* (London), **169**, 263-277.

Chance, B., & Williams, G.R. (1955). Respiratory enzymes in oxidative phosphorylation. *Journal of Biological Chemistry*, **217**, 383-451.

Fleckenstein, A., Janke, J., & Davies, R.E. (1956). Exchange of radioactive phosphate with α β γ-phosphorus of adenylpyrophosphate and phosphocreatine in acetylcholine, nicotine, and succinylcholine induced contraction of frog rectus. *Archives of Experimental Pathology and Pharmacology* (Berlin), **228**, 596-614.

Gyulai, L., Roth, Z., Leigh, J.S., Jr., & Chance, B. (1984). *Biophysical Journal*, **45**, 90.

Gyulai, L., Roth, Z., Leigh, J.J., Jr., & Chance, B. (1985). Bioenergetic studies of mitochondrial oxidative phosphorylation using ^{31}P NMR. *The Journal of Biological Chemistry*, **260**, 3947-3954.

Discussion

In reply to Dr. Bárány, who wanted information regarding changes in ATP, phosphocreatine, and phosphate in the patients with reduced leg blood flow, Dr. Chance replied that Dr. Wilkie had shown that calibration of NMR signals may be achieved by comparing the phosphocreatine area to the ATP area; the measurements had shown that the phosphocreatine reaction maintains ATP concentration. He emphasized the importance of ratios, both from a theoretical point of view in considering metabolic kinetics and an analytical point of view. In the patients whom he had studied, those with severe vascular insufficiency in the legs, the resting PCr/P_i ratio was not maintained even at resting values, and could fail from a maximum of over 20 to 5 or even less in the case of a mitochondrial disease (1.5).

Dr. Stein wondered about the phosphate in other tissues, in influencing the PCr/P_i ratio, particularly in an atrophied limb. Dr. Chance replied that most of the patients did have atrophied legs, with an increased fat/water content; although fat cells contain functioning mitochondria, they are sparse. As ATP concentration is normal, conversion of fast twitch fibers into slow twitch fibers might tend to maintain the phosphate potential. Dr. Wilkie felt Dr. Stein had raised a good point; in normal muscle one can obtain good calibration values, making use of the determinations of Dr. Hultman and his colleagues, but it is more difficult in muscles from patients with neuromuscular disorders such as Duchenne dystrophy, in which the muscle is infiltrated with fatty and fibrous tissue. However, a method was being developed to obtain absolute calibration in diseased states, which is purely orientated towards NMR. The absolute signals from water are compared to those from phosphorous, a method which his group has found works well in investigations of the brains of new born infants.

Dr. Wilkie pointed out that in the interesting plots of P_i/PCr that Dr. Chance showed and that correlated with characteristics such as athletic ability, the linear relationships between this ratio and power output indicated that the reciprocal plot against PCr/P_i could not be linear. Dr. Chance replied that the linear relationship between work and P_i/PCr is obtained in a wide variety of exercise tests and was obtained in experiments on isolated mitochondria. The entire profile is a Michaelis-Menten rectangular hyperbola, and here is represented at its initial straight limb; the curvature is consistent with a hyperbolic function of the form V/Vmax = $1/\{1 + km /(P_i/PCr)\}$.

Dr. Green was interested in the 5 to 1 differences between fast and slow twitch muscles in PCr; he felt that although some differences had been established in some species, such as rat, this did not apply to humans. Dr. Chance mentioned that he was quoting the work of R.E. Davies; as an example of a type II muscle, Dr. Chance cited the barnacle muscle in which the ratio was over 10:1, but of course in this animal it is arginine, not phosphocreatine, that is found in white muscle.

Dr. Newsholme asked if the relationships between PCr/P_i were simply a function of the observations or if they provided evidence of a control system for PCr and the ATP transfer system in muscle. Dr. Chance replied that the P_i/PCr work relationship is the Michaelis-Menten "transfer function" for ADP control. He described the initial experiments in which he and Klingenberg used the fact that ATP will activate the reversal of the electron transport chain, enabling them to solve the equation for the dynamics of DPNH oxidation. For the ATP/ADP ratio in the equation PCr/Cr could be substituted, and complete profiles were obtained for mitochondria mixed with CPK, PCr, Cr, and P_i in steady state conditions, which lasted several minutes; the relationships confirmed the initial linear part of the PCr/P_i relationship, with a strong influence of the pH.

There was also considerable discussion with regard to the effects of changes in pH and in ion concentrations on excitation-contraction coupling, particularly as it related to the site of fatigue. Dr. McComas pointed out that for brief efforts Bigland-Ritchie had shown that the site was peripheral rather than in the central nervous system, and did not involve the action potential in the sarcolemma (Bigland-Ritchie, Jones, Hosking, & Edwards, 1978). Although there was a tacit assumption that it was the contractile machinery that was impaired in fatigue, it may be that excitation-contraction coupling is at fault. Eberstein and Sandow (1963) stimulated amphibian muscle to the point that it could not develop any tetanic tension, but when the muscle was placed in a bath and caffeine was applied, an appreciable contraction tension was developed. The observations of Bigland-Ritchie in low frequency fatigue suggest the possibility of uncoupling. Saltin had pointed out that serum K during exercise became high; if interstitial K increased to the same extent, the K in transverse tubules might become very high.

Dr. Bigland-Ritchie did not want to leave the impression that changes in surface action potential did not occur in fatigue. A slowing of conduction velocity occurs, and after voluntary fatigue the muscle is much more susceptible to failure in response to high frequency stimulation; this may be the external manifestation of profound changes taking place in the transverse tubule system, in which changes in Na and K may play a major part. Dr. Chance indicated that K movement from cortical neurons is linked to the energy state reaching 30 m mol when the PCr/P_i ratio is 1.0. He wondered what the levels of K are in muscles and what fraction of the metabolic energy was required to maintain K equilibration. Dr. Stein pointed out that the emphasis during the symposium has been on the magnitude of force or power output, which is closely related to the PCr/P_i ratios; however, the rate constants of the decay and rise in force may be important in giving information regarding the effects of ion changes. For example, the rate of decay of force is related to the rate of Ca uptake in the sarcoplasmic reticulum in many conditions; on the other hand, the rate of rise is reported to be very slow and probably related quite closely to the rate of release of Ca, which would be slowed if Ca was depleted from the sarcoplasmic reticulum during fatigue.

Dr. Wilkie felt this was an important and interesting question that was approached by Lüttgau in Cambridge in 1965 with some elegant experiments that have not yet been repeated. He took a single isolated muscle fiber and repeatedly stimulated it, measuring the force and action potential with an intracellular electrode. He found a gradually declining twitch response to the stimulation and, surprisingly, a decline in the action potential; when contraction failed completely, as it did after a few hundred twitches, the action potential suddenly increased to its original value and remained there for thousands of responses. This was a perplexing result because the size of the action potential in millivolts is supposed to depend not on metabolic factors, but on ionic gradients that are established a long time before by the Na-K pump. The experiments left no doubt, but the explanation remains nonexistent after nearly 20 years; it suggests some connection in a single muscle fiber between the action potential and the metabolite levels. Dr. Bárány commented that in even earlier experiments Lundsgaard (1930) had shown that the last traces of ATP had to be used in order for the muscle to go into rigor. On performing the same experiment in frog muscle and following ATP concentration, it was surprising to find that contraction stops at a point when ATP is still present. Very little ATP is needed to keep ionic pumps alive, and he felt that this was the reason that action potentials still occur when the muscle cannot contract.

References

Bigland-Ritchie, B., Jones, D.A., Hosking, G.P., & Edwards, R.H.T. (1978). Central and peripheral fatigue in sustained maximum voluntary contractions of human quadriceps muscle. *Clinical Science and Molecular Medicine, 54*, 609-614.

Davies, R.E. (1983). Skeletal muscle. In *Handbook of physiology, Sec. 10* (p. 566, Table 2). Bethesda, MD: American Physiological Society.

Eberstein, A., & Sandow, A. (1963). Fatigue mechanisms in muscle fibres. In *The effect of use and disuse on neuromuscular functions* (pp. 515-526). Prague, Czechoslovakia: Academy of Science.

Lundsgaard, E. (1930). Werter Untersuchungen über Muskelkontraktionen ohnl Milchsaurebildung, *Biochem Z, 227*, 51.

Lüttgau, H.C. (1965). The effect of metabolic inhibitors on the fatigue of the action potential in single muscle fibres. *Journal of Physiology* (London). **178**, 45-67.

Section $\overline{6}$

Adaptation/Maladaptation

16

Biochemical Training Adaptations and Maximal Power

Philip D. Gollnick and Warwick M. Bayly
Washington State University

The consequences of training-induced biochemical adaptations in skeletal muscle are broad and cover all aspects of muscular function. We will consider the basic aspects of the proteins involved in muscular contraction and ATP production, and the substrate stores in the muscle that serve as fuels for metabolism.

"Maximal power" may be considered as the maximal work a muscle can perform in unit time, and in a strict sense this is the work performed over a very short period of time. However, if considered from another point of view, it may be interpreted as the maximal work performed in any defined period. With this definition, maximal power can be assessed for a wide variety of physical activities and sporting events. We will consider maximal power for a variety of work conditions, and the effects of biochemical changes associated with training on power output under each condition. For the purpose of this discussion, "training" refers to participation in programs of chronic exercise resulting in increases in strength, speed, or endurance.

Maximal Instantaneous Power Per Unit Muscle

Maximal "instantaneous power," in one or two muscular contractions, is produced by a maximal rate of cross-bridge cycling at the level of actin and myosin. The concentration of myosin and actin per unit of cross-sectional area for normal and enlarged muscle (Carney & Brown, 1967), and thus the number of cross-bridges per unit area of muscle, is constant. As it has never been demonstrated that physical training alters the ATP required to produce contraction for a given fiber type, it may be assumed that the energy demand and maximal power production per contractile unit of muscle are constant. The quantity of ATP needed to maximally activate cross-bridge cycling for a few contractions is contained in muscle and can be replenished from creatine phosphate to support the contractions for a few seconds. Thus, it does not appear that any type of physical training will influence the maximal power production capacity per unit cross-sectional area of skeletal muscle.

The maximal realizable external work, and thus the power, that a muscle can produce depends upon the speed of the contraction as demonstrated by Hill, Long, and Lupton (1924). The linear decline in force with increasing velocity of muscle contraction may be attributed to loss of force due to the internal resistance that develops during high speed contractions and is measurable in activities such as pedalling a cycle ergometer (Dickinson, 1929).

Because the energy required for such power developments is stored in muscle and such efforts do not rely upon an immediate energy production by the metabolic pathways, expansion of the capacities of these pathways would be of no consequence. However, there are reports (Eriksson, Gollnick, & Saltin, 1973; Karlsson, Nordesjö, Jorfeldt, & Saltin, 1972) of increased ATP and CP in muscle after training that could be important for short-term maximal power production by muscle.

Total Maximal Instantaneous Power

The total power that can be developed by a muscle or group of muscles acting synergistically is a function of the total cross-sectional area of the muscle that can be activated (the sum of the cross-sections of the constituent fibers and not the cross-sectional area of a muscle measured at its point of greatest girth). This capacity can be increased by any factor that increases the total available cross-sectional area of the muscle. Such increases have been produced by heavy resistance training through synthesis of additional contractile units (Gollnick, Parsons, Riedy, Moore, & Timson, 1983) in both man and animals (Edström & Ekblom, 1972; Goldspink, 1983; Ianuzzo, Gollnick, & Armstrong, 1976; MacDougall, Sale, Moroz, Elder, Sutton, & Howald, 1979; Prince, Hikida, & Hagerman, 1976). The increases in size are not accompanied by changes in the contractile properties (Freeman & Luff, 1982; Lesch, Parmley, Hamosh, Kaufman, & Sonnenblick, 1968) or in the sarcoplasmic reticulum (Baldwin, Valdez, Herrick, MacIntosh, & Roy, 1982). Thus, it can be concluded that with heavy resistance training in which total muscle cross-sectional area is increased, there is a concomitant increase in the capacity for maximal power development.

The composition of muscle that enlarges in response to a functional overload is similar to that of normal muscle (Ianuzzo & Chen, 1979). During the early stages of enlargement when rapid growth occurs, there may be a reduction in the concentration of enzymes for terminal oxidation. In the enlarged muscle of persons who have engaged in heavy resistance training, the concentration of such enzymes is lower, or at least not higher, than that of sedentary individuals (Costill, Coyle, Fink, Leemes, & Witzmann, 1979; Gollnick, Armstrong, Saubert, Piehl, & Saltin, 1972). However, such muscle does retain the capacity to increase its oxidative potential with endurance training (Baldwin, Cheadle, Martinez, & Cooke, 1977; Riedy, Moore, & Gollnick, 1985).

Frequently, however, the total increase in power development capacity does not increase linearly with total muscle bulk. This may be due to biomechanical aspects of force development, as the increase in cross-section of the individual fibers may require a change in the angle of pennation within the muscle to avoid a change in the overall muscle length (Binkhorst & van't Hoff, 1973; Gollnick, Timson, Moore, & Riedy, 1981; Meara, 1947). This can alter the angle of pull of the fibers within the muscle (Lindhard, 1931) so that the effective force exerted at the point of insertion is not a linear function of the total change in cross-sectional area. The conclusion, however, remains that the maximal instantaneous power that can be developed by a muscle can be altered by training and that the biochemical mechanism responsible for such a change is an increase in the total contractile material contained in the muscle.

Ultra Short-Term Maximal Power Production

"Ultra short-term" refers to work that can be accomplished in 1 min or less. As the maximal oxygen uptake capacity $\dot{V}O_2$max is exceeded, it is commonly referred to as "supramaximal." This type of effort requires the expenditure of energy from the immediate store of ATP within muscle and its replenishment from the CP stored in muscle, activation of the Embden-Meyerhof pathway with the production of lactate, and the terminal oxidation of substrate by mitochondria to carbon dioxide and water. It has been estimated that under these conditions more than 60% of the energy is derived from anaerobic processes with the remainder coming from aerobic processes (Gollnick & Hermansen, 1973). During such work, the CP, ATP, pH, and glycogen of skeletal muscle are reduced, whereas lactate, glucose-6-phosphate, and free glucose accumulate (Chance, 1983; Dawson, 1983; Jacobs, Tesch, Bar-Or, Karlsson, & Dotan, 1983; Saltin, Gollnick, Eriksson, & Piehl, 1971; Hermansen and Osnes, 1971). Due to the delay in the response of the cardiorespiratory system at the onset of exercise, the total body oxygen consumption during these supramaximal efforts may rise to only about 80% of the maximum (Saltin et al., 1971). Such data illustrate the need to derive energy from all sources to support the contractile process during this type of exercise, resulting in a post-exercise oxygen consumption that is most frequently referred to as an "oxygen debt."

Individuals whose athletic events require efforts such as those described in the previous paragraph commonly engage in high intensity "sprint" training programs that mimic the events and are designed to increase the ability to work at supramaximal levels. This training may produce, at most, small increases in the enzymes from terminal oxidation (Davies, Packer, & Brooks, 1981; Saltin, et al., 1976; Saubert, Armstrong, Shepherd, & Gollnick, 1973; Staudte, Exner, & Pette, 1973). The $\dot{V}O_2$ max can be increased by sprint-type training (Saltin et al., 1976), and the enzymes in the Embden-Meyerhof pathway may increase or not change (Saltin & Gollnick, 1983). If the concentration of these enzymes is increased with sprint training, the magnitude of this change is relatively small.

It is not clear that sprint training has a major effect on the concentrations of glycogen or CP in skeletal muscle. An increase in CP would provide an immediate energy reserve for use during power outputs that could by sustained only for very short periods of time, but it is questionable whether an increase in the concentration of glycogen or of enzymes of the Embden-Meyerhof pathway would be of any benefit. The basis for this conclusion is the observation that in most cases the glycogen of muscle is not emptied at the point when exercise can no longer be sustained. Similarly, in most sedentary individuals the concentration of the enzymes in muscle for lactate production is greater than that needed to degrade the muscle glycogen to lactate in a very short time, should this system be activated to even half maximal—a level normally assumed to be that at which enzymes function in vivo. When considered from the standpoint of providing energy to the contractile complex, it does not appear that any major changes in the biochemical aspect for energy production would alter the capacity for short-term power production. However, when repeated bouts of such work are performed, it is advantageous to increase the store of glycogen within the muscle because the capacity to perform short-term, high-intensity exercise diminishes when the glycogen stores of muscle are depleted (Åstrand, Hallback, Hedman, & Saltin, 1963; Heigenhauser, Sutton, & Jones, 1983).

Short-Term Maximal Power Production

"Short-term maximal power production" is defined as that which can be sustained for 5 to 6 min. It has been estimated that for this type of endeavor about 20% of the total energy production comes from the anaerobic metabolic pathways, with the remainder produced by terminal oxidation (Gollnick &

Hermansen, 1973). These efforts can be at or above the $\dot{V}O_2$max and require activation of all methods for ATP synthesis.

Training for this type of power production can involve elements of endurance, strength, and sprint training. It produces increases in the total body $\dot{V}O_2$ max and in the concentrations of glycogen and enzymes for terminal oxidation. There may also be a small change in the CP concentration (see above). As illustrated by Åstrand and Saltin (1961), the rate of increase in the $\dot{V}O_2$ during exercise is a function of the intensity of the exercise. Thus, in this type of exercise there is a moderately rapid rise in the $\dot{V}O_2$ reaching a value of close to maximal between the 4th and 5th minute. One effect of endurance training is to increase the rate of rise in the $\dot{V}O_2$ after the onset of exercise (Hagberg, Hickson, Ashani, & Holloszy, 1980; Whipp & Wasserman, 1972). This may be a response related to the biochemical changes that occur in muscle (Gollnick, Riedy, Quintinskie, & Bertucci, 1985). Exercise at this intensity is usually terminated by the subject before exhaustion of the glycogen stores, suggesting that factors other than the availability of fuel must be responsible for the inability to continue the exercise. However, a depletion of glycogen produces a decrease in the power output, and so it cannot be dismissed as unimportant for short periods of high power output.

Moderately Long-Term Maximal Power

This type of exercise requires a $\dot{V}O_2$ of about 75% of the $\dot{V}O_2$ max and can be sustained by man for 1 to 3 hr (Gollnick et al., 1973) depending upon the state of training. The glycogen of the active muscle declines during the course of such exercise until it is nearly emptied at the point of exhaustion (Bergström, Hermansen, Hultman, & Saltin, 1967; Gollnick et al., 1973; Hermansen, Hultman, & Saltin, 1967). Training for this type of exercise is mainly endurance in nature. Endurance training increases the maximal cardiac output, $\dot{V}O_2$ max, the glycogen content of muscle, and the concentration of enzymes for terminal oxidation of carbohydrates and fats, but causes little or no change in the concentration of enzymes of the Embden-Meyerhof pathway (Saltin & Gollnick, 1983). During such exercise there is a slower rate of glycogen depletion from the exercising muscle, a greater reliance on fat as fuel (evidenced by a lower respiratory exchange ratio), and lower concentrations of lactate in the blood and muscle in the trained state (Karlsson et al., 1972). This adaptive response to training has been demonstrated for one leg during two-legged exercise in which only one leg was endurance trained (Henriksson, 1977). Trained subjects (both man and animals) are able to perform such exercise at higher percentages of their $\dot{V}O_2$ max and to sustain it longer that nontrained subjects after training.

How then are the biochemical changes that occur with training related to the maximal power production that can be sustained under this exercise condition? First, it is an old observation that the onset of exhaustion during this type of exercise is closely associated with the depletion of glycogen in the active muscle. The greater storage of glycogen that occurs with training will prolong the total time that moderately intense, long-term exercise can be continued (Bergström et al., 1967; Hermansen et al., 1967), thereby increasing the maximal power output for this exercise condition. The second major biochemical change is the large increase that occurs in the concentration of enzymes of terminal oxidation of carbohydrates and fats. This adaptation, produced by an elevation in the concentration of mitochondria per unit of skeletal muscle, occurs in all types of muscle when the training is of appropriate intensity and duration. When considered from the nontrained to trained state it is clear that the increase in oxidative potential that occurs with training exceeds the change in the $\dot{V}O_2$ max. It may, however, be related to a greater use of fats during exercise and the lower concentration of lactate in both muscle and blood after training. It has been proposed that this shift to a greater reliance upon fat as a fuel is the result of a more rapid translocation of the ADP produced by contraction into the mitochondria. This would have the effect of maintaining the ATP/ADP ratio higher, thereby more tightly controlling glycolytic flux.

An elevated use of fat as a fuel during exercise can be induced in the rat by the prolonged feeding of a low carbohydrate diet (Miller, Bryce, & Conlee, 1984), accompanied by increases in the concentration of enzymes for fat oxidation, reduced concentrations of glycogen in liver and muscle at rest, and a reduced rate of glycogen depletion during exercise. The endurance, taken as the time to exhaustion while running at 35 m/min, of rats fed a low carbohydrate diet for 5 wks was 33% greater than control animals. These data demonstrate that shifts in the choice of fuel oxidized during exercise can be modified by the type of food consumed. In this regard, a shift towards a greater use of fat during exercise can be induced simply by reducing the concentration of glycogen stored in muscle (Gollnick, Pernow, Essén, Jansson, & Saltin, 1981). In these experiments the low glycogen concentrations were produced in one leg by a previous day's one-legged exercise and the consumption of a low carbohydrate diet. During two-legged exercise on the second day, the respiratory quotient was lower in the leg with low glycogen than that with normal glycogen. Moreover, the rate of glycogen depletion was less. There was an uptake rather than release of lactate from the leg with low glycogen; the uptake of fatty acid and glucose was also greater. Collectively, these data illustrate that numerous factors can alter the choice of fuel used during exercise. The importance of the finding of Miller et al. (1984) is that the chronic consumption of a low carbohydrate diet can produce alterations in the concentrations of key enzymes in muscle that would promote the use of fat during exercise.

Prolonged Power Production

We view "prolonged power production" as that which can be sustained for 6 or more hours. Such power production can be sustained at exercise intensities of about 30% and 50% of the $\dot{V}O_2$ max for sedentary and endurance trained individuals, respectively. Athletic events that require such efforts are the double marathon, some cross-country ski competitions, and a number of bicycle events. Training for such events is primarily the same as that for moderately long-term maximal power production. Thus, there are elevations in the concentrations of mitochondrial enzymes, and there may also be an enhanced storage of glycogen in the muscles.

The significance of the biochemical adaptations to training for these events appears to be primarily that of providing for a greater utilization of fat as a fuel during the exertion. This is important in some events like cross-country skiing, which may expend as many as 1350 kcal/hr (Åstrand et al., 1963). If these energy expenditures were produced by oxidation of the carbohydrate stored in the body, exhaustion would occur in about 2 hr. Therefore, it is important in such events that the mobilization and oxidation of fatty acids contribute as much as possible to the total caloric production. That this does occur is illustrated by the observation that the respiratory exchange ratio of cross-country skiers during an 85 km competition average 0.71, which is consistent with more than 95% of the oxygen uptake used for the combustion of fat (Åstrand et al., 1963). This primary reliance upon fat as fuel during prolonged exercise is similar to that reported by Edwards, Margaria, and Talbott (1934) for men during the last hr of a 6 hr treadmill run. The biochemical adaptations that occur in skeletal muscle in response to endurance training appear to be aimed primarily at increasing endurance capacity, therefore enhancing the maximal power production under these conditions rather than increasing short-term power production.

References

Åstrand, P.-O., Hallback, I., Hedman, R., & Saltin, B. (1963). Blood lactate after prolonged severe exercise. *Journal of Applied Physiology, 18*, 619-622.

Åstrand, P.-O., & Saltin, B. (1961). Maximal oxygen uptake and heart rate in various types of muscular exercise. *Journal of Applied Physiology, 16*, 971-976.

Baldwin, K.M., Cheadle, W.G., Martinez, O.M., & Cooke, D.A. (1977). Effect of functional overload on enzyme levels in different types of muscle. *Journal of Applied Physiology: Respiratory, Environmental and Exercise Physiology, 42*, 312-317.

Baldwin, K.M., Valdez, V., Herrick, R.E., MacIntosh, A.M., & Roy, R.R. (1982). Biochemical properties of overloaded fast twitch skeletal muscle. *Journal of Applied Physiology: Respiratory, Environmental and Exercise Physiology, 52*, 467-472.

Bergström, J., Hermansen, L., Hultman, E., & Saltin, B. (1967). Diet muscle glycogen, and physical performance. *Acta Physiologica Scandinavica, 71*, 140-150.

Binkhorst, R.A., & van't Hoff, M.A. (1973). Force-velocity relationships and contraction time of the rat fast plantaris muscle due to compensatory hypertrophy. *Pflügers Archives, 342*, 145-158.

Carney, J.A., & Brown, A.L. (1967). The morphology of myosin in cardiac hypertrophy. *Lab. Invest., 16*, 36-43.

Chance, B. (1983). Fatigue in retrospect and prospect: ^{31}P NMR studies of exercise performance. In H.G. Knuttgen, J.A. Vogel, & J. Poortmans (Eds.), *Biochemistry of exercise* (pp. 895-908). Champaign, IL: Human Kinetics.

Costill, D.L., Coyle, E.F., Fink, W.F., Leemes, G.R., & Witzmann, F.A. (1979). Adaptation in skeletal muscle following strength training. *Journal of Applied Physiology: Respiratory, Environmental and Exercise Physiology, 46*, 96-99.

Davies, K.J.A., Packer, L., & Brooks, G.A. (1982). Exercise bioenergetics following sprint training. *Archives of Biochemistry and Biophysics, 215*, 260-265.

Dawson, M.J. (1983). Phosphorus metabolites and the control of glycolysis studied by nuclear magnetic resonance. In H.G. Knuttgen, J.A. Vogel, & J. Poortmans (Eds.), *Biochemistry of exercise* (pp. 116-125). Champaign, IL: Human Kinetics.

Dickinson, S. (1929). The efficiency of bicycle pedalling as affected by speed and load. *Journal of Physiology* (London), *67*, 242-255.

Edstrom, L., & Ekblom, B. (1972). Differences in sizes of red and white muscle fibres in vastus lateralis of musculus quadriceps femoris of normal individuals and athletes. *Scandinavian Journal of Clinical Laboratory Investigation.*

Edwards, H.T., Margaria, R., & Talbott, J.H. (1934). Metabolic rate, blood sugar, and the utilization of carbohydrate. *American Journal of Physiology, 108*, 203-209.

Eriksson, B.O., Gollnick, P.D., & Saltin, B. (1973). Muscle metabolism and enzyme activities after training in boys 11-13 years old. *Acta Physiologica Scandinavica, 87*, 485-497.

Freeman, P.L., & Luff, A.R. (1982). Contractile properties of hindlimb muscles in rat during surgical overload. *American Journal of Physiology, 242*, C259-C264.

Goldspink, G. (1983). Alterations in myofibril size and structure during growth, exercise, and changes in environmental temperature. In L.D. Peachy, R.H. Adrian, & S.R. Geiger (Eds.), *Handbook of physiology* (pp. 539-554). Baltimore: Williams and Wilkins.

Gollnick, P.D., Armstrong, R.B., Saubert, C.W., IV, Piehl, K., & Saltin, B. (1972). Enzyme activity and fiber composition in skeletal muscle of untrained and trained men. *Journal of Applied Physiology*, **33**, 312-319.

Gollnick, P.D., Armstrong, R.B., Saubert, C.W., IV, Sembrowich, W.L., Shepherd, R.E., & Saltin, B. (1973). Glycogen depletion patterns in human skeletal muscle during prolonged work. *Pflügers Archives*, **344**, 1-12.

Gollnick, P.D., & Hermansen, L. (1973). Biochemical adaptations to exercise: Anaerobic metabolism. In J.H. Wilmore (Ed.), *Exercise and sports science reviews* (pp. 1-43). New York: Academic Press.

Gollnick, P.D., Parsons, D., Riedy, M., Moore, R.L., & Timson, B.F. (1983). An evaluation of mechanisms modulating muscle size in response to varying perturbations. In K.T. Borer, D.W. Edington, & T.P. White (Eds.), *Frontiers of exercise biology* (pp. 27-50). Champaign, IL: Human Kinetics.

Gollnick, P.D., Pernow, B., Essen, B., Jansson, E., & Saltin, B. (1981). Availability of glycogen and plasma FFA for substrate utilization in leg muscle of man during exercise. *Clinical Physiology*, **1**, 27-42.

Gollnick, P.D., Riedy, M., Quintinskie, J.J., Jr., & Bertocci, L.A. (1985). Differences in metabolic potential of skeletal muscle fibres and their significance for metabolic control. *The Journal of Experimental Biology*, **15**, 191-199.

Gollnick, P.D., Timson, B.F., Moore, R.L., & Riedy, M. (1981). Muscular enlargement and number of fibers in skeletal muscle of rats. *Journal of Applied Physiology: Respiratory, Environmental and Exercise Physiology*, **50**, 936-943.

Hagberg, J.M., Hickson, R.C., Ashani, A.A., & Holloszy, J.O. (1980). Faster adjustment to and recovery from submaximal exercise in the trained state. *Journal of Applied Physiology: Respiratory, Environmental and Exercise Physiology*, **48**, 218-224.

Heigenhauser, G.J.F., Sutton, J.R., & Jones, N.L. (1983). Effect of glycogen depletion on the ventilatory response to exercise. *Journal of Applied Physiology: Respiratory, Environmental and Exercise Physiology*, **54**, 470-474.

Henriksson, J. (1977). Training-induced adaptation of skeletal muscle and metabolism during submaximal exercise. *Journal of Physiology* (London), **270**, 661-690.

Hermansen, L., Hultman, E., & Saltin, B. (1967). Muscle glycogen during prolonged severe exercise. *Acta Physiologica Scandinavica*, **71**, 129-139.

Hermansen, L., & Osnes, J.B. (1972). Blood and muscle pH after maximal exercise in man. *Journal of Applied Physiology*, **32**, 304-308.

Hill, A.V., Long, C.N.H., & Lupton, H. (1924). The effect of fatigue on the relationship between work and speed in the contraction of human arm muscle. *Journal of Physiology* (London), **58**, 334-337.

Ianuzzo, C.D., & Chen, V. (1979). Metabolic character of hypertrophied rat muscle. *Journal of Applied Physiology*, **46**, 738-742.

Ianuzzo, C.D., Gollnick, P.D., & Armstrong, R.B. (1976). Compensatory adaptations of skeletal muscle fiber types to a long-term functional overload. *Life Sciences, 19,* 1517-1524.

Jacobs, I., Tesch, P.A., Bar-Or, O., Karlsson, J., & Dotan, F. (1983). Lactate in human skeletal muscle after 10 and 30 s of supramaximal exercise. *Journal of Applied Physiology: Respiratory, Environmental and Exercise Physiology, 55,* 365-367.

Karlsson, J., Nordesjö, L.-O., Jorfeldt, L., & Saltin, B. (1972). Muscle lactate, ATP, and CP levels during exercise after physical training in man. *Journal of Applied Physiology, 33,* 199-203.

Lesch, M., Parmley, W.W., Hamosh, M., Kaufman, S., & Sonnenblich, E.H. (1968). Effects of hypertrophy on the contractile properties of skeletal muscle. *American Journal of Physiology, 214,* 685-690.

Lindhard, J. (1931). Der Skeletmuskel und seine Funktion. *Ergebnis Physiologisch, 33,* 337-557.

MacDougall, J.D., Sale, D.G., Moroz, J.R., Elder, G.C.B., Sutton, J.R., & Howald, H. (1979). Mitochondrial volume density in human skeletal muscle following heavy resistance training. *Medicine and Science in Sport, 11,* 164-166.

Meara, P.J. (1947). Post-natal growth and development of muscle, as exemplified by the gastrocnemius and psoas muscles of the rabbit. *Onderstepoort J. Vet. Sci. Anim. Ind., 21,* 329-428.

Miller, W.C., Bryce, G.R., & Conlee, R.K. (1984). Adaptations to a high-fat diet that increase exercise endurance in male rats. *Journal of Applied Physiology: Respiratory, Environmental and Exercise Physiology, 56,* 78-83.

Prince, F.P., Hikida, R.S., & Hagerman, F.C. (1976). Human muscle fiber types in power lifters, distance runners, and untrained subjects. *Pflügers Archives, 363,* 19-26.

Riedy, M., Moore, R.L., & Gollnick, P.D. (1985). Adaptive response of hypertrophied skeletal muscle to endurance training. *Journal of Applied Physiology: Respiratory, Environmental and Exercise Physiology, 59,* 127-131.

Saltin, B., & Gollnick, P.D. (1983). Skeletal muscle adaptability: Significance for metabolism and performance. In L.H. Peachy, R.H. Adrian, & S.R. Geiger (Eds.), *Handbook of physiology* (pp. 555-631). Baltimore: Williams & Wilkins.

Saltin, B., Gollnick, P.D., Eriksson, B.O., & Piehl, K. (1971). Metabolic adjustments at the onset of maximal work. In A. Gilbert & P. Guille (Eds.), *Onset of exercise* (pp. 63-76). Toulouse, France: University of Toulouse Press.

Saltin, B., Nazar, K., Costill, D.L., Stein, E., Jansson, E., Essen, B., & Gollnick, P.D. (1976). The nature of the training response: Peripheral and central adaptations to one-legged exercise. *Acta Physiologica Scandinavica, 96,* 289-305.

Saubert, C.W., IV, Armstrong, R.B., Shepherd, R.E., & Gollnick, P.D. (1973). Anaerobic enzyme adaptations to sprint training in rats. *Pflügers Archives,* **341**, 305-312.

Staudte, H.W., Exner, G.U., & Pette, D. (1973). Effects of short-term, high intensity (sprint) training on some contractile and metabolic characteristics of fast and slow muscle of the rat. *Pflügers Archives,* **344**, 159-168.

Whipp, B.J., & Wasserman, K. (1972). Oxygen uptake kinetics for various intensities of constant-load work. *Journal of Applied Physiology,* **33**, 351-356.

Discussion

The discussion following Dr. Gollnick's presentation began with some controversy with regard to the changes in creatine phosphate and glycogen in strength trained athletes. Although MacDougall, Ward, Sale, and Sutton (1977) showed a 20% increase in concentration of CP, coupled with a 25% hypertrophy, Dr. Gollnick's group has not been able to show this. Dr. Hultman reported that he had found slightly higher CP concentration in type II fibers, and he made the point that heavy resistance training will increase the area of these fibers and also increase the overall CP concentration. He felt it was important also to measure total creatine. CP may vary and the measurement of creatine allows a check to be made on whether CP was broken down at the time of the biopsy.

In reply to a question from Dr. Newsholme, Dr. Gollnick confirmed that there was an increase in mitochondrial concentration, his own studies having shown increases in both number and size (Gollnick & King, 1969). However, the studies of Kirkwood, Munn, Packer, and Brooks (1984) suggest that mitochondria may be a network of tubules within the muscles and not isolated structures as commonly thought; of course, what is really important is the surface area for the adenine nucleotide translocase to move ADP into the mitochondria at a high rate. Behind Dr. Newsholme's question was the idea that CPK may be important in the transport of phosphate from the mitochondria to the myofibrils. If training increased CPK activity, at least in the mitochondrial system, this could be potentially important; he felt that the role of CPK as a phosphate shuttle is not discussed often enough.

Dr. Gollnick was asked what is known about the total redox state in muscle and the extent to which it might be modified by training; he replied that the most recent data he knew was that of Connett, Gayeski, and Honig (1984), who examined oxidative states at different degrees of electrical stimulation and found that in heavy states of contraction the muscle was very oxidative. They also showed that a high rate of lactate production occurred at low levels of stimulation when the muscles were still oxidative, and the findings were probably due to early activation of glycolytic muscle before the rest of the system had had time to down-regulate it. Dr. Chance said that the redox potential of resting muscle is very positive and the state remains oxidative up to the point at which the NADH and ubiquinone pools are activated; the rate-limiting step is the translocase reaction, which results in a delay of about 70 msec. In recent studies (Honig & Connett) the redox state of the working gracilis muscle is measured by NMR to show that these muscles go through a peak of oxidation, but there is then a subsequent decline that appears to coincide with the accumulation of lactic acid.

Dr. MacDougall felt that in activities in which maximal power is required for less than 2 min, a logical adaptation would be the development of mechanisms that minimize increases in hydrogen ion concentration. He wondered what evidence there was that trained athletes improve their performance partly because they are able to handle a heavy acid load and minimize changes in intramuscular pH, perhaps through increases in myoglobin. Dr. Gollnick replied that training may increase the buffering capacity of muscle, but changes in myoglobin were unlikely to be large enough to have much of an effect. Dr. MacDougall countered that Holloszy had shown some impressive increases in myoglobin concentration in trained animals, but Dr. Gollnick pointed out that studies both in dystrophic animals (Booth, 1978) and (Svedenhag, Henriksson, & Slyven, 1983) in electrically stimulated animals had not shown such impressive changes and he preferred not to speculate. Peter LaChance asked whether the observation of Gonyea of hypertrophy-induced reduction in contractile speed after resistance training indicated that this type of training would not be appropriate in developing muscle power for sport events. Dr. Gollnick replied that data also existed that showed no changes in power output and contractile speed in hypertrophied muscle (Binkhorst, & van't Hoff, 1973; Carney & Brown, 1967; Freeman & Luff, 1982; Lesch, Parmley, Hamosh, Kaufman, & Sonnenblick, 1968). He was disinclined to discourage the use of high resistance work for power athletes.

References

Binkhorst, R.A., & van't Hoff, M.A. (1973). Force-velocity relationships and contraction time of the rat fast plantaris muscle due to compensatory hypertrophy. *Pflügers Archives, 342*, 145-158.

Booth, F.W. (1978). Inability of myoglobin to increase in dystrophic skeletal muscle during daily exercise. *Pflügers Archives, 373*, 175-178.

Carney, J.A., & Brown, A.L. (1967). The morphology of myosin in cardiac hypertrophy. *Laboratory Investigation, 16*, 36-43.

Connett, R.J., Gayeski, T.E.J., & Honig, C.R. (1984). Lactate accumulation in fully aerobic, working, dog gracilis muscle. *American Journal of Physiology, 246*, H120-H128.

Freeman, P.L., & Luff, A.R. (1982). Contractile properties of hindlimb muscles in rat during surgical overload. *American Journal of Physiology*, **242**, C259-C264.

Gollnick, P.D., & King, D.W. (1969). Effect of exercise and training on mitochondria of rat skeletal muscle. *American Journal of Physiology*, **216**, 1502-1509.

Kirkwood, S.P., Munn, E.A., Packer, L., & Brooks, G.A. (1984). Mitochondrial reticulum in rat skeletal muscle. *Medicine and Science in Sports and Exercise*, **16**, 120, (Abstract).

Lesch, M., Parmley, W.W., Hamosh, M., Kaufman, S., & Sonnenblick, E.H. (1968). Effects of hypertrophy on the contractile properties of skeletal muscle. *American Journal of Physiology*, **214**, 685-690.

MacDougall, J.D., Ward, G.R., Sale, D.G., & Sutton, J.R. (1977). Biochemical adaptation of human skeletal muscle to heavy resistance training and immobilization. *Journal of Applied Physiology: Respiratory, Environmental and Exercise Physiology*, **43**, 700-703.

Svedenhag, J., Henriksson, J., & Slyven, C. (1983). Dissociation of training effects on skeletal muscle mitochondrial enzymes and myoglobin in man. *Acta Physiologica Scandinavica*, **117**, 213-218.

17

Morphological Changes in Human Skeletal Muscle Following Strength Training and Immobilization

J.D. MacDougall
McMaster University

An athlete undergoes physical training in order to effect biological changes that will improve his performance in a specific task. Thus, training may include an almost infinite variety of combinations of intensity and frequency of muscle contractions. For example, at one extreme the endurance training of the marathon runner entails many thousands of low resistance contractions in a single training session. By contrast, a typical training session for a powerlifter would normally include fewer than 20 contractions of a particular muscle group but at maximal or near-maximal strength.

The effects of endurance training on oxygen transport and on muscle structure and function have been well documented, but there have been relatively few investigations of the effects of strength training. This presentation will attempt to focus on those adaptations that occur in skeletal muscle in response to brief but high-intensity training, known as strength or power training.

Methods

The structural changes accompanying training-induced hypertrophy and disuse atrophy were investigated by application of the needle biopsy procedure to a series of studies with human volunteer subjects. In general, these investigations were of two types:

1. A series of longitudinal training studies in which groups of previously untrained subjects underwent 4-6 months of heavy resistance training of either the elbow extensors or elbow flexor muscle groups. The training program that subjects followed was similar to that used by bodybuilders and strength athletes, in that 3 or 4 sets of 6-8 maximal repetitions were performed for each exercise, 3 times per week. In addition to undergoing training, 11 subjects in one study had their arms immobilized in elbow casts for a period of 6 weeks so that the effects of disuse atrophy could also be examined. Needle biopsy samples were taken from either triceps or biceps brachii muscles before and after the training or immobilization periods.

2. A series of studies where muscle ultrastructure from elite and intermediate calibre bodybuilders and powerlifters was compared with that of age-matched controls. The effects of chronic (6-8 yr) intensive training was thus inferred by comparison of such examples of extreme hypertrophy with skeletal muscle from untrained and short-term (6 months) trained subjects.

Tissue was prepared for histochemical and ultrastructural analysis as described previously (MacDougall, Ward, Sale, & Sutton, 1977; MacDougall et al., 1979; MacDougall, Elder, Sale, Moroz, & Sutton, 1980; MacDougall, Sale, Elder, & Sutton, 1982) and photographed under the light and electron microscopes. At the light microscope level a minimum of 150 fibers were analyzed from each biopsy sample, and at the electron microscope level a minimum of 80 fibers were photographed and analyzed.

For ultrastructural analysis, tissue was photographed at a low magnification (290x) and at two higher magnifications as follows: for each of the 80 fibers selected, 10 random non-overlapping micrographs were made of the interior of the fiber at a magnification of 10,260x and 10 at a magnification of 51,300x. No attempt was made to control whether or not the section had been made at the A or the I band, but since tissue obtained by needle biopsy is almost always fully contracted, the vast majority of micrographs were found to occur at the A band. Area measurements were made with a computerized digitizer, and stereological analysis was performed by means of a 168-point short line test system (Weibel, 1972).

Results and Discussion

Changes in Fiber Area

Heavy resistance training results in an increase in cross-sectional area of both Type I and Type II fibers, with a greater degree of hypertrophy occurring in the Type II fibers (Thorstensson, 1976; MacDougall et al., 1980). Immobilization also affects both fiber types but with a greater degree of atrophy occurring in the Type II fibers (MacDougall et al., 1980).

In a study where triceps brachii was trained for a period of 5-6 months, the area of the Type II fibers was found to have increased by approximately 33% whereas that of the Type I fibers had increased by only 27% (see Figure 1). Immobilization in elbow casts for 6 weeks resulted in a reduction in cross-sectional area of 38% for the Type II fibers and 31% for Type I fibers.

The greater degree of hypertrophy that occurred in the Type II fibers (see Figure 1) indicates a greater relative involvement of these units in the adaptive response to training. The selective atrophy of the Type II units with immobilization is in contrast to a study by Sargeant, Davies, Edwards, Maunder, and Young (1977), who found greater atrophy in the Type I fibers in the thigh; this may reflect functional differences between triceps brachii and postural muscles of the lower limb.

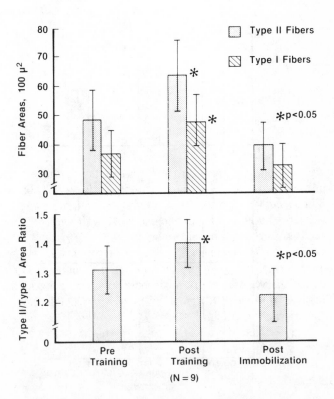

Figure 1. Cross-sectional area for Type I and Type II fibers in the control condition and following training and immobilization. The lower figure illustrates this data as Type II/Type I area ratios. Values are means ± 1SD. See text for further explanation.

Myofibril Changes

The results of 6 months of strength training and 6 weeks immobilization on the ultrastructure of triceps brachii in 6 subjects are illustrated in Figure 2. Training resulted in an increase in cross-sectional fiber area by approximately 31%, whereas immobilization resulted in a decrease in fiber area by approximately 40%.

Measurement of more than 3,500 myofibrils for each condition indicated that, despite wide variations in size, myofibril cross-sectional area increased significantly (p<0.01) by approximately 16% following training and decreased by a similar amount following immobilization. The number of myofibrils that were considered to have one or more "splits" in them (see Figure 3) was also recorded. Because of the subjectivity of such a measurement and the fact that results could easily be influenced by fixation or handling artifact, these mea-

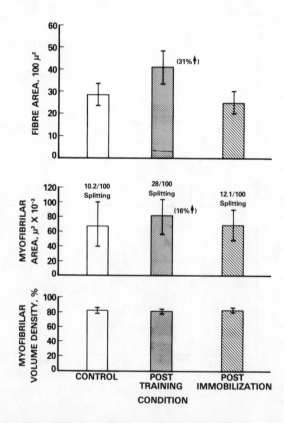

Figure 2. Changes in fiber area, myofibrilar area, and myofibrillar volume density following training and immobilization (N=6). The proportion of myofibrils considered as having "splits" in them is also included. Values are means ± 1SD. See text for further explanation.

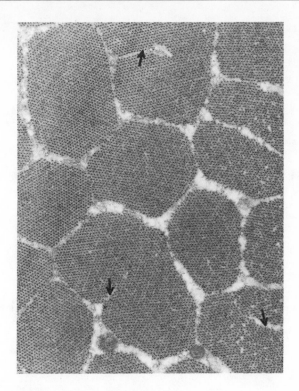

Figure 3. Examples of what were considered to be "splitting" myofibrils. The "splits" are indicated by the arrows. Photographed at 10,260x.

sures were made "blind," without the investigator's knowledge of which condition was being examined. Following training, there was an almost threefold increase in the number of myofibrils having "splits" in them, when compared to the control state.

The packing density of the myosin filaments was estimated from the high magnification micrographs at the A band by counting the number of filaments within an enclosed area (see Figure 4). Measurements were made at both the interior and exterior of approximately 500 myofibrils for each subject randomly chosen from a minimum of 50 fibers per subject per biopsy. The spacing of the myosin filaments (approximately $280/\mu m^2$) was found to be extremely consistent within each subject and between conditions, and was identical at the interior of the myofibril and at the exterior.

The increase in myofibril cross-sectional area with strength training is thus the result of the addition of actin and myosin filaments. Because the packing density of the myosin filaments remains the same at the interior of the myofibril as at the exterior, it is apparent that the contractile proteins are added to the outside of the myofibril and thus do not alter the cross-bridge configurations.

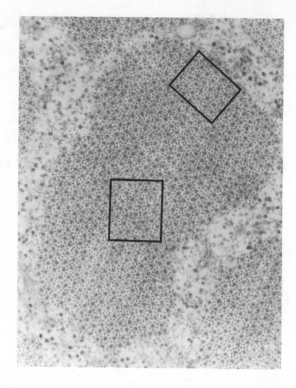

Figure 4. Illustration of the method used for estimating myosin filament packing density. Photographed at 51,300x.

Similarly, the decrease in myofibril size following immobilization is due to a loss of contractile protein from the periphery of the myofibril.

Because the volume density of the myofibrils in the fiber remains unaltered by training or immobilization (see Figure 5), changes in fiber size with these conditions are largely due to changes in myofibril size (or number). The finding that total fiber area increased by a greater proportion than did myofibril area (see Figure 5) indicates an increase in myofibril number as well as myofibril size. Presumably, this proliferation of myofibrils is the result of a longitudinal splitting process, as has been shown to occur in normal postnatal growth in animals (Goldspink, 1970, 1974; Rowe & Goldspink, 1969). This is supported by the apparent increase in the number of "splitting" myofibrils in the training state.

Goldspink (1970) has suggested several mechanisms by which this splitting process might occur, including a mechanical possibility related to discrepancies between the A and I band lattice spacing. Because of this discrepancy, with contraction, the peripheral I filaments (actin) are pulled at an angle slightly oblique to the myofibril axis. As more filaments are added to the myofibril,

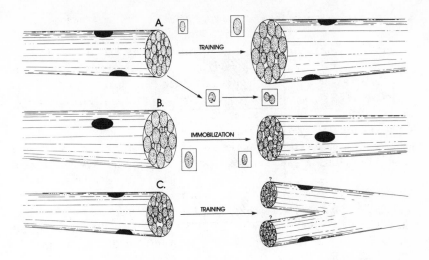

Figure 5. A possible model for the changes in muscle size that occur in response to strength training and immobilization. A. With training, cross-sectional fiber area increases in direct proportion to the increase in myofibril size and number. B. With immobilization fiber area decreases in direct proportion to the decrease in myofibril area. C. The possibility of training-induced fiber splitting is discussed later in this chapter.

the girth and strength are increased and the strain causes the center of the Z discs to rupture, resulting in two or more "daughter" myofibrils of the same sarcomere length.

The correlation between the increase in Type I or Type II fiber area and the increase in maximal voluntary strength following training was low and non-significant. Also, there was a poor correlation between the decrease in fiber size and the decline in strength following immobilization. Thus, it is apparent that changes in the quantity of contractile protein only partially account for the changes in maximal voluntary strength that occur with training or disuse. Other adaptations, most notably those within the central nervous system, may be as important as fiber size in the expression of maximal voluntary contractile strength. These adaptations are discussed in the subsequent chapter by Dr. Sale.

Mitochondrial Volume Density

Heavy resistance training results in a reduction in mitochondrial volume density (Vv_{mit}) and the mitochondrial/myofibrillar volume ratio (Vmit/Vmyof). In a study in which subjects trained their elbow extensor muscles for 6 months, morphometric analysis indicated that Vv_{mit} decreased by approximately 26% and Vmit/Vmyof by approximately 25% (see Figure 6).

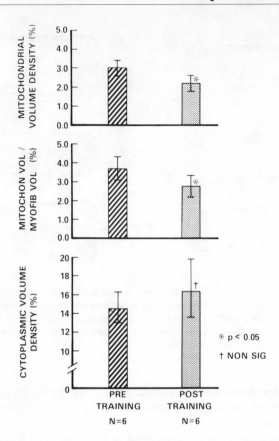

Figure 6. Mean (± 1 SD) mitochondrial and cytoplasmic volume density and mitochondrial-to-myofibrillar volume ratio before and after training (MacDougall et al., 1979).

The decrements in Vv_{mit} showed a high correlation with the increase in Type II fiber area that occurred with training (MacDougall et al., 1979). This indicates that heavy resistance training does not result in an increase in mitochondria in proportion to the increase in contractile protein, and thus the relative volume density for mitochondria is diluted. These findings have also been confirmed by comparison of tissue from powerlifters and bodybuilders with that of untrained subjects (MacDougall et al., 1982).

Assuming that mitochondrial volume density reflects the oxidative potential of the muscle, it would seem that this form of training not only fails to enhance the endurance characteristics of skeletal muscle, but also may even be detrimental to endurance performance by decreasing oxidative potential per total muscle mass.

Sarcoplasmic Reticulum

Although our sample size is too small to draw any conclusions, we have tentative evidence that the sarcoplasmic reticulum/myofibrillar volume ratio in gastrocnemius of bodybuilders (N=4) is less than that of untrained subjects (N=4). Whether or not this dilution of SR in hypertrophied fibers is sufficient to affect the mechanics of Ca^{2+} release and uptake is not known. It may, however, provide a partial explanation for our previous findings of prolonged twitch contraction time in triceps surae of a group of bodybuilders and weightlifters (Sale, Upton, McComas, & MacDougall, 1983).

Capillary Supply

Unlike endurance training, which has been reported to result in an increase in capillary supply (Anderson, 1975; Ingjer, 1979), strength training appears to have no effect on the capillary-to-fiber ratio. We have recently calculated capillarization from biopsy samples of biceps brachii in a group of 8 subjects before and after 3-4 months of heavy weight training of the elbow flexors. The capillary counts were made from photographs of tissue prepared with the amylase-PAS stain.

Although training resulted in a 17% increase in Type II fiber area and a 13% increase in Type I area, the capillary-to-fiber ratio remained unchanged (see Figure 7). When counts were expressed as capillary density (capillaries per mm^2), values showed a 13% decrease. It thus appears that, as with mitochondrial volume density, capillary density is also diluted by the increase in contractile protein that occurs with strength training. These findings are in agreement with a recent study by Tesch, Thorsson, and Kaiser (1984), who found an approximately 35% lower capillary density in weight and power lifters compared to untrained controls.

Fiber Hyperplasia

Controversy exists as to whether or not heavy resistance training results in an increase in fiber numbers in humans, as has been shown to occur in certain animal species (Gonyea, Erickson, & Bonde-Peterson, 1977; Gonyea, 1980; Sola, Christensen, & Martin, 1973). We think not. We have recently estimated fibers numbers in biceps brachii in 25 male subjects. Mean fiber area and collagen volume density were calculated from needle biopsies and muscle cross-sectional area by CT scans of the upper arm (see Figure 8). The sample comprised a group of 5 elite bodybuilders, 7 intermediate-calibre bodybuilders, and 13 untrained controls.

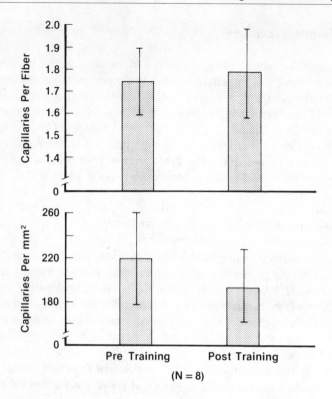

Figure 7. Capillary supply to biceps brachii before and after training. Values are expressed as a capillary-to-fiber ratio as well as capillary density (capillaries per mm²). Values are means (±1 SD).

Our results indicated that there was a wide inter-individual range for fiber numbers in biceps (172,000-419,000), but despite large differences in muscle size, both bodybuilder groups possessed the same number of muscle fibers as the group of control subjects (see Figure 9). The extremely large muscle size of the bodybuilders is primarily the result of their large fiber size and large absolute amounts of connective tissue. We therefore conclude that in humans heavy resistance training directed towards achieving maximum size in skeletal muscles does not result in an increase in fiber numbers (MacDougall, Sale, Alway, & Sutton, 1984).

Other Changes

Connective Tissue. In the preceding investigation of biceps brachii in bodybuilders and controls, the volume density for collagen and other non-contractile tissue was estimated by means of a point-counting technique (Weibel, 1972) applied to light micrographs of tissue that had been stained with

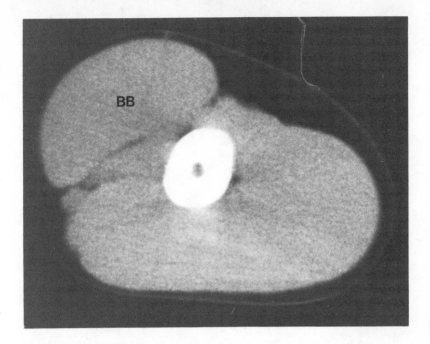

Figure 8. CT scan of upper arm showing biceps brachii (BB).

a modified Gomori trichrome stain. This proportion was found to be extremely consistent among all individuals, constituting approximately 13% of the total tissue sample. Of this, approximately 6% was identified as collagen and 7% as other tissue (MacDougall et al., 1984).

Our finding of a constant proportion of collagen and other noncontractile tissue, regardless of muscle size or state of training, indicates that the absolute amount of connective tissue is considerably greater in bodybuilders than in untrained subjects. Thus, training-induced hypertrophy of muscle fibers is accompanied by a proportional increase in connective tissue.

Biochemical Adaptation. In an investigation of 9 previously untrained subjects who trained their triceps brachii for 5 months, we found significant increases in resting concentrations of muscle glycogen (by 66%), creatine (by 39%), CP (by 22%), and ATP (by 18%). Presumably the increase in CP and ATP concentration in muscle homogenate could be caused by a greater relative hypertrophy of the Type II fibers, which are generally considered to have higher phosphagen stores than Type I fibers. When these same subjects underwent immobilization of their arms for 5 weeks, muscle glycogen concentration declined by approximately 40% and CP by approximately 25% (MacDougall et al., 1977). Because there was also a significant increase in muscle size with training, the observed elevations in the high-energy phosphate pool and glycogen concentrations indicate even greater changes in their absolute mus-

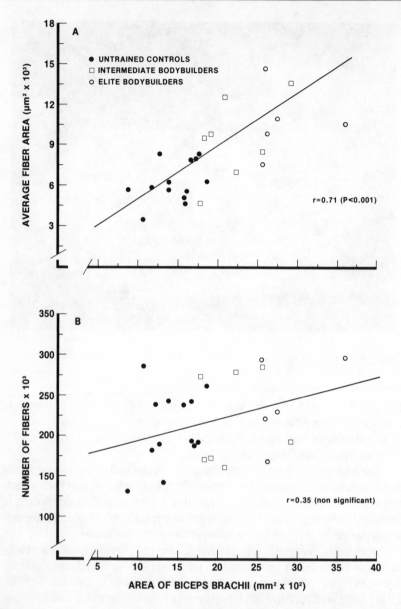

Figure 9. A. The correlation between cross-sectional area of biceps brachii and average fiber area. B. The correlation between cross-sectional area of biceps brachii and estimated fiber number. Data is presented for 13 control subjects, 7 intermediate, and 5 elite calibre bodybuilders.

cle content. Moreover, because the process was reversed with immobilization, it is likely that the phenomenon was indeed a training response.

The functional significance of this increase in resting concentration of ATP and CP is somewhat difficult to interpret. It is unlikely that it would contribute to the increase in strength (as measured by a single maximal voluntary contraction) observed following a period of strength training. Similarly, an increase in muscle concentration of CP would not be expected to affect the maximal rate of energy production in the trained muscle. It would, however, increase the total amount of energy available from this source and thus prolong the time that this maximal rate of power output could be maintained. It could therefore be advantageous in events such as the 200 m in track, which calls for a maximal power output over approximately 20 s.

The Stimulus

The mechanisms by which a program of near-maximal contractions results in enhanced protein synthesis and larger muscle fibers are not known. It may be the amount of tension a muscle develops that is the key that somehow provides the signal for increased uptake of amino acids and enhanced synthesis of contractile protein (Goldberg, Etlinger, Goldspink, & Jablecki, 1975; Booth, Nicholson, & Watson, 1982). In support of this, it has been shown that mechanisms exist that link passive stretch of a muscle with both decreased protein degradation and increased protein synthesis (Sola et al., 1973; Goldberg, 1979). Although it has been demonstrated that increased synthesis of RNA is an essential requirement for the hypertrophy process, the stimulus for increased muscle uptake of amino acids apparently occurs before there is any evidence of increased RNA synthesis (Goldberg & Goodman, 1969).

A second possible mechanism and one that can be found in popular strength and bodybuilding lore is what might be termed the "break down and build up theory." Bodybuilders tend to visualize their intensive training as "breaking down" muscle protein, which is "rebuilt" between training sessions, leading to a supercompensation of muscle size. As simplistic as this may sound, there may also be some evidence to support it. Forceful muscular contractions, especially those involving an eccentric component, are well known to result in delayed muscle soreness and to yield indirect evidence of actual muscle damage (Abraham, 1977; Tiidus & Ianuzzo, 1983). Elevations in serum enzymes such as CPK (Tiidus & Ianuzzo, 1983) and the presence of myoglobin in the urine (Abraham, 1977) suggest that the damage has occurred to contractile protein, whereas elevations in urinary hydroxyproline (Abraham, 1977) suggest that it also occurs to connective tissue.

Such damage has been confirmed by electron microscopic analysis of tissue following intense eccentric exercise carried out by Friden, Sjostrom, and Ekblom (1983). These authors have noted marked disturbances in the arrangement of the myofilaments and disruptions in the Z discs in biopsy samples taken immediately following exercise. Maximal strength and especially maximal power were also reduced following the exercise, suggesting greater damage to the Type II units. These structural abnormalities and decrements in strength were found to persist for several days before returning to normal.

It is thus possible that the hypertrophy process in skeletal muscle in response to training is simply a repair process. Lifting (and lowering) of heavy weights during a training session may result in damage to contractile elements and connective tissue, which are repaired over the several days that normally elapse between training sessions. This repeated process of damage and repair may result in an overshoot of protein synthesis somewhat similar to the over-compensation of muscle glycogen that occurs in response to endurance training. In partial support of this theory, it is known that strength athletes and bodybuilders achieve the greatest increases in muscle size and strength if they allow 3 days between training sessions for any one muscle group and that more frequent training, such as daily training, will actually result in decline in muscle size and strength.

Whatever the mechanism is for stimulating increased protein synthesis, it is known that hypertrophy will occur in starving animals in the absence of most pituitary hormones and insulin (Goldberg et al., 1975; Booth et al., 1982) and even in denervated muscles (Sola et al., 1973). It is also known that it is the intensity of the loading on the muscle that is the main determinant of whether or not increments in strength and size will occur. Training at low resistance (less than 60% of maximal voluntary strength) is ineffective for in-creasing strength, even though the athlete may perform hundreds of such con-tractions in a training session. On the other hand, 5-6 contractions at 90% of maximal strength (5-6 RM) will prove effective in increasing both the size and the strength of a muscle group (Atha, 1981). This direct relationship between the intensity of the load and the training effect does not appear to hold at very high percentages of maximal strength, however, because it has been shown that training at 5-6 RM is more effective than training at 1-2 RM, despite the fact that the load is higher in the 1-2 RM program (Atha, 1981).

Summary

Resistance training at high percentages of one's maximal strength results in an increase in cross-sectional area of both Type I and Type II fibers, with a greater degree of hypertrophy occurring in the Type II fibers. This increase in fiber size is directly related to an increase in both the size and the number of myofibrils within the fiber. The change in myofibril size is the result of the addition of actin and myosin filaments to the periphery, and the increase in number is apparently due to a longitudinal splitting of myofibrils. The decrease in fiber area that occurs when healthy muscle is immobilized involves the rever-sal of this process; that is, there is a loss of contractile protein from the periphery of the myofibril and a corresponding shrinkage in myofibril, and fiber size. A low correlation between the increase in average fiber area and the increase in strength with training indicates the importance of adaptations within the central nervous system in the expression of maximal voluntary strength.

Mitochondrial volume density and capillary density decrease with a program of strength training due to the diluting effect of increased contractile protein. On the other hand, the proportion of the muscle that is composed of connective tissue remains constant, thus indicating that increases in fiber area are accompanied by a parallel increase in connective tissue. Other adaptations to strength training include increases in high-energy phosphate stores and glycogen within the trained muscles. The mechanisms linking heavy resistance training with enhanced protein synthesis are not yet known but are apparently related to the amount of tension that the muscle develops during the training contractions.

Acknowledgment

Much of the work described in this chapter was supported by grants from the Muscular Dystrophy Association of Canada and the Natural Sciences and Engineering Research Council of Canada. The work was done in collaboration with Drs. D.G. Sale, G. Elder, and J.R. Sutton. I would also like to acknowledge the valuable assistance of J.R. Moroz and S.E. Alway.

References

Abraham, W.M. (1977). Factors in delayed muscle soreness. *Medicine and Science in Sports, 9*, 11-20.

Anderson, P. (1975). Capillary density in skeletal muscle of man. *Acta Physiologica Scandinavica, 95*, 203-205.

Atha, J. (1981). Strengthening muscle. In D.I. Miller (Ed.), *Exercise and sport sciences reviews* (Vol. 9, pp. 1-73). American College of Sports Medicine Series.

Booth, F.W., Nicholson, W.F., & Watson, P.A. (1982). Influence of muscle use on protein synthesis and degradation. In R.L. Terjung (Ed.), *Exercise and Sport Sciences Reviews* (Vol. 10, pp. 927-948). American College of Sports Medicine Series.

Friden, J., Sjöstrom, M., & Ekblom, B. (1983). Myofibrillar damage following intense eccentric exercise in man. *The International Journal of Sports Medicine, 3*, 170-176.

Goldberg, A.L. (1979). Influence of insulin and contractile activity on muscle size and protein balance. *Diabetes,* Supplement 1, 18-24.

Goldberg, A.L., Etlinger, J.D., Goldspink, D.F., & Jablecki, C. (1975). Mechanisms of work-induced hypertrophy of skeletal muscle. *Medicine and Science in Sports, 7*, 248-261.

Goldberg, A.L., & Goodman, H.M. (1969). Amino acid transport during work-induced growth of skeletal muscle. *American Journal of Physiology, 216*, 1111-1115.

Goldspink, G. (1970). The proliferation of myofibrils during muscle fibre growth. *Journal of Cell Science, 6*, 593-603.

Goldspink, G. (Ed.). (1974). *Differentiation of growth of cells in vertebrate tissue.* London: Chapman and Hall.

Goldspink, G., & Howells, K.F. (1974). Work-induced hypertrophy in exercised normal muscles of different ages and the reversibility of hypertrophy after cessation of exercise. *Journal of Physiology* (London), *239*, 179-193.

Gonyea, W.J. (1980). Role of exercise in inducing increases in skeletal muscle fiber number. *Journal of Applied Physiology: Respiratory, Environmental and Exercise Physiology, 48*, 421-426.

Gonyea, W.J., Erickson, G.C, & Bonde-Peterson, F. (1977). Skeletal muscle fiber splitting induced by weight-lifting exercise in cats. *Acta Physiologica Scandinavica, 99*, 105-109.

Ingjer, F. (1979). Capillary supply and mitochondrial content of different skeletal muscle fiber types in untrained and endurance trained men: A histochemical and ultrastructural study. *European Journal of Applied Physiology and Occupational Physiology, 40*, 197-209.

MacDougall, J.D., Elder, G.C.B., Sale, D.G., Moroz, J.R., & Sutton, J.R. (1980). Effects of strength training and immobilization on human muscle fibers. *European Journal of Applied Physiology, 43*, 25-34.

MacDougall, J.D., Sale, D.G., Elder, G.C.B., & Sutton, J.R. (1982). Muscle ultrastructural characteristics of elite powerlifters and bodybuilders. *European Journal of Applied Physiology, 48*, 117-126.

MacDougall, J.D., Sale, D.G., Alway, S.E., & Sutton, J.R. (1984). Muscle fiber number in biceps brachii in bodybuilders and control subjects. *Journal of Applied Physiology: Respiratory, Environmental and Exercise Physiology, 57*, 1399-1403.

MacDougall, J.D., Sale, D.G., Moroz, J.R., Elder, G.C.B., Sutton, J.R., & Howald, H. (1979). Mitochondrial volume density in human skeletal muscle following heavy resistance training. *Medicine and Science in Sports, 11*, 164-166.

MacDougall, J.D., Ward, G.R., Sale, D.G., & Sutton, J.R. (1977). Biochemical adaptation of human skeletal muscle to heavy resistance training and immoblization. *Journal of Applied Physiology: Respiratory, Environmental and Exercise Physiology, 43*, 700-703.

Rowe, R.W.D., & Goldspink, G. (1969). Muscle fibre growth in five different muscles in both sexes of mice. *Journal of Anatomy, 104*, 519-530.

Sale, D.G., Upton, A.R.M., McComas, A.J., & MacDougall, J.D. (1983). Neuromuscular function in weight-trainers. *Experimental Neurology, 82*, 521-531.

Sargeant, A.J., Davies, C.T.M., Edwards, R.H.T., Maunder, C., & Young, A. (1977). Functional and structural changes after disuse of human muscle. *Clinical Science and Molecular Medicine, 52*, 337-342.

Sola, O.M., Christensen, D.L., & Martin, A.W. (1973). Hypertrophy and hyperplasia of adult chicken latissimus dorsi muscles following stretch with and without denervation. *Experimental Neurology*, **41**, 76-100.

Tesch, P., Thorsson, A., & Kaiser, P. (1984). Muscle capillary supply and fibre type characteristics in weight and power lifters. *Journal of Applied Physiology: Respiratory, Environmental and Exercise Physiology*, **56**, 35-38.

Thorstensson, A. (1976). Muscle strength, fibre types and enzyme activities in man. *Acta Physiologica Scandinavica*, (supplement) **443**, 1-44.

Tiidus, P.M., & Ianuzzo, C.D. (1983). Effects of intensity and duration of muscular exercise on delayed soreness and serum enzyme activities. *Medicine and Science in Sports and Exercise*, **15**, 461-465.

Weibel, E.R. (1972). A stereological method for estimating volume and surface of sarcoplasmic reticulum. *Journal of Microscopy*, **95**, 229-242.

Discussion

Dr. Gonyea opened the discussion by suggesting that a longitudinal study of muscle fiber type changes was needed for several reasons. He felt it was important to know the size and number of muscle fibers initially, in relation to their increase following training, for two reasons: First, it may not be valid to assume that someone with large muscles will have more fibers; and second, a large scatter in the data may be misleading when trained versus untrained individuals are compared. Dr. MacDougall felt that the large differences in muscle size between the three groups he described could not be explained in that way; because one group had some individuals with muscles that were four to five times the size of the untrained group, yet the average number of muscle fibers for each group was within a few thousand of each other. He agreed that the starting point was important and that individuals with large numbers of fibers may have an advantage in terms of their capacity for training. There was a weak relationship between the number of fibers and the muscle size, and within each group the individuals tending to have the largest areas also tended to have the most fibers. To become a world champion body builder then, it was best to inherit a large number of fibers and then train them.

Dr. Stauber felt that while the data were impressive, he felt they should be considered in the context of the total muscle development; that is, we start out life with a fiber size of 10 μm and have a sixfold increase by the age of 16 or 17 and then at best a twofold increase in later years. It was extraordinary that these individuals were able to increase size to the extent reported by Dr. MacDougall. Dr. MacDougall reminded the audience that much of the total muscle volume is connective tissue, and although with training the relative amount remains constant, the absolute amount increases. Also, he pointed out that photographs of body builders tend to exaggerate the real muscle size because body builders like to be photographed after they have used the technique known as "pumping," in which they will do 30 to 40 contractions at low resistance and, through hyperemia or edema, make the muscles appear larger than they really are.

Dr. Jacobs questioned whether the CAT scan measurements were really precise enough to draw any conclusions; the correlation coefficient between the mean fiber area from the biopsies and the total muscle area from the CAT scan was only 0.7, indicating that less than 50% of the variation was accounted for by the two variables. He wondered what made up the additional variance. Dr. MacDougall agreed that the increase in fiber area only partially accounted for the increased muscle size, some of it being related to the number of fibers. However, within each group the average fiber number was the same and individuals with the largest muscles tended to have the largest number of fibers. On average, 13% of the muscle was composed of connective tissue. Dr. MacDougall also pointed out that the technique was validated by estimating fiber numbers in the right and left arm and that these results showed that the standard error of this estimate was 10%. The CAT scan was standardized by taking the scan at the largest circumference, together with a few distal and proximal cuts in order to get the largest area. Dr. Saltin supported this approach and described a different one in which the biceps muscles were removed within a few hours of death in some otherwise healthy individuals who had died suddenly; a large range in the number of fibers was also found, but the total number of fibers was close to that found by Dr. MacDougall.

Dr. Ianuzzo made a number of points that he prefaced by stating his bias that hyperplasia may not necessarily be occurring in these muscles. There is some evidence in the literature that myofibrillar splitting may occur in heavy resistance training, but Eugene Morkin (1970) had shown that in the periphery of muscle during normal growth there was also a synthesis of fibers that may be an additional mechanism for increasing fiber number other than the splitting of fibers. Also, the volume density changes in mitochondria found by Dr. MacDougall were relatively small, amounting to only about 0.5% change in the total volume of muscle. That may mean very little in terms of oxidative capacity and the functional capacity of muscle. Finally, he felt that very little was known regarding the stimulus for the changes; everyone appeared to be looking at the input stimulus and the phenotypic expression to the exclusion of other mechanisms. Dr. Heigenhauser enquired what the performance ability of these individuals was when expressed per unit of cross-sectional area. Dr. MacDougall replied that the increase in strength did not occur linearly with bulk. Dr. Howald did not feel that this meant that the muscles of body builders were not strong. If one considered the weights they lifted, they are very high, although perhaps not in terms of elite weight lifting athletes. Dr. Heigenhauser agreed that the muscles are strong, but his comment had to do with the relative strength per unit of cross-sectional area.

Dr. Stauber took up the question of tension as the proposed stimulus for hypertrophy, and pointed out that Vandenburgh and Kaufman (1979) had shown that a high degree of tension caused a hyperpolarization of the muscle cell that is similar to the effects of insulin and possibly mediates amino acid transport. Also, prostaglandin F2 is released from muscle in heavy contraction; this protein accelerates protein synthesis and decreases protein degradation. Even in cells without neural stimuli in culture, there is evidence that when the cell is stretched, a direct effect occurs on the cell membrane. Dr. Ianuzzo commented that in culture the cells that were stretched did not hypertrophy in cross-sectional area but elongated; protein synthesis occurred and membrane changes associated with the sodium pump increased. Thus, these findings are not the same as those reported by Dr. MacDougall because the muscle has not become stronger in terms of the parallel arrangement of muscle fibers normally seen.

Dr. Ethel Cosmos entered the discussion to give information obtained in a model that had many advantages over the ones already presented. This was the avian embryo in which the neural tubes are removed. The muscles are grown in vivo in an aneurogenic condition; they appear to develop similarly to normal muscles except in size, but if artificial stimulation is added to this preparation a large increase in size is found. After hatching, massive damage to the muscle is produced by allowing it to contract and then stretching it. In electron microscopic studies a great deal of destruction with cellular infiltration is followed by a regeneration process that occurs along the periphery of each of the muscle fibers, with regeneration adding to the outside of the fiber. These findings may explain what the stimuli are in body builders if injury is produced, and she wondered what happened to the muscle appearance if the muscle atrophies during detraining in these athletes. Dr. MacDougall replied that many fibers from body builders who take steroids are found to be very angulated and triangular in shape; most pathologists suggest that this appearance is characteristic of denervation atrophy. Whatever the stimulus to hypertrophy, it appears to be very powerful as it can occur in starving muscles and also without the presence of pituitary hormones, insulin, and a nerve supply.

Dr. Gonyea wanted to know to what extent glycogen storage and steroids might influence the storage of water in muscle to increase muscle size. Dr. MacDougall replied that there was an increase in glycogen concentration, but he felt that the total duration of the training sessions was probably not sufficient to deplete glycogen; for this reason the enhanced storage of glycogen was a minor factor. Of both groups of body builders, about half were on steroids; in a previous study he had found that body builders on steroids had slightly lower contractile tissue per cross-sectional area.

Dr. Lewis was interested in the high blood pressure values recorded in Dr. MacDougall's study; Dr. MacDougall said that these occur only during the concentric phase of the lift and then decrease as the weight is being lowered, staying high for only about 2 sec. The pulse pressures were also elevated, suggesting that cardiac output was maintained with a brisk venous return and a great increase in arterial resistance.

Dr. Newsholme pointed out that anecedotally body builders eat large amounts of protein, which they believe to be essential. He wondered whether there were any studies on other fuels in these subjects, such as the use of branched chain amino acids, glucose tolerance, and adipose tissue fat use. Dr. MacDougall was not aware of any metabolic studies, but in terms of adipose tissue they have very small amounts because the body builders are trying to obtain very good muscle definition under the skin. Studies of protein requirements in weight lifters have shown a higher protein intake amounting to about 20%, but he knew of no data in body builders.

References

Vandenburg, H., & Kaufman, S. (1979). In vitro model for stretch-induced hypertrophy of skeletal muscle. *Science, 203*, 265-268.

Morkin, E. (1970). Postnatal muscle fiber assembly: Localization of newly synthesised myofibrillar proteins. *Science, 167*, 1499-1501.

18

Neural Adaptation in Strength and Power Training

Digby G. Sale
McMaster University

Strength and power performance is determined not only by the quantity and quality of the involved muscle mass, but also by the extent to which the muscle mass may be activated by voluntary effort. Further, the expression of voluntary strength and power may be likened to a skilled act, in which prime movers must be fully activated, synergists appropriately activated, and antagonists suitably inhibited. Strength and power training may cause changes within the nervous system that allow an individual to better coordinate the activation of muscle groups, thereby effecting a greater net force, even in the absence of adaptation within the muscles themselves. The possible changes within the nervous system that enhance strength and power performance may be referred to as "neural adaptation." The purpose of this paper is to review the evidence that suggests neural adaptation occurs in response to strength and power training, and to discuss the possible underlying mechanisms.

Evidence for Neural Adaptation: Training Studies

Rapid Increases in Strength

The initial increases in strength in a training program occur rapidly, and it is unlikely that muscle adaptation could account for these rapid gains

(Delorme, West, & Shriber, 1950; Hellebrandt & Houtz, 1956; Moritani & de Vries, 1979). In fact, improvement in strength has been demonstrated within the first training session (Whitley & Elliot, 1968).

Increased Voluntary But Not Evoked Contraction Strength

Following short periods (5-8 wk) of strength training, voluntary strength may increase without an increase in evoked (by electrical stimulation) maximal twitch and tetanic tension (Davies & Young, 1983; McDonagh, Hayward, & Davies, 1983). These findings may be interpreted to indicate that training does not increase the intrinsic contractile force of the muscles; rather, the trainees may learn to activate the muscles more fully or improve coordination of the voluntary contraction. A longer period of training is associated with an increase in evoked as well as voluntary strength; however, in the study of Liberson and Asa (1959), the percentage increase in voluntary strength was twice the percentage increase in evoked contraction strength, suggesting that "extra muscular" adaptation occurred.

Increased Voluntary Strength Without Hypertrophy

Short-term training studies have demonstrated increases in voluntary strength without increases in muscle size (Dons, Bollerup, Bonde-Petersen, & Hancke, 1979; Komi, Viitasalo, Rauramaa, & Vihko, 1978; Liberson & Asa, 1959; Moritani & de Vries, 1979; Rose, Radzyminski, & Beatty, 1957; Tanner, 1952; Tesch, Hjort, & Balldin, 1983; Thorstensson, Hulten, Von Doblen, & Karlsson, 1976) or muscle fibre size (Costill, Coyle, Fink, Lesmes, & Witzmann, 1979; Tesch et al., 1983; Thorstensson et al., 1976). When increases in muscle and muscle fibre size have occurred, the magnitude of the increases have been considerably less than the increase in voluntary strength (Houston, Froese, Valeriote, Green, & Ranney, 1983; Ikai & Fukunaga, 1970; MacDougall, Elder, Sale, Moroz, & Sutton, 1980; Moritani & de Vries, 1979). Thus, in studies in which muscle cross-sectional area has been measured, training has resulted in an increase in the ratio of voluntary strength to muscle cross-sectional area (Dons et al., 1979; Ikai & Fukunaga, 1970). Although an increase in voluntary strength per unit muscle cross-sectional area (MVC/CSA) with training has usually been interpreted as indicating that neural adaptation has occurred, an alternative explanation is that muscle "quality" increased; that is, the intrinsic strength of muscle per unit cross-sectional area (specific tension) increased after training. However, this interpretation is improbable in the light of two findings. In the study (Ikai & Fukunaga, 1970) in which MVC/CSA increased in the trained limb, it also increased in the contralateral untrained limb, suggesting that the increase in both limbs was caused by a neural adaptation rather than by qualitative changes in the muscles. In a second study (Dons et al., 1979), MVC/CSA increased when measurement of strength was specific to the training (weight lifting); however, when the same muscle group was tested with a nonspecific test (isometric contractions), there was no significant change in MVC/CSA.

In contrast to the observation that short-term strength training causes an increase in MVC/CSA, observations made on subjects who have strength trained over a period of years indicate that those individuals do not have increased MVC/CSA in relation to untrained control subjects (Ikai & Fukunaga, 1968; Maughan, Watson, & Weir, 1982; Schantz, Randall-Fox, Hutchison, Tyden, & Åstrand, 1983). These apparently contradictory observations may be explained by considering, first, that the trained groups (usually weight lifters) were tested for voluntary strength with methods (isometric or isokinetic dynamometers) unfamiliar to them. Consequently, part of any "neural" advantage they might have enjoyed with a specific test (weight lifting) was not fully revealed. Second, if neural adaptation in the trained groups did tend to increase MVC/CSA, even with unfamiliar methods, this increase may be counterbalanced by adaptive changes within the muscles that decrease the specific tension. Such changes have been observed in animal muscles that have undergone extreme hypertrophy (Roy, Meadows, Baldwin, & Edgerton, 1982). There are no specific tension data available on greatly hypertrophied human muscles; however, a reduced myofibrillar volume density has been reported in hypertrophied human muscle (MacDougall, Sale, Elder, & Sutton, 1982). A reduced myofibrillar volume density indicates a dilution of contractile protein within the muscle fibres and may contribute to a decrease in specific tension. Thus, the increase in MVC/CSA that occurs in the early weeks and months of training may be due to a predominance of neural as opposed to muscle adaptation (Hakkinen & Komi, 1983; Moritani & de Vries, 1979). As training is prolonged and muscle adaptation (hypertrophy) predominates, the decrease in specific tension may cause MVC/CSA to decrease toward the pretraining level.

Cross-Training Effect

Training of one limb is associated with increased voluntary strength in the contralateral untrained limb (Coleman, 1969; Darcus & Salter, 1955; Hellebrandt, Parrish, & Houtz, 1947; Houston et al., 1983; Ikai & Fukunaga, 1970; Komi et al., 1978; Mathews, Shay, Godin, & Hogdon, 1956; Moritani & de Vries, 1979; Rasch & Morehouse, 1957; Slater-Hamel, 1950; Yasuda & Miyamura, 1983); the effects of skill training may also be transferred in this manner (Hellebrandt, 1951). In these studies the increase in voluntary strength in the untrained limb has been attributed to neural adaptation. Support for this interpretation comes from those studies that demonstrated no increase in muscle size (Ikai & Fukunaga, 1970; Moritani & de Vries, 1979), muscle fibre size (Houston et al., 1983; Krotkiewski, Aniansson, Grimby, Bjorntorp, & Sjostrom, 1979) or evoked contraction strength (Duchateau & Hainaut, 1984) in the untrained limb.

The Specificity of Training Effects

At least four kinds of specificity of training can be identified. First, increases in voluntary strength with training are largely specific to the type of contraction used in the training. Thus, training a muscle group by lifting weights (concentric and eccentric contractions) causes a large increase in weight lifting strength but only a small increase in isometric contraction strength (Dons et al., 1979; Thorstensson et al., 1976) or isokinetic (constant velocity) concentric contraction strength (Fahey & Brown, 1973). Isokinetic concentric contraction training leads to an increase in dynamic strength (power) without an increase in isometric strength (Kanehisa & Miyashita, 1983a), whereas isometric training significantly improves isometric strength but not isokinetic concentric contraction strength (Lindh, 1979).

Second, in isometric strength training, increases in voluntary strength are greatest at the joint positions trained, and there may be no significant increases at "unfamiliar" joint angles (Bender & Kaplan, 1963; Gardner, 1963; Lindh, 1979; Meyers, 1967; Raitsin, 1974).

Third, strength training effects may be specific to the velocity of contraction used in training. Training with low velocity isokinetic concentric contractions causes relatively large increases in low velocity strength but relatively small increases in high velocity strength; similarly, training with high velocity contractions causes specifically larger increases in high velocity strength (Caiozzo, Perrine, & Edgerton, 1981; Coyle et al., 1981; Kanehisa & Miyashita, 1983a, 1983b; Moffroid & Whipple, 1970).

Finally, strength training may be specific according to whether limb exercises are performed unilaterally or bilaterally. For example, training with synchronous, bilateral knee extensions caused a greater increase in bilateral than unilateral knee extension strength (Coyle et al., 1981).

All of these examples of specificity of training might be attributed to neural adaptation; however, in the cases of specificity of contraction type and velocity, there is evidence that training has specific effects on the contractile properties of muscle as well. Isometric and rapid weight lifting exercises have differential effects on evoked isometric tetanic and twitch contractile properties, and upon evoked maximal shortening velocity (Duchateau & Hainaut, 1984).

Electromyographic Changes with Training

Electromyographic studies have attempted to monitor possible increases in motor unit activation (increased recruitment and/or firing frequency) following strength training. The most common method has been to observe the integrated EMG (IEMG) in brief maximal voluntary contractions. The IEMG has been shown to increase with strength training (Hakkinen & Komi, 1983; Komi & Buskirk, 1972; Komi et al., 1978; Moritani & de Vries, 1979). Most of the increase in IEMG occurs in the first 3-4 weeks of training; thereafter, increased voluntary strength is associated with muscle hypertrophy (Hakkinen & Komi, 1983; Moritani & de Vries, 1979). A study of leg training by weight lifting showed significant increases in weight lifting strength and to a lesser extent isometric leg "press" strength. Isolated isometric knee extension strength did not increase, but in this movement there was also no increase in IEMG. Had IEMG been recorded in the other movements, an increase might have been observed in conjunction with the increased voluntary strength (Thorstensson, Karlsson, Viitasalo, Luhtanen, & Komi, 1976). In one of the cross-training experiments (Moritani & de Vries, 1979), the increase in voluntary strength in the untrained limb was associated with an increase in IEMG without evidence of hypertrophy.

A second electromyographic technique that has been used to monitor motor unit activation is the measurement of the potentiation of reflex EMG responses by maximal voluntary contractions (Upton, McComas, & Sica, 1971). In this method, the responses to supramaximal nerve stimulation at rest and during voluntary contractions are compared, and "potentiation ratios" can be calculated. Strength training caused an increase in reflex potentiation in some (Sale, MacDougall, Upton, & McComas, 1983) but not all (Sale, McComas, MacDougall, & Upton, 1982) muscle groups investigated. Cross-sectional studies have shown reflex potentiation to be enhanced in weight lifters (Milner-Brown, Stein, & Lee, 1975; Sale, Upton, McComas, & MacDougall, 1983) and in elite sprinters (Upton & Radford, 1975). With this method, it is assumed that the degree of reflex potentiation is correlated to the degree of motor unit activation achieved by voluntary effort. It is of interest in this regard that reflex potentiation is greatly reduced in patients suffering from upper motoneurone lesions (Sica, McComas, & Upton, 1971).

A third electromyographic method used to observe the effects of training has been to determine the degree of sychronization of discharge of motor units during voluntary contractions. Longitudinal training studies have shown an increase in motor unit synchronization, and cross-sectional studies have shown motor unit synchronization to be enhanced in weight lifters and in others who regularly perform brief, maximal contractions (Milner-Brown, Stein, & Lee, 1975). Unlike the first two electromyographic methods discussed above, in which it is easy to appreciate how an increase in the values obtained might increase the force of voluntary contraction, it is not readily apparent how an increase in motor unit synchronization could increase the force of voluntary contractions. On the contrary, at submaximal firing frequencies force output is greater with asynchronous motor unit activation, and at firing frequencies similar to the maximum observed in voluntary contractions, there is no difference in force attained between synchronous and asynchronous discharge (Lind

& Petrofsky, 1978; Rack & Westbury, 1969). If synchronization of motor unit firing cannot increase the peak force of voluntary contractions, perhaps it may increase the rate of force development in brief, maximal contractions. However, in experiments in which maximal voluntary contractions of the first dorsal interosseous muscle were compared to evoked tetanic contractions at frequencies as high as 200 Hz, a greater rate of force development was observed in the voluntary contractions (Miller, Mirka, & Maxfield, 1981). In interpreting these results, it must be remembered that the rate of force development in voluntary contractions is facilitated by appropriate co-contraction of synergists, which is difficult to duplicate with evoked (nerve stimulation) contractions. Nevertheless, the role of increased motor unit synchronization in enhancing the performance of brief maximal voluntary contractions remains unclear.

The three electromyographic methods discussed previously have documented increases as a result of training. The validity of the results is strengthened by observation of decreases following detraining and periods of extreme inactivity, such as in joint immobilization. A decrease in both the integrated EMG (Hakkinen & Komi, 1983) and motor unit synchronization (Milner-Brown, Stein, & Lee, 1975) has been observed following detraining, and a period of limb immobilization has caused a decrease in both integrated EMG (Funglsang-Frederiksen & Scheel, 1978) and reflex potentiation (Sale et al., 1982).

Possible Mechanisms of Neural Adaptation

Strength and power training causes an increased voluntary contraction force (MVC) in the intended direction of movement. Apart from the effect of muscle hypertrophy, the increased MVC could result from increased activation of prime movers, more appropriate co-contraction of synergists, and increased inhibition of antagonists. In a training experiment the relative importance of these three mechanisms could be determined only by an electromyographic investigation of all the involved muscles. To the author's knowledge, only the first of the possible mechanisms, increased activation of prime movers, has been examined in training studies. The EMG studies reviewed previously were devoted to this mechanism and indicated an increased prime mover activation after training. Increased prime mover activation reflects an increased net excitation of prime mover motoneurones. This in turn could result from increased excitatory input, reduced inhibitory input, or both. An obvious implication is that many untrained people cannot activate their muscles fully under normal conditions. There appears to be a functional reserve that is not readily available for use, despite presumed maximal voluntary effort. Additional evidence in support of this view will now be considered.

Influence of Hypnosis and Sensory Stimuli on MVC

It was reported by Ikai and Steinhaus (1961) that hypnosis and specific sensory stimuli may enhance voluntary strength performance. These investigators proposed that some form of inhibition limits performance but that the inhibition may be overcome in unusual circumstances. It is of interest that the subject whose strength was least enhanced by hypnosis or sensory stimulation was a trained weight lifter, whereas the subject who demonstrated the greatest effect was a person who had always avoided exertion because of childhood asthma (Ikai & Steinhaus, 1961).

Assessment of Motor Unit Activation Using the Interpolated Twitch Technique

If, during a maximal voluntary contraction, a single supramaximal shock is delivered to the motor nerve of the contracting muscle, a small increment in force would be expected if not all motor units were recruited or made to fire at the optimal frequency for tension development (Denny-Brown, 1928). On the other hand, if full motor unit activation was achieved, no increment would appear. The twitch interpolation technique has been applied to the adductor pollicis (Merton, 1954), the dorsiflexors and plantarflexors of the ankle (Bélanger & McComas, 1981), and more recently to the quadriceps (Chapman, Edwards, Grieg, & Rutherford, 1984). The results have demonstrated that even untrained but well-motivated subjects are able to achieve full motor unit activation (Chapman et al., 1984; Merton, 1954). The degree of activation appears to vary with different muscle groups. The 17 men and 11 women tested by Bélanger & McComas (1981) were all able to achieve full activation of the dorsiflexors, whereas 60% of the men and 36% of the women were unable to achieve full activation of the plantarflexors. The technique has not been applied to multijoint movements often used in strength and power training. Nevertheless, the available data indicated substantial variability among muscles and between subjects in the extent of motor unit activation during effort. Moreover, this variability may not account for the variable response to short-term training regimens (Brown & Wilmore, 1974; Jones, 1966; Mathews & Kruse, 1957; Rose et al., 1957; Hettinger & Muller, 1953; Muller, 1962).

Comparison of MVC with Evoked Tetanic Contractions

Another method of measuring the extent of motor unit activation is to compare the force of a maximal voluntary contraction (MVC) with the force produced by tetanic stimulation of the same muscles. One difficulty with this technique is selecting a muscle or muscle group that is solely responsible for a joint action and that can be selectively stimulated. Another difficulty is the extreme discomfort usually associated with tetanic stimulation. Despite these problems, the method has been applied to small muscles of the hand (Bigland & Lippold, 1954; Bigland-Ritchie, Johansson, Lippold, & Woods, 1983; Ikai, Yabe, & Ischii, 1967; Merton, 1954), the triceps surae (Dietz, Schmidtbleicher, & Noth, 1979), and the quadriceps femoris (Edwards, Hill, & Jones, 1975). The number of subjects investigated has been small, but in several studies (Bigland & Lippold, 1954; Bigland-Ritchie et al., 1983; Edwards et al., 1975; Merton, 1954), the force of MVC did match the force produced by tetanic stimulation. Once again, the method has not been applied to large muscle group, multijoint movements, but in the muscles investigated there is also evidence that some apparently untrained individuals can fully activate their muscles by voluntary effort.

Unilateral vs. Bilateral Contractions

Conventional strength and power training often involves exercises in which the same muscle groups of both limbs contract simultaneously. It has been observed in these bilateral contractions that the force produced is less than the sum of forces produced by the right and left limbs contracting singly (Coyle et al., 1981; Henry & Smith, 1961; Kroll, 1965; Ohtsuki, 1981, 1983; Secher, Rorsgaard, & Secher, 1978; Vandervoort, Sale, & Moroz, 1984). In two of these studies the reduced force in the bilateral condition was associated with a reduction in the integrated EMG (Ohtsuki, 1983; Vandervoort et al., 1984), suggesting that there was reduced activation of prime movers.

Various mechanisms have been advanced to explain the bilateral deficit. Dispersion of concentration to two limbs rather than one may not allow full excitation of motoneurones to occur in the bilateral condition (Vandervoort et al., 1984). Alternatively the bilateral deficit may result from interaction between the cerebral hemispheres, or spinal reflexes, but at the present time the mechanisms underlying this finding cannot be identified (Ohtsuki, 1983).

Four additional observations relating to this phenomenon are of interest. First, the bilateral deficit in force and EMG is present in isometric and also rapid "ballistic" dynamic contractions (Vandervoort, Sale, & Moroz, 1984), suggesting that higher centers involved in programming the movement contribute to the underlying mechanism. Second, the bilateral deficit is minimized or abolished when contraction of a muscle group in one limb is simultaneous with contraction of the antagonists of the contralateral limb (Ohtsuki, 1983). This observation suggests that simple dispersion of concentration is not the major underlying mechanism. Third, the bilateral condition is associated with greater EMG activity in the antagonists (Ohtsuki, 1983); increased activity of antagonists would reduce force in the bilateral contraction by opposing the agonists and perhaps, by reciprocal inhibition, reducing the net excitation of the agonists. Finally, training with bilateral contractions reduces the bilateral deficit (Secher, 1975), possibly a form of neural adaptation to training.

Some strength training equipment manufacturers have sought to avoid the bilateral deficit problem by producing machines that permit the performance of reciprocating movements (i.e., flexors of one limb contracting simultaneously with the extensors of the contralateral limb). Such an approach would be specific to sports that involve reciprocal movements (e.g., sprinting, jumping). However, athletes in sports that require simultaneous bilateral contraction of the same muscle groups (e.g., rowing) should train with similar contractions in order to reduce or eliminate the bilateral deficit (Secher, 1975).

Effect of Precontractions of Antagonists

The force and EMG produced by a muscle group in a MVC are increased when the contraction is immediately preceded by a MVC of the antagonists. In isokinetic concentric contractions, this enhancement is greatest in the low velocity—high force region of the in-vivo force-velocity relationship (Caiozzo, Barnes, Prietto, & McMaster, 1981); it has been proposed that a tension-dependent, neural mechanism limits the excitation of agonist motoneurones during MVC's against high resistance (Perrine & Edgerton, 1978). The precontraction of antagonists in some way counters the inhibitory influence and allows greater activation of the agonists in the subsequent contraction. It has been hypothesized that the increases in low velocity isokinetic strength that have been observed in the absence of hypertrophy (Costill et al., 1979; Thorstensson, 1977) are the result of a neural adaptation that overcomes or modifies the inhibitory influence (Caiozzo, Perrine, & Edgerton, 1981). A strength training program that employs the precontraction technique is more effective for increasing low velocity strength than a program consisting only of prime mover contractions (Caiozzo, Laird, Chow, Prietto, & McMaster, 1982). Some strength training equipment manufacturers provide equipment that allows the precontraction method to be used.

Motor Unit Recruitment Thresholds and Firing Rates

The recruitment threshold of a motor unit is generally related to its size. The highest threshold motor units possess the largest and fastest twitch contractions (for a review, see Freund, 1983), and may be the units that many untrained people cannot recruit or raise to the optimal firing rates. Evidence in support of the latter possibility was provided by DeLuca, LeFever, McCue, and Xenakis (1982), who noted that high threshold motor units had a lower firing frequency than low threshold motor units during maximal or near maximal voluntary contractions. The authors suggested that the potentially higher firing rates of the high threshold motor units were not achieved because the subjects could not sufficiently excite those motoneurones by voluntary effort. Sufficient excitation might be possible only in unusual circumstances such as stress and hypnosis.

The relative role of recruitment and changes in firing rate in grading the force of voluntary contractions may vary in different muscles. In two small muscles of the hand, most motor units are recruited at thresholds less than 50% MVC; thereafter, force is increased further almost exclusively by increasing the firing rate of motor units (DeLuca et al., 1982; Kukulka & Clamann, 1981; Milner-Brown, Stein, & Yemm, 1973a). However, in larger, more proximal muscles such as the deltoid and biceps, recruitment of additional motor units appears to occur throughout the force range up to 100% MVC (DeLuca et al., 1982; Kukulka & Clamann, 1981). It has been suggested that a predominance of firing rate over recruitment in contractions requiring more than 30%-40% MVC is most suitable in the small hand muscles for producing smooth, accurate movements of the fingers (DeLuca et al., 1982; Milner-Brown, Stein, & Yemm, 1973b). On the other hand, in large muscles with many motor units, each newly recruited unit may add a sufficiently small force increment so that the production of smooth contractions is not compromised; thus, recruitment is an appropriate means of grading force up to 100% MVC (DeLuca et al., 1982). The question arises whether the arrangement seen in the large proximal muscles may make it more difficult to achieve full motor unit activation during voluntary effort. If so, then increased motor unit activation may be part of the neural adaptation that is apparently observed when large muscle groups are engaged in strength and power training.

The recruitment order of motor units is rather fixed for a muscle involved in a specific movement, even if the rate of force development or speed of contraction varies (Desmedt & Godaux, 1977). However, in the case of a change in position (Person, 1974) or in the case of a multifunction muscle performing different movements (Desmedt & Godaux 1981; Haar Romeny, Dernier Van Der Gon, & Gielen, 1982; Schmidt & Thomas, 1981), recruitment order can be altered. Thus, some motor units within a muscle might have a low threshold for one movement and a higher threshold for another movement. The variation in recruitment order according to movement may be partially responsible for the specificity of training that has been observed (Sale & MacDougall, 1981) and may support the notion long held by strength trainers that full development of a muscle is possible only when it is exercised in all its possible movements.

Conclusion

A question that is often raised in connection with neural adaptation to strength and power training is why humans are designed so that some motor units are so difficult or impossible to activate fully unless diligent training is performed or a crisis situation is faced. The answer usually given is that protection is provided by inhibitions that prevent the making of truly maximal contractions frequently and at a whim; the muscles might not withstand repeated maximal forces or infrequent maximal contractions in the untrained state. Even after training, athletes face the risk of injury because of their ability to achieve full activation of their muscles. Athletes have been known to tear muscles from their attachments during maximal efforts. The use of anabolic steroids by strength and power athletes is usually associated with muscular adaptation; however, athletes also claim it affects their nervous system, allowing them to become more aggressive and focused in training. The greater concentration may lead to more complete neural activation of muscles and partly accounts for the apparent increased incidence of muscle avulsions in athletes as the use of anabolic steroids becomes more widespread.

References

Bélanger, A.Y., & McComas, A.J. (1981). Extent of motor unit activation during effort. *Journal of Applied Physiology: Respiratory, Environmental and Exercise Physiology*, **53**, 419-424.

Bender, J., & Kaplan, H. (1963). The multiple angle testing method for the evaluation of muscle strength. *Journal of Bone and Joint Surgery*, **45A**, 135-140.

Bigland, B., & Lippold, O.C.J. (1954). Motor unit activity in the voluntary contraction of human muscle. *Journal of Physiology*, **125**, 322-335.

Bigland-Ritchie, B., Johansson, R., Lippold, O.C.J., & Woods, J.J. (1983). Contractile speed and EMG changes during fatigue at sustained maximal voluntary contractions. *Journal of Neurophysiology*, **50**, 313-324.

Brown, C.H., & Wilmore, J.H. (1974). The effects of maximal resistance training on the strength and body composition of women athletes. *Medicine and Science in Sports*, **6**, 174-178.

Caiozzo, V.J., Barnes, W.S., Prietto, C.A., & McMaster, W.C. (1981). The affect of isometric precontractions on the slow velocity-high force region of the in-vivo force-velocity relationship. *Medicine and Science in Sports and Exercise*, **13**, 128.

Caiozzo, V.J., Laird, T., Chow, K., Prietto, C.A., & McMaster, W.C. (1982). The use of precontractions to enhance the in-vivo force-velocity relationship. *Medicine and Science in Sports and Exercise*, **14**, 162.

Caiozzo, V.J., Perrine, J.J., & Edgerton, V.R. (1981). Training-induced alterations of the in-vivo force-velocity relationship of human muscle. *Journal of Applied Physiology: Respiratory, Environmental and Exercise Physiology*, **51**, 750-754.

Chapman, S.J., Edwards, R.H.T., Grieg, C., & Rutherford, O. (1984). Practical application of the twitch interpolation technique for the study of voluntary contraction of the quadriceps in man. *Journal of Physiology*, **353**, 3 P.

Coleman, A.E. (1969). Effect of unilateral isometric and isotonic contractions on the strength of the contralateral limb. *Research Quarterly*, **40**, 490-495.

Costill, D.L., Coyle, E.F., Fink, W.F., Lesmes, G.R., & Witzmann, F.A. (1979). Adaptation in skeletal muscle following strength training. *Journal of Applied Physiology: Respiratory, Environmental and Exercise Physiology*, **46**, 96-99.

Coyle, E.F., Feiring, D.C., Rotkis, T.C., Cote III, R.W., Roby, F.B., Lee, W., & Wilmore, J.H. (1981). Specificity of power improvements through slow and fast isokinetic training. *Journal of Applied Physiology: Respiratory, Environmental and Exercise Physiology*, **51**, 1437-1442.

Darcus, H.D., & Salter, N. (1955). The effect of repeated muscular exertion on muscle strength. *Journal of Physiology*, **129**, 325-336.

Davies, C.T.M., & Young, K. (1983). Effects of training at 30% and 100% maximal isometric force (MVC) on the contractile properties of the triceps surae in man. *Journal of Physiology*, **336**, 31 P.

Delorme, T.L., West, F.E., & Shriber, W.J. (1950). Influence of progressive resistance exercise on knee function following femoral fractures. *Journal of Bone and Joint Surgery*, **32A**, 910-924.

DeLuca, C.J., Le Fever, R.S., McCue, M.P., & Xenakis, A.P. (1982). Behavior of human motor units in different muscles during linearly varying contractions. *Journal of Physiology*, **329**, 113-128.

Denny-Brown, D. (1928). On inhibition as a reflex accompaniment of the tendon jerk and of other forms of active muscular response. *Proceedings of the Royal Society of London. Series B.*, **103**, 321-336.

Desmedt, J.E., & Godaux, E. (1977). Ballistic contractions in man: Characteristic recruitment pattern of single motor units of the tibialis anterior muscle. *Journal of Physiology*, **264**, 673-694.

Desmedt, J.E., & Godaux, E. (1981). Spinal motoneuron recruitment in man: Rank deordering with direction but not with speed of voluntary movement. *Science*, **214**, 933-936.

Dietz, V., Schmidtbleicher, D., & Noth, J. (1979). Neuronal mechanisms of human locomotion. *Journal of Neurophysiology*, **42**, 1212-1222.

Dons, B., Bollerup, K., Bonde-Petersen, F., & Hancke, S. (1979). The effect of weight-lifting exercise related to muscle fiber composition and muscle cross-sectional area in humans. *European Journal of Applied Physiology*, **40**, 95-106.

Duchateau, J., & Hainaut, K. (1984). Isometric or dynamic training: Differential effects on mechanical properties of a human muscle. *Journal of Applied Physiology: Respiratory, Environmental and Exercise Physiology*, **56**, 296-301.

Edwards, R.H.T., Hill, D.K., & Jones, D.A. (1975). Heat production and chemical changes during isometric contractions of the human quadriceps muscle. *Journal of Physiology*, **251**, 301-315.

Fahey, T.D., & Brown, C.H. (1973). The effects of an anabolic steroid on the strength, body composition and endurance of college males when accompanied by a weight training program. *Medicine and Science in Sports, 5,* 272-276.

Freund, H. -J. (1983). Motor unit and muscle activity in voluntary motor control. *Physiological Reviews, 63,* 387-436.

Fuglsang-Frederiksen, A., & Scheel, U. (1978). Transient decrease in number of motor units after immobilization in man. *Journal of Neurology, Neurosurgery and Psychiatry, 41,* 924-929.

Gardner, G. (1963). Specificity of strength changes of the exercised and nonexercised limb following isometric training. *Research Quarterly, 34,* 98-101.

Haar Romeny, B.M., Denier Van Der Gon, J.J., & Gielen, C.C.A.M. (1982). Changes in recruitment order of motor units in the human biceps muscle. *Experimental Neurology, 78,* 360-368.

Hakkinen, K., & Komi, P.V. (1983). Electromyographic changes during strength training and detraining. *Medicine and Science in Sports and Exercise, 15,* 455-460.

Hellebrandt, F.A. (1951). Cross education: Ipsilateral and contralateral effects of unimanual training. *Journal of Applied Physiology, 4,* 136-143.

Hellebrandt, F.A., & Houtz, S.J. (1956). Mechanisms of muscle training in man: Experimental demonstration of the overload principle. *Physical Therapy Review, 36,* 371-383.

Hellebrandt, F.A., Parrish, A.M., & Houtz, S.J. (1947). Cross-education: The effect of unilateral exercise on the contralateral limb. *Archives of Physical Medicine and Rehabilitation, 28,* 76-85.

Henry, F.M., & Smith, L.E. (1961). Simultaneous vs. separate bilateral muscular contractions in relation to neural overflow theory and neuromotor specificity. *Research Quarterly, 32,* 42-46.

Hettinger, T.L., & Muller, E.A., (1953). Muscular performance and training. *Arbeitsphysiologie, 15,* 111-126.

Houston, M.E., Froese, E.A., Valeriote, St. P., Green, H.J., & Ranney, D.A. (1983). Muscle performance, morphology and metabolic capacity during strength training and detraining: A one leg model. *European Journal of Applied Physiology, 51,* 25-35.

Ikai, M., & Fukunaga, T. (1968). Calculation of muscle strength per unit cross-sectional area of human muscle by means of ultrasonic measurement. *European Journal of Applied Physiology, 26,* 36-32.

Ikai, M., & Fukunaga, T. (1970). A study on training effect on strength per unit cross-sectional area of muscle by means of ultrasonic measurement. *European Journal of Applied Physiology, 28,* 173-180.

Ikai, M., & Steinhaus, A.H. (1961). Some factors modifying the expression of human strength. *Journal of Applied Physiology, 16,* 157-163.

Ikai, M., Yabe, K., & Ischii (1967). Muskelkraft und muskulane ermudung bei willkurlicher Anspannung und elektrischer reizung des muskels. *Sportarzt Sportmedicine, 5,* 1973.

Jones, R.E. (1966). *A neurological interpretation of maximum isometric training and its relationship to individual training variability.* Unpublished doctoral dissertation, University of Wisconsin.

Kanehisa, H., & Miyashita, M. (1983a). Effect of isometric and isokinetic muscle training on static strength and dynamic power. *European Journal of Applied Physiology,* **52,** 104-106.

Kanehisa, H., & Miyashita, M. (1983b). Specificity of velocity in strength training. *European Journal of Applied Physiology,* **52,** 104-106.

Komi, P.V., & Buskirk, E. (1972). Effect of eccentric and concentric muscle conditioning on tension and electrical activity of human muscle. *Ergonomics,* **15,** 417-434.

Komi, P.V., Viitasalo, J., Rauramaa, R., & Vihko, V. (1978). Effect of isometric strength training of mechanical, electrical and metabolic aspects of muscle function. *European Journal of Applied Physiology,* **40,** 45-55.

Kroll, W. (1965). Isometric cross-transfer effects under conditions of central facilitation. *Journal of Applied Physiology,* **20,** 297-300.

Krotkiewski, M., Aniansson, A., Grimby, G., Bjorntorp, P., & Sjostrom, L. (1979). The effect of unilateral isokinetic strength training on local adipose and muscle tissue morphology, thickness and enzymes. *European Journal of Applied Physiology,* **42,** 271-281.

Kukulka, C.G., & Clamann, H.P. (1981). Comparison of the recruitment and discharge properties of motor units in human brachial biceps and adductor pollicis during isometric contractions. *Brain Research,* **219,** 45-55.

Liberson, W.T., & Asa, M.M. (1959). Further studies of brief isometric exercises. *Archives of Physical Medicine and Rehabilitation,* **40,** 330-336.

Lind, A.R., & Petrofsky, J.S. (1978). Isometric tension from rotary stimulation of fast and slow cat muscle. *Muscle & Nerve,* **1,** 213-218.

Lindh, M. (1979). Increase of muscle strength from isometric quadriceps exercise at different knee angles. *Scandinavian Journal of Rehabilitation Medicine,* **11,** 33-36.

MacDougall, J.D., Elder, G.C.B., Sale, D.G., Moroz, J.R., & Sutton, J.R. (1980). Effects of strength training and immobilization on human muscle fibres. *European Journal of Applied Physiology,* **43,** 25-34.

MacDougall, J.D., Sale, D.G., Elder, G.C.B., & Sutton, J.R. (1982). Muscle ultrastructural characteristics of elite powerlifters and bodybuilders. *European Journal of Applied Physiology,* **48,** 117-126.

Mathews, D.K., & Kruse, R. (1957). Effects of isometric and isotonic exercises on elbow muscle groups. *Research Quarterly,* **28,** 26-37.

Mathews, D.K., Shay, C.T., Godin, F., & Hogdon, R. (1956). Cross-transfer effects of training on strength and endurance. *Research Quarterly,* **27,** 206-212.

Maughan, R.J., Watson, J.S., & Weir, J. (1982). Strength and cross-sectional area of the knee extensor muscles in man: Effects of strength training. *Journal of Physiology,* **336,** 21-22 P.

McDonagh, M.J.N., Hayward, C.M., & Davies, C.T.M. (1983). Isometric training in human elbow flexor muscles. *Journal of Bone and Joint Surgery,* **65,** 355-358.

Merton, P.A. (1954). Voluntary strength and fatigue. *Journal of Physiology,* **123,** 553-564.

Meyers, C. (1967). Effects of two isometric routines on strength, size, and endurance in exercised and non-exercised arms. *Research Quarterly,* **38,** 430-440.

Miller, R.G., Mirka, A., & Maxfield, M. (1981). Rate of tension development in isometric contractions of a human hand muscle. *Experimental Neurology,* **73,** 267-285.

Milner-Brown, H.S., Stein, R.B., & Lee, R.G. (1975). Synchronization of human motor units: Possible roles of exercise and supraspinal reflexes. *Electroencephalography and Clinical Neurophysiology,* **38,** 245-254.

Milner-Brown, H.S., Stein, R.B., & Yemm, R. (1973a). The orderly recruitment of human motor units during voluntary isometric contractions. *Journal of Physiology,* **270,** 350-370.

Milner-Brown, H.S., Stein, R.B., & Yemm, R. (1973b). Changes in firing rate of human motor units during linearly changing voluntary contractions. *Journal of Physiology,* **230,** 371-390.

Moffroid, M., & Whipple, R.H. (1970). Specificity of speed of exercise. *Physical Therapy,* **50,** 1693-1699.

Moritani, T., & de Vries, H.A. (1979). Neural factors vs hypertrophy in time course of muscle strength gain. *American Journal of Physical Medicine and Rehabilitation,* **58,** 115-130.

Muller, E.A. (1962). Physiology of muscle training. *Revue Canadienne de Biologie,* **21,** 303-313.

Ohtsuki, T. (1981). Decrease in grip strength induced by simultaneous bilateral exertion with reference to finger strength. *Ergonomics,* **24,** 37-48.

Ohtsuki, T. (1983). Decrease in human voluntary isometric arm strength induced by simultaneous bilateral exertion. *Behavioral Brain Research,* **7,** 165-178.

Perrine, J.J., & Edgerton, V.R. (1978). Muscle force-velocity and power-velocity relationships under isokinetic loading. *Medicine and Science in Sports,* **10,** 159-166.

Person, R.S. (1974). Rhythmic activity of a group of human motoneurons during voluntary contraction of a muscle. *Electroencephalography and Clinical Neurophysiology,* **36,** 585-595.

Rack, P.M.H., & Westbury, D.R. (1969). The effects of length and stimulus rate on tension in the isometric cat soleus muscle. *Journal of Physiology,* **204,** 443-460.

Raitsin, L. (1974). The effectiveness of isometric and electro-stimulated training on muscle strength at different joint angles. *Yessis Review,* **11,** 35-39.

Rasch, P.J., & Morehouse, C.E. (1957). Effect of static and dynamic exercises on muscular strength and hypertrophy. *Journal of Applied Physiology*, **11**, 29-34.

Rose, D.L., Radzyminski, S.F., & Beatty, R.R. (1957). Effect of brief maximal exercise on strength of the quadriceps femoris. *Archives of Physical Medicine and Rehabilitation*, **38**, 157-164.

Roy, R.R., Meadows, I.D., Baldwin, K.M., & Edgerton, V.R. (1982). Functional significance of compensatory overloaded rat fast muscle. *Journal of Applied Physiology: Respiratory, Environmental and Exercise Physiology*, **52**, 473-478.

Sale, D., & MacDougall, D. (1981). Specificity in strength training: A review for the coach and athlete. *Canadian Journal of Applied Sports Sciences*, **6**, 87-92.

Sale, D.G., MacDougall, J.D., Upton, A.R.M., & McComas, A.J. (1983). Effect of strength training upon motoneuron excitability in man. *Medicine and Science in Sports and Exercise*, **15**, 57-62.

Sale, D.G., McComas, A.J., MacDougall, J.D., & Upton, A.R.M. (1982). Neuromuscular adaptation in human thenar muscles following strength training and immobilization. *Journal of Applied Physiology: Respiratory, Environmental and Exercise Physiology*, **53**, 419-424.

Sale, D.G., Upton, A.R.M., McComas, A.J., & MacDougall, J.D. (1983). Neuromuscular function in weight-trainers. *Experimental Neurology*, **82**, 521-531.

Schantz, P., Randall-Fox, E., Hutchison, W., Tyden, A., & Åstrand, P.-O. (1983). Muscle fibre type distribution, muscle cross-sectional area and maximal voluntary strength in humans. *Acta Physiologica Scandinavica*, **117**, 219-226.

Schmidt, E.M., & Thomas, J.S. (1981). Motor unit recruitment order: Modification under volitional control. In J.E. Desmedt (Ed.), *Progress in clinical neurophysiology* (Vol. 9, pp. 145-148). Basel: Karger.

Secher, N.H. (1975). Isometric rowing strength of experienced and inexperienced oarsmen. *Medicine and Science in Sports*, **7**, 280-283.

Secher, N.H., Rorsgaard, S., & Secher, O. (1978). Contralateral influence on recruitment of curarized muscle fibers during maximal voluntary extension of the legs. *Acta Physiologica Scandinavica*, **103**, 456-462.

Sica, R.E.P., McComas, A.J., & Upton, A.R.M. (1971). Impaired potentiation of H-reflexes in patients with upper motoneuron lesions. *Journal of Neurology, Neurosurgery and Psychiatry*, **34**, 712-717.

Slater-Hammel, T.A. (1950). Bilateral effects of muscular activity. *Research Quarterly*, **21**, 203-209.

Tanner, J.M. (1952). The effect of weight lifting on physique. *American Journal of Physical Anthropology*, **10**, 427-461.

Tesch, P.A., Hjort, H., & Balldin, U.I. (1983). Effects of strength training on G tolerance. *Aviation, Space, and Environmental Medicine*, **54**, 691-695.

Thorstensson, A., Hulten, B., Von Doblen, W., & Karlsson, J. (1976). Effect of strength training on enzyme activities and fibre characteristics in human skeletal muscle. *Acta Physiologica Scandinavica, 96,* 392-398.

Thorstensson, A., Karlsson, J., Viitasalo, J.H.T., Luhtanen, P., & Komi, P.V. (1976). Effect of strength training on EMG of human skeletal muscle. *Acta Physiologica Scandinavica, 98,* 232-236.

Upton, A.R.M., McComas, A.J., & Sica, R.E.P. (1971). Potentiation of 'late' responses evoked in muscles during effort. *Journal of Neurology, Neurosurgery and Psychiatry, 34,* 699-711.

Upton, A.R.M., & Radford, P.F. (1975). Motoneuron excitability in elite sprinters. In P.V. Komi (Ed.), *Biomechanics V-A* (pp. 82-87). Baltimore: University Park Press.

Vandervoort, A.A., Sale, D.G., & Moroz, J. (1984). Comparison of motor unit activation during unilateral and bilateral leg extension. *Journal of Applied Physiology: Respiratory, Environmental and Exercise Physiology, 56,* 46-51.

Whitley, J.D., & Elliott, G. (1968). Learning component of repetitive maximal static contractions. *Perceptual Motor Skills, 27,* 1195-1200.

Yasuda, Y., & Miyamura, M. (1983). Cross-transfer effects of muscular training on blood flow in the ipsilateral and contralateral forearms. *European Journal of Applied Physiology, 51,* 321-329.

Discussion

Dr. Sale was asked if training led to increased synchronization of motor units. He replied that there was some evidence of this (Milner-Brown, Stein, & Lee, 1975), but it was difficult to see how this would increase strength if time was not a constraint. It might increase the rate of force development in ballistic contractions, but in studies of the small hand muscles, the rate of force development evoked by synchronized stimuli could not match the rate of force development of voluntary contractions (Miller, Mirka, & Maxfield, 1981). Dr. Sale asked Dr. Stein for his view on this question; he replied that synchronization was probably a by-product of training that involved repetitive maximum force development, perhaps through increasing strength of descending neural inputs, so as to activate more securely the high threshold units that may be activated experimentally only for brief periods and with small margins of safety. The effect would tend to drive motor units together, but it could conceivably be detrimental, as an increased clustering of motor unit activity might lead to tremor. Incidentally, Dr.Stein expressed a reservation regarding the use of the word "adaptation" in the context of training; this had come to have a very specific meaning in neurophysiology related to a decreasing firing rate for a given force production. In the present context, adaptation appeared to be used to mean increasing force production through a variety of mechanisms. Dr. Sale replied that in exercise physiology the word "adaptation" has come to mean the effects of training. Here the term is distinguished from the term "adjustment," which is commonly used to refer to the acute effects of a single bout of exercise.

Dr. Komi emphasized that the force-time relationships in investigating training effects are important because in most athletic events there is a limited time in which to produce force. This may be studied by EMG techniques, in which the raw EMG is obtained during repeated contractions, and the signal rectified and averaged. A group in Freiburg studying well-trained athletes compared the rate of force development with the EMG signal and found differences between untrained and trained individuals that might be due to better synchronization of motor units in the trained, but also might be due to different rates of motor unit activation at the onset of contractions. This is a difficult topic to study because in any joint movement the position may exert a large effect on the maximum EMG signal related to maximal activation of the muscle.

Dr. Green asked if post-tetanic potentiation was changed with training. Dr. Sale replied that to his knowledge the effect of training on post-activation potentiation had not been investigated. In reply to another question regarding the possibility that subjects able to recruit all motor units are a separate population, he pointed out that Upton and Radford (1975) studied seven elite sprinters and found reflex potentiation to be extremely high even in muscles not involved in the subject's events; they appeared to have inherited a particularly excitable nervous system. On the other hand, a reflex potentiation, and hence motor unit activation, may be modified by training and immobilization.

Dr. Bigland-Ritchie pointed out that one could never sustain maximum activation when synergists were used among a group of muscles. This may affect the ability to activate muscle maximally and may also be affected by training. Using the superimposed twitch technique, they had studied the biceps, soleus, adductor policis, and quadriceps and found that most subjects needed practice before recordings of maximal force were obtained.

Dr. Gonyea wondered if precontraction of antagonists might have an effect on maximum force production by stretching the synergists. Dr. Sale replied that this could not be ruled out when the precontractions were concentric; however, potentiation may also occur when the precontraction of antagonists is isometric. In this case little stretching of the prime movers would occur. Dr. Gonyea mentioned the work of Willis on the connections between la motor neurons supplying antagonists, which suggested that antagonists were "wired up" to produce a precontraction effect.

Mr. LaChance wondered about the mechanism underlying the velocity specific effect of adaptations to isokinetic training. If improvement was produced by training at 180° per sec, why can't the effect be demonstrated at 300° per sec. Dr. Sale pointed out that the specificity applied only to the two extremes of velocities. Specificity of velocity in training has usually been attributed to a learning effect; however, recently Duchateau and Hainaut (1984) demonstrated velocity-specific effects of training upon evoked contractile properties.

Dr. Komi pointed out that most of the studies carried out were all working in a narrow and low velocity range and that other methods needed to be developed in order to study the force velocity characteristics. The stretch-shortening cycle is crucial in isometric performance, and it seemed possible that this might be trained if prestretching could be controlled and the force-time curve moved upwards.

References

Duchateau, J., & Hainaut, K. (1984). Isometric or dynamic training: Differential effects on mechanical properties of human muscle. *Journal of Applied Physiology: Respiratory, Environmental and Exercise Physiology,* **56**, 296-301.

Miller, R.G., Mirka, A., & Maxfield, M. (1981). Rate of tension development in isometric contractions of a human hand muscle. *Experimental Neurology,* **73**, 267-285.

Milner-Brown, H.S., Stein, R.B., & Lee, R.G. (1975). Synchronization of human motor units: Possible roles of exercise and supraspinal reflexes. *Electroencephalography and Clinical Neurophysiology,* **38**, 245-254.

Upton, A.R.M., & Radford, P.F. (1975). Motoneuron excitability in elite sprinters. In P.V. Komi (Eds.), *Biomechanics, V-A* (pp. 82-87). Baltimore: University Park Press.

19

Muscle Performance in Neuromuscular Disorders

Alan J. McComas, Alain Y. Bélanger, Scott Garner,
Neil McCartney
McMaster University Medical Centre

Measurements of muscle strength and power may be applied to the study of patients with neuromuscular disorders. Isometric contractions indicate the maximum strength that a muscle can produce, and they may be used to investigate the rate of fatigue. The twitch and compound action potential (M-wave) obtained by indirect muscle stimulation provide information of value in answering fundamental questions concerning the pathophysiology of muscle weakness. Finally, measurements of dynamic force generation may be used in the assessment of overall disability.

Isometric Strength Measurement

Maximum strength, expressed as either tension or torque, depends on the number of activated myofibrils. The latter, in turn, will be proportional to the number of muscle fibres, the square of the mean diameter of the fibres, and the packing density of myofibrils within the fibres. Strength will also depend upon the mean sarcomere length (Gordon, Huxley, & Julian, 1966) and upon the proportions of type I and type II fibres present because the type II moiety

Supported by grants from the Muscular Dystrophy Association of Canada and the Medical Research Council of Canada.

appear to develop more tension per unit cross-sectional area (Burke, 1981). Of these parameters, the packing density of the myofibrils may be ignored in health because there is no evidence that this is influenced by the size or histochemical type of the muscle fibers (Schmalbruch, 1979). In disease, however, the overall packing density of myofibrils within the fibre may be very abnormal; for example, myofibrils are absent from the innermost part of the fibre in central core disease and, to a lesser extent, in myotubular myopathy. Similarly, in some patients with myotonic dystrophy, myofibrils are excluded from the periphery of the fibres by the presence of subsarcolemmal masses of degenerated material (Engel & Brooke, 1966).

The various factors influencing maximum strength may also be arranged in the form of a simple equation,

$$P = f \, (N.D^2.K.L.T.)$$

in which N represents the number of fibres, D the mean fibre diameter, K the mean packing density of the myofibrils, L muscle length related to its optimum value, and T a factor for fibre type. For a single twitch, P would also depend on the active state duration and would be diminished by the series elastic component within the fibres and tendinous elements. For voluntary or tetanic contractions, the tensions developed depend on the firing frequency of the motoneurones. In disease states an additional factor is introduced to account for the completeness of excitation of the myofibrils. In myasthenia gravis, Lambert-Eaton myasthenic syndrome, familial periodic paralysis, and myotonia congenita, excitation is known to be defective; the same is obviously true for denervating disorders and for some myopathies.

In practice, the contributions of the extrinsic factors determining strength can be controlled, or at least monitored. In relation to sarcomere length, the degree of overlap of the actin and myosin filaments will vary along the length of the fibre during an isometric contraction (Edman & Reggiani, 1984). From a practical standpoint it is customary to determine the optimum length of the muscle, corresponding to maximal twitch torque, and to use this for all subsequent measurements of strength. In passing, it should be noted that, in at least some human muscles, the optimum length does not correspond to the length of the muscle when the limb is at rest (Marsh, Sale, McComas, & Quinlan, 1981; Sale, Quinlan, Marsh, McComas, & Bélanger, 1982).

So far as excitation is concerned, it is necessary to ensure that the stimulus intensity is supramaximal for evoking twitch or tetanic tensions and to monitor the amplitude of the muscle compound action potential (M-wave) during repetitive stimulation. For maximum voluntary contractions, we have employed an interpolated twitch technique to ascertain if all motor units have been recruited and are firing at optimal frequencies for tension development (Bélanger & McComas, 1981). If these extrinsic determinants of strength are controlled, it follows that measurements of strength will be governed by the intrinsic factors, that is, the numbers and sizes of fibres and the myofibrillar packing density.

Questions Concerning Contractile Behavior in Neuromuscular Disorders

What are the questions that may usefully be considered in the study of contractile behavior in muscular dystrophy, or, for that matter, in any other type of neuromuscular disorder? The most fundamental one is undoubtedly whether or not the muscles are weak, and, if so, whether the loss of strength affects different muscles equally. Because, on the basis of clinical observations, the answer to this question is likely to be in the affirmative, it is worth refining the question to enquire if there is any evidence within the same muscle group of preferential involvement of fibres of one type or another by the disease process. To answer this question, evidence is sought of any change in the contraction and half-relaxation times of the maximum isometric twitch or in the degree of post-activation potentiation. The third question is whether the data provide any evidence of excitation-contraction uncoupling. If present, such a defect would be expected to yield a twitch that was disproportionately small in relation to the M-wave. The final question is whether the patient is able to activate his/her remaining muscle tissue maximally during a voluntary contraction; this aspect is tested by the interpolated twitch technique.

Methods and Results

Our selection of human muscles for assessments of maximum strength was influenced by a number of variables; these included susceptibility to disease, ease of measuring torque, and accessibility of motor nerves for stimulation. The majority of human studies have employed either the quadriceps femoris or the adductor pollicis, but we have preferred to use the dorsiflexors and plantarflexors of the ankle. Being "intermediate" muscles, that is, neither proximal nor distal, the ankle flexors are likely to become involved in both myopathic and neuropathic disorders. A further advantage is that the respective nerves can be readily stimulated for twitch studies and the M-waves recorded. The tibialis anterior, gastrocnemii, and soleus are sufficiently large for muscle biopsies to be taken by needle if necessary. Finally, the fact that the dorsiflexor and plantarflexor muscles normally differ from each other in their physiological properties (Bélanger, McComas, & Elder, 1983) adds an additional dimension to the interpretation of results in investigations of disease. The apparatus employed in our laboratory permits determinations of isometric torque to be made with the ankle joint adjusted to correspond to the optimum muscle length (Marsh et al., 1981).

The present study was conducted on 25 patients with myotonic dystrophy (Bélanger & McComas, 1983) and on 20 patients with limbgirdle muscular dys-

Table 1. Contractile properties of ankle dorsiflexor and plantarflexor muscles in patients with myotonic dystrophy (MyD) and limbgirdle dystropy (LGMD) and in controls

Measurement	Plantarflexors			Dorsiflexors		
	Controls	My D	LGMD	Controls	My D	LGMD
P_t (Nm)	17.8 ± 4.3	10.2 ± 6.9*	11.2 ± 7.3*	1.9 ± 1.7	0.7 ± 0.7*	1.1 ± 0.8*
M (mV)	14.2 ± 5.2	8.6 ± 6.1*	8.8 ± 5.4	2.0 ± 1.2	0.7 ± 0.7*	1.4 ± 1.5
$P_t \backslash M$	1.5 ± 1.0	1.7 ± 1.9	1.5 ± 1.0	1.1 ± 1.0	1.2 ± 0.9	0.5 ± 0.3
CT(ms)	135 ± 17	112 ± 16*	124 ± 22	85 ± 10	76 ± 11*	88 ± 21
½RT(ms)	122 + 21	114 + 28	126 + 27	99 + 24	92 ± 18	97 ± 30
PAP (%)	17 + 14	11 + 26	40 + 58	134 + 66	90 + 58	100 + 52
MVC (Nm)	129 + 35	74 + 49*	67 + 56*	40 + 12	22 + 15*	20 + 14*
MUA(%)	95 ± 8.3	84 ± 22	93 ± 11	100 ± 0	100 ± 0	100 ± 0
n	45	25	20	45	25	20

CT, contraction time; *M-wave*; *MVC*, maximum voluntary contraction torque; *MUA*, motor unit activation; P_t, twitch torque; *PAP*, post-activation potentiation; *½RT*, half-relaxation time. Values shown are means ± SD. Astrisks mark significant differences from control values (p<.05).

trophy. In each patient group the findings were compared with those of the same number of controls matched for age, sex, and height. Although in both studies maximum voluntary torque was measured in the entire dorsiflexor muscle group, the analysis of twitch properties was performed on the tibialis anterior alone. For convenience the two samples of normative data have been combined in Table 1.

Table 1 shows that, as might have been anticipated, the mean twitch and maximum voluntary torques were significantly smaller than the respective

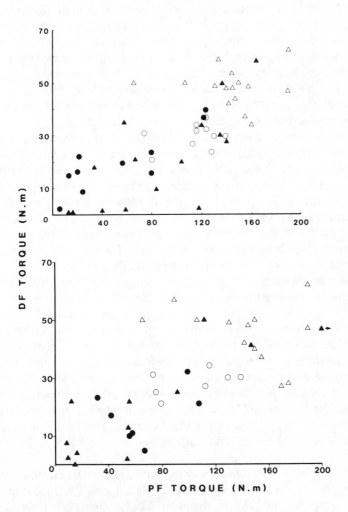

Figure 1.   Maximum voluntary torques compared in the dorsiflexor (*DF*) and plantarflexors (*PF*) muscles of patients with myotonic dystrophy (*upper*) and limbgirdle muscular dystrophy (*lower*). Values for patients and controls are shown by filled and open symbols, respectively; males and females are represented by triangles and circles, respectively.

values for controls. This finding applied to both myotonic and limbgirdle dys-
trophies and to dorsiflexors and plantarflexors alike. Within both populations
of patients, however, there were some individuals who had normal strength,
even though the diagnosis of dystrophy could be made with confidence. Six
patients with myotonic dystrophy had dorsiflexor and plantarflexor torques
within the control ranges and six patients with limbgirdle dystrophy also fell
into this category (see Figure 1). Indeed one of the latter patients actually developed greater voluntary torque of his plantarflexors (235 Nm) than any of
the 13 male controls. There were 5 men who had total, or almost total, paralysis of the dorsiflexors, while retaining moderate strength in the plantarflexors
(see Figure 1), the most striking instance being a patient in whom voluntary
dorsiflexion and plantarflexion were 5% and 90% of the respective control mean
values (see arrowed point in Figure 1). The twitch data confirmed these findings; all the myotonic dystrophy patients had detectable plantarflexor twitches,
but there were eight in whom a dorsiflexor response was not observed. In limbgirdle dystrophy, by contrast, there tended to be more uniformity in the degrees
of involvement of the dorsiflexor and plantarflexor muscles.

The measurement of twitch contraction times was of importance in indicating whether or not, within the same muscle or muscle group, fibres of one
type were more susceptible to the disease process than another. In limbgirdle
dystrophy there was no evidence of such a difference, but in myotonic dystrophy the contraction times of both the dorsiflexors and the plantarflexors
were significantly shorter than those of controls (see Figure 2). This finding
is compatible with the observation by Engel and Brooke (1966) that some
patients, at a relatively early stage of myotonic dystrophy, develop subsarcolemmal masses of non-myofibrillar material in type I fibers.

The possibility that there is some form of uncoupling of the excitatory and
contractile events in dystrophic muscle fibres is one that was raised by Desmedt
(1976) in a study of patients with limbgirdle and facioscapulohumeral
dystrophy. Some of our patients with myotonic dystrophy showed surprisingly
little voluntary strength in the intrinsic muscles of their hands despite pos-
sessing M-waves of normal amplitude. In four patients with myotonic dystrophy there was evidence of excitation-contraction uncoupling,—a normal
M-wave with a small or absent twitch response. In the remaining patients,
however, the decreases in M-wave amplitude were approximately proportional
to the diminutions in twitch torque; thus, it appeared that either uncoupling
was temporary or it was not an invariable step in the natural history of dystrophy.

The completeness of voluntary motor unit activation was examined by the
response to a maximal indirect stimulus applied during a brief bout of maximal effort. In healthy subjects, the interpolated stimulus fails to evoke any
additional torque in the dorsiflexor muscles (Bélanger & McComas, 1981),
indicating that all motor units are recruited during a voluntary contraction and
fire at optimal frequencies for tension development. Similar results have re-

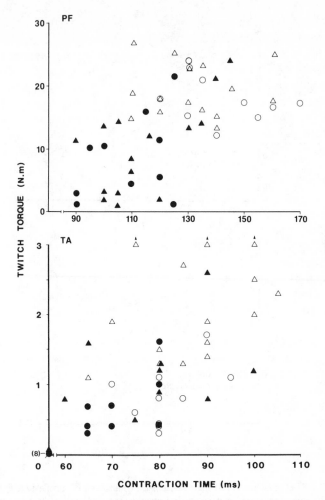

Figure 2. Contraction time as a function of twitch torque in plantarflexor (PF) and tibialis anterior (TA) muscles of patients with myotonic dystrophy and controls. Symbols are the same as those for Figure 1. Reprinted with permission for Bélanger and McComas (1983) by courtesy of the editor and publishers of the *Journal of Neurology, Neurosurgery and Psychiatry.*

cently been obtained for the human quadriceps femoris (Chapman, Edwards, Greig, & Rutherford, 1984). In the case of the ankle plantarflexors, some normal subjects cannot achieve full motor unit activation (Bélanger & McComas, 1981); in myotonic dystrophy, however, twice as many individuals fell into this category (see Table 1). It was also noticed that with both types of dystrophy, patients often required several attempts before developing maximal voluntary torque, whereas control subjects were more likely to be successful at their initial attempt. These observations suggested that the descending motor pathways had become less effective in exciting lumbo sacral motoneurons,

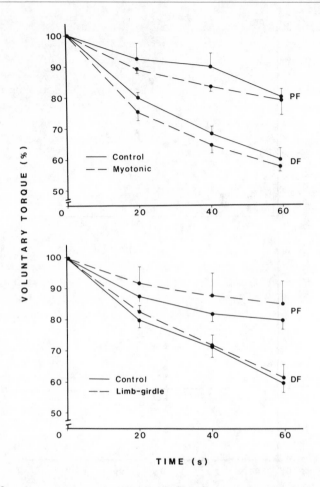

Figure 3. Rates of fatigue during maximal isometric contractions of dorsiflexor (DF) and plantarflexor (PF) muscles in patients with myotonic dystrophy (upper) and limbgirdle dystrophy (lower) and in controls. Values shown are means with 1 SEM; patient curves do not differ significantly from those of controls.

perhaps because of reduced physical activity. Similar findings have been noted in healthy subjects after immobilization of muscles by plaster casts (Fuglsang-Frederiksen & Scheel, 1978; Sale et al., 1982). The improvement in strength with repetition during the same testing session indicated that the inability to activate motoneurones fully was "functional" rather than the result of any degenerative process in the descending motor pathways. These observations are of practical significance in two respects. First, they indicate that voluntary muscle strength may be underestimated in dystrophic patients unless several repetitions are made. Second, by the institution of appropriate physiotherapy, it should be possible to enhance the physical capacity of patients irrespective of any change in the muscle fibres.

The apparatus used for maximum strength measurements (Marsh et al., 1981) may be used to study the rates of fatigue in the dorsiflexor and plantarflexor muscles of the ankle during a maximal contraction sustained for 60 sec; the fall in torque is normalized with respect to the initial maximal value. The pooled results were remarkable in that, despite the presence of severe weakness in many of the patients, the mean rate of decline of torque did not differ significantly from that of the corresponding control population. This finding suggested that surviving fibres had a nomal susceptibility to fatigue.

Muscle Power Measurement: Methods and Results

More recently we have extended our investigations of fatigue in neuromuscular disorders by measuring dynamic power generated during cycle ergometry in an incremental progressive exercise test (Jones & Campbell, 1982), an endurance test at 80% of maximal aerobic power and a short-term maximal power output test, in which central circulatory adaptation is theoretically less important than the other tests. The first two tests are well known, but the third may be less familiar. In this test the subject pedals on an isokinetic cycle ergometer (McCartney, Heigenhauser, Sargeant, & Jones, 1983) at a controlled angular velocity of 60 rpm for 30 sec, and the forces exerted on the pedal cranks are detected by foil strain gauges and transmitted on-line to a laboratory computer. Torque, work, and power are calculated for each leg in every pedal stroke to obtain data on maximal power and the decline in power during 30 sec, which is expressed as a fatigue index. Despite losses of strength in leg muscles on clinical examination and obvious difficulties in walking, all of the patients we have studied have been able to maintain the required pedalling rate with ease, probably because of a slipping clutch that minimizes initial inertial resistance to movement and allows the subject to attain a pedalling rhythm quickly. It is the short-term isokinetic ergometry that has provided the best indication of residual muscle power in neuromuscular disorders. The patient data are compared with normal standards previously established in more than 100 healthy subjects of both sexes between the ages of 15 and 70 years (Makrides, McCartney, & Jones, 1985).

In patients with established neuromuscular disease, both the maximal power (achieved early in the test) and the total work generated in 30 sec were invariably low, usually 2-6 standard deviations below the respective age and sex matched population means, ranging from 20% to 60% of the predicted values. However, despite the markedly low maximal power the extent of fatigue in 30 sec was usually within the normal range, a finding in keeping with those of the isometric torque studies described above. The diminished work performance may be attributed to reduced effective muscle mass secondary to dener-

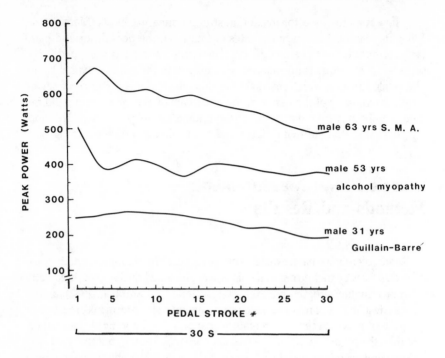

Figure 4. Short-term (30s) isokinetic cycle ergometry results in three male patients with different neuromuscular disorders.

vation or muscle fibre degeneration, but the observation of normal fatigue suggests that the residual muscle fibers were able to sustain dynamic tension in the normal manner. Figure 4 contrasts the findings in three male patients with strikingly different work capacities but similar fatigue characteristics. The findings are also consistent with a dominant degeneration of fast twitch muscle fibres in many neuromuscular disorders.

Although a normal fatigue pattern is a common finding in the majority of patients that we have tested, this is not always the case. For example, a patient with the neural form of a facioscapulohumeral syndrome (see Figure 5) generated maximal power and total work that were 5.5 and 6.5 SD below the respective control values; however, the fatigue at the end of the 30 sec was clearly excessive, power having fallen to 36% of its initial value, compared to 75% in the control subject. It could be argued that the application of volitional exercise tests to a patient such as this is of limited value because it is impossible to determine if the effort was truly maximal. However, the shape of the power output curve in maximal isokinetic ergometry is uniform and reproducible in the majority of subjects, allowing reduced or variable effort to be recognized.

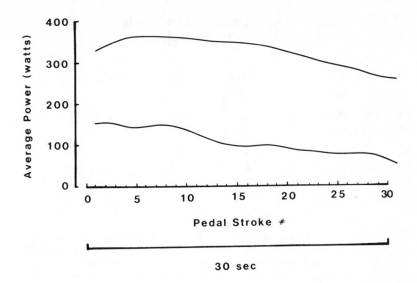

Figure 5. Short-term (30s) isokinetic cycle ergometry results in a 37-year-old woman with a neural form of the facioscapulohumeral syndrome (lower curve) and in a female control subject (upper curve).

The application of these techniques to patients with neuromuscular disorders has emphasized that measurement of isometric strength in one group of muscles should not be used to predict dynamic performance in the same or other leg muscles. Also muscle strength, power, and susceptibility to fatigue may not correspond to gross estimates of muscle mass, and the contractile behavior may differ markedly in individuals with the same diagnosis.

These points are illustrated by a comparison of two patients with the clinical, EMG, and muscle biopsy findings of spinal muscular atrophy (see Table 2). Both patients exhibited weakness of voluntary plantarflexion under isometric conditions, but when the torques were expressed in relation to the cross-sectional areas of the triceps surae muscles, determined from CT scans, it was evident that these muscles were more effective in producing force in patient 1 than in patient 2. The discrepancy noted between the two patients in the force generating capacity of their plantarflexor muscles was also evident for the quadriceps, which are mainly responsible for the downward thrust of the cycle pedals associated with the development of peak instantaneous power. When tested on the isokinetic cycle ergometer, patient 1 was able to develop 90% of the peak power predicted for a man of his age, but patient 2 could manage only 30%. Thus, in relation to cross-sectional area, patient 1 generated 2.7 times as much power as patient 2 (see Table 2). A similar disparity in maximal power was noted in the progressive incremental exercise test; however, in the submaximal endurance test, patient 1 was able to continue pedalling

Table 2. Isometric strength, power, and rate of fatigue contrasted in two patients with spinal muscular atrophy.

Measurement	Patient 1	Patient 2	Muscles
MVC (% control)	44	55	Ankle Plantarflexors
MVC (Nm/cm²)	2.7	1.5	
Max power (watts)	827	294	
Max power (% control)	90	30	Quadriceps
Max power (watts/cm²)	12.5	4.7	
Fatigue time (min)	7.4	25.7	Quadriceps

Maximal power was recorded during isokinetic cycle ergometry and related to measures of muscle cross-sectional area derived from CT scans. The fatigue studies were carried out with patients cycling at 80% of the maximum power achieved in a progressive incremental exercise test. MVC, maximum voluntary contraction torque.

at 80% of maximal power for 7.4 min, whereas patient 2 was not fatigued after more than 25 min. The increased contraction times of the plantarflexors in this patient together with the resistance to fatigue are compatible with the presence of a high proportion of slow-twitch fatigue-resistant (type 1) fibres.

Conclusions

Our studies have shown that patients with the same type of neuromuscular disorder may have widely varying degrees of weakness in different muscles, ranging from none to total paralysis. In an individual patient the strength in one muscle group cannot be predicted from the observations made in another one, nor is strength necessarily related to muscle size. There is also a wide variation in the susceptibility to fatigue, but most patients with chronic neuropathies or myopathies have normal fatigue properties. In myotonic dystrophy, the fast-twitch fibres are more resistant than slow-twitch fibres to the dystrophic process, although other interpretations of the twitch data are possible. Some patients with dystrophy have evidence of excitation-contraction uncoupling, and moderately disabled patients with dystrophy often have difficulty in activating their motor units fully.

References

Bélanger, A.Y., & McComas, A.J. (1981). Extent of motor unit activation during effort. *Journal of Applied Physiology: Respiratory, Environmental and Exercise Physiology*, **51**, 160-167.

Bélanger, A.Y., & McComas, A.J. (1983). Contractile properties of muscles in myotonic dystrophy. *Journal of Neurology, Neourosurgery and Psychiatry*, **46**, 625-631.

Bélanger, A.Y., McComas, A.J., & Elder, G.C.B. (1983). Physiological properties of two antagonistic human muscle groups. *European Journal of Applied Physiology*, **51**, 381-393.

Burke, R.E. (1981). Motor units: Anatomy, physiology and functional organization. In V.C. Brooks (Ed.), *Handbook of physiology: Sec. 1. Motor control: Vol. 11 (pp. 345-422)*. Baltimore: Williams & Wilkins.

Chapman, S.J., Edwards, R.H.T., Greig, C., & Rutherford, O. (1984). Practical application of the twitch interpolation technique for the study of voluntary contraction of the quadriceps muscle in man. *Journal of Physiology* (London), **353**, 3.

Desmedt, J.E. (1967). The isometric twitch of human muscle in the normal and dystrophic states. In A.J. Milhorat (Ed.), *Exploratory concepts in muscular dystrophy and related disorders* (pp. 224-230). New York: Excerpta Medica.

Edman, K.A.P., & Reggiani, C. (1984). Redistribution of sarcomere length during isometric contraction of frog muscle fibres and its relation to tension creep. *Journal of Physiology* (London), **351**, 169-198.

Engel, W.K., & Brooke, M.H. (1966). Histochemistry of the myotonic disorders. In E. Kuhn (Eds.), *Progressive muskeldystrophie, myotonie, myasthenie* (pp. 203-22). Heidelberg: Springer.

Fuglsang-Frederiksen, A., & Scheel, U. (1978). Transient decrease in number of motor units after immobilization in man. *Journal of Neurology, Neurosurgery and Psychiatry*, **41**, 924-929.

Gordon, A.M., Huxley, A.F., & Julian, F.J. (1966). The variation of isometric tension with sarcomere length in vertebrate muscle fibers. *Journal of Physiology* (London), **184**, 170-192.

Jones, N.L., & Campbell, E.J.M. (1982). *Clinical exercise testing* (2nd ed.). Philadelphia: W.B. Saunders.

Makrides, L., Heigenhauser, G.J.F., McCartney, N., & Jones, N.L. (1985). Maximal short-term exercise capacity in healthy subjects aged 15-70 years. *Clinical Science*, **69**, 197-205.

Marsh, E., Sale, D., McComas, A.J., & Quinlan, J. (1981). Influence of joint position on ankle dorsi-flexion in humans. *Journal of Applied Physiology: Respiratory, Environmental and Exercise Physiology,* **51,** 160-167.

McCartney, N., Heigenhauser, G.J.F., Sargeant, A.J., & Jones, N.L. (1983). A constant-velocity cycle ergometer for the study of dynamic muscle function. *Journal of Applied Physiology: Respiratory, Environmental and Exercise Physiology,* **55,** 212-217.

Sale, D., McComas, A.J., MacDougall, J.D., & Upton, A.R.M. (1982). Neuromuscular adaptation in human thenar muscles following strength training and immobilization. *Journal of Applied Physiology: Respiratory, Environmental and Exercise Physiology,* **53,** 419-424.

Sale, D., Quinlan, J., Marsh, E., McComas, A.J., & Bélanger, A.Y. (1982). Influence of joint position on ankle plantarflexion in humans. *Journal of Applied Physiology: Respiratory, Environmental and Exercise Physiology,* **52,** 1636-1642.

Schmalbruch, H. (1971). "Rote" Muskelfasen. *Z. Zellrorsch. Mikrosk. Anatomy,* **119,** 120-146.

Vandervoort, A.A. (1984). *Aging and human neuromuscular function.* Unpublished doctoral dissertation, McMaster University, Hamilton, Canada.

Discussion

Dr. McComas was asked about the use of muscle training techniques for patients with neuromuscular disorders. He replied that some formal training was undoubtedly helpful; however, rather than starting with a heavy resistance programme, it was better to employ a less strenuous regimen that could be increased over a period of months, and he favored the use of isometric contractions for each muscle group, lasting several seconds and repeated three to four times a day. Apart from inducing hypertrophy, such exercise may encourage the production of healthy "daughter" fibers from split "parent" fibers. A further benefit of an exercise programme was that patients could more readily activate their motor unit populations maximally, thereby discouraging the disuse phenomenon noted not only in patients (Bélanger & McComas, in press) but also in healthy subjects after temporary limb immobilization (Fuglsang-Frederiksen & Scheel, 1978; Sale, McComas, MacDougall, & Upton, 1982). Dr. Green enquired whether the short twitch contraction times in myotonic dystrophy might be caused by reduced activity. Dr. McComas was aware of animal experiments that would support such a hypothesis, but use and disuse appear to be less important in determining contraction and relaxation times in man (Sale et al., 1982). Also, if disuse led to briefer twitches, such results should be found in limbgirdle dystrophy, but that was not the case (Bélanger & McComas, in press).

Discussion followed on the possible part played by excitation-contraction uncoupling in disuse and neuromuscular disorders. Dr. McComas observed that some patients with myotonic dystrophy showed maximal evoked muscle action potentials (M-waves) that were large in relation to the associated twitch torque. This finding provided indirect evidence of uncoupling, but there was no sign of similar dissociation between twitch torque and the M-wave in simple disuse (Sale et al., 1982). In hereditary muscular dysgenesis in the mouse, the developing muscle fibers were able to fire action potentials, but the latter were incapable of eliciting contractions (Powell & Fambrough, 1973). Malignant hyperthermia, a genetic disorder of humans and swine, could be regarded as a condition in which excitation and contraction were too tightly coupled so that muscles might go into contracture during certain types of physical or chemical stress.

Dr. Faulkner wondered if the apparently normal fatigue properties of diseased muscle might be an artefact; if a small fraction of the motor unit population was recruited at any given instant, the time for the whole muscle to become fatigued might be prolonged. Dr. McComas pointed out that the twitch interpolation technique (Bélanger & McComas, 1981) had been employed to verify that motor unit activation was as complete in dystrophic patients as in normal subjects during fatigue testing. Furthermore, even when stimulation was restricted to a single motor unit, as in the cat medial gastrocnemius muscle, fatigue could still be induced readily, especially if the unit was of the fast twitch glycolytic (FF) type (Burke, 1967). This was an important observation because, unlike the situation during maximal muscle activation, the circulation to the muscle would not be compromised by high intramuscular pressures (Barcroft & Millen, 1939).

Dr. Gonyea asked Dr. Faulkner if his technique of force-velocity measurements in small bundles of fibers might be applied to patients with suspected neuromuscular disorder. Dr. Faulkner replied that Dr. Edwards and his group had shown large dissociations between histochemical characteristics and physiological properties in developing or degenerating muscles.

References

Barcroft, H., & Millen, J.L.E. (1939). The blood flow through muscle during sustained contraction. *Journal of Physiology* (London), **97**, 17-31.

Bélanger, A.Y., & McComas, A.J. (1981). Extent of motor unit activation during effort. *Journal of Applied Physiology: Respiratory, Environmental and Exercise Physiology, **51**, 160-167.

Bélanger, A.Y., & McComas, A.J. (1983). Contractile properties of muscles in myotonic dystrophy. *Journal of Neurology, Neurosurgery and Psychiatry, **46**, 625-631.

Bélanger, A.Y., & McComas, A.J. (in press). Neuromuscular function in limb-girdle dystrophy. *Journal of Neurology, Neurosurgery and Psychiatry.*

Burke, R.E. (1967). Motor unit types of cat triceps surae muscle. *Journal of Physiology* (London), **193**, 141-160.

Fuglsang-Frederiksen, A., & Schell, U. (1978). Transient decrease in number of motor units after immobilization in man. *Journal of Neurology, Neurosurgery and Psychiatry,* **41**, 924-929.

Powell, J.A., & Fambrough, D.M. (1973). Electrical properties of normal and dysgenic mouse muscle in culture. *Journal of Cell Physiology,* **82**, 21-38.

Sale, D., McComas, A.J., MacDougall, J.D., & Upton, A.R.M. (1982). Neuromuscular adaptation in human thenar muscles following strength training and immobilization. *Journal of Applied Physiology: Respiratory, Environmental and Exercise Physiology,* **53**, 419-424.

Author Index

* denotes leading author

Subject Index